Advances in Pain Research and Therapy
Volume 10

PAIN AND MOBILITY

ADVANCES IN PAIN RESEARCH AND THERAPY
John J. Bonica, Series Editor

Pain and Mobility
Mario Tiengo, John Eccles, A. Claudio Cuello, and David Ottoson, Editors

Proceedings of the Fourth World Congress on Pain, Seattle
Howard L. Fields, Ronald Dubner, and Fernando Cervero, Editors; Louisa E. Jones, Associate Editor

Opioid Analgesics in the Management of Clinical Pain
Kathleen M. Foley and Charles E. Inturrisi, Editors

Recent Advances in the Management of Pain
Costantino Benedetti, C. Richard Chapman, and Guido Moricca, Editors

Proceedings of the Third World Congress on Pain, Edinburgh
John J. Bonica, Ulf Lindblom, Ainsley Iggo, Louisa E. Jones, and Costantino Benedetti, Editors

Management of Superior Pulmonary Sulcus Syndrome (Pancoast Syndrome)
John J. Bonica, Vittorio Ventafridda, Carlo A. Pagni, Costantino Benedetti, and Louisa E. Jones, Editors

Advances in Pain Research and Therapy
Volume 10

Pain and Mobility

Editors

Mario Tiengo, M.D.
Cattedra di Fisiopatologia
e Terapia del Dolore
Universita degli Studi di Milano
Milan, Italy

John Eccles, M.D.
CH6611 Contra (TI)
Switzerland

A. Claudio Cuello, M.D.
Department of Pharmacology
and Therapeutics
McGill University
Montreal, Canada

David Ottoson, M.D.
Department of Physiology
Karolinska Institute
Stockholm, Sweden

Raven Press ⬧ New York

Raven Press, 1185 Avenue of the Americas, New York, New York 10036

Made in the United States of America

Library of Congress Cataloging-in-Publication Data

Pain and mobility.

   (Advances in pain research and therapy; v. 10)
   Based on the International Conference on Pain and Motility held in
Milan, Italy, on Mar. 18–21, 1986.
   Includes bibliographies and index.
   1. Pain—Congresses. 2. Intractable pain—Congresses. 3. Movement
disorders—Congresses. I. Tiengo, Mario. II. International Conference on
Pain and Motility (1986 : Milan, Italy) III. Series. [DNLM: 1. Movement
Disorders—congresses. 2. Pain—physiopathology—congresses.
W1 AD706 v.10 / WL 704 P14436 1986]
RB127.P33215 1987   616′.0472   86-42923
ISBN 0-88167-319-6

   The material contained in this volume was submitted as previously
unpublished material, except in the instances in which credit has been
given to the source from which some of the illustrative material was
derived.
   Great care has been taken to maintain the accuracy of the information
contained in the volume. However, neither Raven Press nor the editors
can be held responsible for errors or for any consequences arising from
the use of the information contained herein.

9 8 7 6 5 4 3 2 1

Preface

This tenth volume of *Advances in Pain Research and Therapy* explores the physiological and psychological connections between pain and motor activity.

Anything that causes pain has some effect on movement. Crying out, trying to escape the cause of pain, grimacing, respiratory alterations: all are responses of the voluntary musculative, while changes in blood pressure and heart rate are responses of the smooth muscles. These reactions are all commonly used in laboratory and clinical practice to assess the modulating effects produced by drugs or other therapeutic agents on the pain system.

Movement is also inhibited when chronic pain is present, both directly and indirectly. Direct inhibition of movement occurs, for example, in the case of joint or muscular pain, which obviously limit movement. Indirect inhibition may take place through more complex circuits that also may impinge upon the psychic centers.

Immobility is typical of patients afflicted by chronic pain; in fact, its opposite, that is, activity, is considered proof of the analgesic efficacy of the therapy used.

A few years ago, I took these simple concepts as a foundation for a definition of the pain phenomenon that comprises its three major physiological phases: the transmission pathway from the periphery to the nociceptive center; the psychological interpretation in terms of suffering; and the proportionally related behavioral response.

> Pain is an alarm mechanism that relevantly alters the psychological state of the individual, and causes a behavioral response.

As with all attempts to define pain, this definition does not pretend to be unerring, but it perhaps has the merit of giving an objective and basic description of the pain phenomenon.

Pain is a neurophysiological event related to other neurophysiological processes such as learning, sleep, and memory, but which we not only for practical but also for qualitative reasons tend to consider as separate entities. That which we familiarly call pain is a complex protection system that all living things—probably including vegetable life—have in common. It clearly recognizes an input and an output.

The chapters in this volume attempt to measure and describe the input (cause of pain) and output responses (in terms of electrical or biochemical events or vegetative motor activity), not unlike what the neurophysiologist or pharmacologist usually describes. Yet everything that lies between input and output is shrouded largely still in mystery. Little is yet known about the refinements of the mechanism whereby a painful (or noxious) stimulus arriving at the higher centers is perceived, produces a state of suffering, and evokes a response.

A decade or so ago we thought we were closer to a solution to certain problems than we have since realized. Our problem is probably that our observations and measurements are still too rudimentary and our models too elementary and biased to enable us to understand a system that seems increasingly complex. As in the game of Chinese boxes, opening one box reveals yet another. We are still in this stage as far as these studies are concerned.

By bringing together the diverse contributions of an international, multi-disciplinary group of experts, this book seeks to lay the foundation for further research and understanding of pain. It will be of interest to both researchers and clinicians concerned with chronic pain syndromes and the cognitive and emotional aspects of pain.

Mario Tiengo

Acknowledgments

The chapters in this book were prepared by participants at the International Conference on Pain and Motility held in Milan, Italy, on March 18 to 21, 1986.

I would like officially to thank Sir John Eccles, to whom we are all indebted. I also wish to thank my colleagues, Antonio Cuello and David Ottoson, for having accepted the roles of Editors, and all the contributors who have honored us with their papers.

Last, but not least, I wish to thank our friend John Bonica, who accepted this text for the prestigious *Advances in Pain Research and Therapy* series.

Mario Tiengo

Contents

ix

Contributors

Goffredo Acampora
Ospedale Fondazione Senatore Pascale
Istituto per la Diagnosi e Cura dei Tu-
* mori*
Naples, Italy

Bruno Amantea
Istituto di Anestesia e Rianimazione e
* Terapia Intensiva*
II Falcoltà di Medicina e Chirurgia
Università degli Studi di Napoli
80131 Naples, Italy

L. Azzarà
Department of Anesthesiology and Re-
* animation*
University of Turin
Turin, Italy

Francesco Belfiore
Istituto di Anestesia e Rianimazione e
* Terapia Intensiva*
II Facoltà di Medicina e Chirurgia
Università degli Studi di Napoli
80131 Naples, Italy

Mauro Bianchi
Department of Pharmacology
University of Milan
20129 Milan, Italy

G. Biella
Centro Studi Analgesia
University of Milan
20129 Milan, Italy

R. Bortolami
Institute of Veterinary Anatomy
University of Bologna
40100 Bologna, Italy

P. C. Braga
Department of Pharmacology, Chemo-
* therapy, and Toxicology*
University of Milan
20129 Milan, Italy

Anna Brini
Department of Pharmacology
University of Milan
20129 Milan, Italy

Corrado Bucherelli
Department of Physiological Science
University of Florence
50134 Florence, Italy

E. Callegari
Institute of Veterinary Anatomy
University of Bologna
40100 Bologna, Italy

L. Calzà
Department of Pathophysiology and
* Pain Therapy*
University of Milan
20129 Milan, Italy

E. Campailla
Department of Traumatology
University of Trieste
Trieste, Italy

S. Candeletti
Institute of Pharmacology
University of Bologna
40126 Bologna, Italy

Augusto Caraceni
Istituto Nazionale per lo Studio e la
* Cura dei Tumori*
Servizio di Terapia del Dolore
20133 Milan, Italy

M. Carbone
*Department of Anesthesiology and Re-
animation*
University of Turin
Turin, Italy

Giancarlo Carli
Institute of Human Physiology
53100 Siena, Italy

Roberto Casale
*Foundation "Clinica del Lavoro", Pa-
via*
*Rehabilitation Medical Center of Mon-
tescano*
Service of Neurophysiology
27040 Montescano, Italy

E. Cavicchini
Institute of Pharmacology
University of Bologna
40126 Bologna, Italy

R. Cavallo
*Department of Anesthesiology and Re-
animation*
University of Turin
Turin, Italy

Carlo Lorenzo Cazzullo
State University of Milan
Institute of Psychiatry
20122 Milan, Italy

L. Ceretto
*Department of Anesthesiology and Re-
animation*
University of Turin
Turin, Italy

G. Cerutti
*Department of Anesthesiology and Re-
animation*
University of Turin
Turin, Italy

Ennio Cocco
Department of Pharmacology
University of Milan
20129 Milan, Italy

Beatrice Crespi
Department of Neurology
"Clinica del Lavoro" Foundation
Medical Center of Rehabilitation
28010 Veruno (No), Italy

A. C. Cuello
*Department of Pharmacology and
Therapeutics*
McGill University
Montreal, Quebec H3G 1Y6, Canada

U. Cugini
Department of Pain Therapy
University of Trieste
Trieste, Italy

Renato Cuocolo
*Istituto di Anestesia e Rianimazione e
Terapia Intensiva*
II Facoltà di Medicina e Chirurgia
Università degli Studi di Napoli
80131 Naples, Italy

Giuseppe De Benedittis
Pain Research and Treatment Unit
Institute of Neurosurgery
University of Milan
20122 Milan, Italy

Franco De Conno
*Istituto Nazionale per lo Studio e la
Cura dei Tumori*
Servizio di Terapia del Dolore
20133 Milan, Italy

Ciro Esposito
*Istituto di Anestesia e Rianimazione e
Terapia Intensiva*
II Facoltà di Medicina e Chirurgia
Università degli Studi di Napoli
80131 Naples, Italy

S. Ferri
Institute of Pharmacology
University of Bologna
40126 Bologna, Italy

A. Formenti
Istituto di Fisiologia Umana II
Università degli Studi di Milano
20133 Milan, Italy

Gianfranco Formicola
Clinica Urologica
II Facoltà di Medicina e Chirurgia
Università degli Studi di Napoli
80131 Naples, Italy

Costanzo Gala
State University of Milan
Institute of Psychiatry
20122 Milan, Italy

Aldo Giachetti
Department of Physiological Science
University of Florence
50134 Florence, Italy

M. A. Giamberardino
Institute of Medical Physiopathology
University of Chieti
Chieti, Italy

L. Giardino
Department of Pathophysiology and
  Pain Therapy
University of Milan
20125 Milan, Italy

Ji-Sheng Han
Department of Physiology
Beijing Medical University
Beijing 100083, China

L. Imeri
Istituto di Fisiologia Umana II
Università degli Studi di Milano
20133 Milan, Italy

Olle Johansson
Department of Histology
Karolinska Institute
S-104 01 Stockholm, Sweden

D. A. Jones
Department of Medicine
University College London
London, England

Carlo Ambrogi Lorenzini
Department of Physiological Science
University of Florence
50134 Florence, Italy

M. L. Lucchi
Institute of Veterinary Anatomy
University of Bologna
40100 Bologna, Italy

M. Mancia
Istituto di Fisiologia Umana II
Università degli Studi di Milano
20133 Milan, Italy

E. Manni
Institute of Human Physiology
Catholic University Medical School
00168 Rome, Italy

E. Manno
Department of Anesthesiology and Re-
  animation
University of Turin
Turin, Italy

Marco Maresca
Institute of Medical Clinic
Pain Center
University of Florence
50134 Florence, Italy

I. Marini
Institute of Medical Physiopathology
University of Chieti
Chieti, Italy

M. Mariotti
Istituto di Fisiologia Umana II
Università degli Studi di Milano
20133 Milan, Italy

G. Mocavero
Department of Pain Therapy
University of Trieste
Trieste, Italy

V. Moschini
Cattedra di Fisiopatologia e Terapia del
*   Dolore*
Università degli Studi di Milano
20122 Milan, Italy

D. J. Newham
Department of Medicine
University College London
London, England

G. Obletter
Institute of Medical Physiopathology
University of Chieti
Chieti, Italy

Alberto E. Panerai
Department of Pharmacology
University of Milan
20129 Milan, Italy

V. Paladini
Department of Pain Therapy
University of Trieste
Trieste, Italy

M. Palestini
Faculty of Medicine
University of Chile
Santiago, Chile

G. C. Pastorino
Servizio di Neurofisiopatologia
Emanuela dalla Chiesa Setti Carraro
Istituti Clinici di Perfezionamento
20122 Milan, Italy

Giovanni Peretti
Clinica Ortopedica dell' Università
*   degli Studi di Milano*
III Cattedra
Milan, Italy

V. E. Pettorossi
Institute of Human Physiology
Catholic University Medical School
00168 Rome, Italy

Paolo Pinelli
First Neurological Clinic
University of Milan
20129 Milan, Italy

Paolo Procacci
Institute of Medical Clinic
Pain Center
University of Florence
50134 Florence, Italy

M. Rigoli
Department of Pathophysiology and
*   Pain Therapy*
University of Milan
20125 Milan, Italy

M. Riva
Department of Anesthesiology and Re-
*   animation*
University of Turin
Turin, Italy

P. Romualdi
Institute of Pharmacology
University of Bologna
40126 Bologna, Italy

Lucio Rovati
Department of Pharmacology
University of Milan
20129 Milan, Italy

Paola Sacerdote
Department of Pharmacology
University of Milan
20129 Milan, Italy

Luigi Saita
Istituto Nazionale per lo Studio e la
  Cura dei Tumori
Servizio di Terapia del Dolore
20133 Milan, Italy

Antonio Savenelli
Clinica Chirurgica Pediatrica
II Facoltà di Medicina e Chirurgia
Università degli Studi di Napoli
80131 Naples, Italy

Gennaro Savoia
Istituto di Anestesia e Rianimazione e
  Terapia Intensiva
II Facoltà di Medicina e Chirurgia
Università degli Studi di Napoli
80131 Naples, Italy

Alberto Sbanotto
Istituto Nazionale per lo Studio e la
  Cura dei Tumori
Servizio dei Terapia del Dolore
20133 Milan, Italy

M. Scalia
Department of Pain Therapy
University of Trieste
Trieste, Italy

M. Sciuto
Department of Anesthesiology and Re-
  animation
University of Turin
Turin, Italy

S. Spampinato
Institute of Pharmacology
University of Bologna
40126 Bologna, Italy

E. Speroni
Institute of Pharmacology
University of Bologna
40126 Bologna, Italy

Elio Spoldi
Istituto Nazionale per lo Studio e la
  Cura dei Tumori

Servizio di Terapia del Dolore
20133 Milan, Italy

Lars Terenius
Department of Pharmacology
University of Uppsala
Uppsala, Sweden

Mario Tiengo
Cattedra di Fisiopatologia e Terapia del
  Dolore
Università degli Studi di Milano
20122 Milan, Italy

M. Trompeo
Reanimation and Intensive Care Unit
University of Turin
Turin, Italy

Eldon Tunks
Chedoke-McMaster Hospital
Hamilton, Ontario L8N 325, Canada

L. Vecchiet
Institute of Medical Physiopathology
University of Chieti
Chieti, Italy

Vittorio Ventafridda
Istituto Nazionale per lo Studio e la
  Cura dei Tumori
Servizio di Terapia del Dolore
20133 Milan, Italy

Angelo Villani
Department of Neurology
"Clinica del Lavoro" Foundation
Medical Center of Rehabilitation
28010 Veruno (No), Italy

Roberto Villani
Pain Research and Treatment Unit
Institute of Neurosurgery
University of Milan
20122 Milan, Italy

M. Zanni
Department of Pathophysiology and
  Pain Therapy
University of Milan
20125 Milan, Italy

Advances in Pain Research and Therapy
Volume 10

PAIN AND MOBILITY

Advances in Pain Research and Therapy,
Vol. 10. Edited by M. Tiengo et al.
Raven Press, Ltd., New York © 1987.

Synaptic Organization of Peptide-Containing Sensory Neurons

A.C. Cuello

Department of Pharmacology and Therapeutics, McGill University,
Montreal, Quebec H3G 1Y6, Canada

PEPTIDES AS TRANSMITTER CANDIDATES

In recent years, a number of peptides have been associated with subsets of primary sensory neurons. Some of these peptides have also been shown to display "neurotransmitter properties." Although the list of peptides as candidates for a neurotransmitter role in primary sensory neurons is growing steadily, the best candidates at present are: substance P and related tachykinins, vasoactive intestinal peptide, somatostatin, colecystokinin, bombesin, and angiotensin. The best established case is that of substance P and related tachykinins. The main criteria for which substance P is regarded as a transmitter candidate are summarized as follows:

1. Substance P immunoreactive material is present in the central nervous system (CNS) and peripheral neuronal system (PNS) and absent in glial cells (12,13,33).
2. Substance P immunoreactive material has been found in cellular fractions of synaptic vesicles (11,15), and located in synaptic boutons with the aid of electron microscopy (2,47).
3. The peptide is synthesized in neuronal cell bodies (19) and transported by axonal flow to nerve terminal fields (1,17,18). Precursor molecules have been described (see later).
4. It is released from nerve terminal areas following electrical (43), high potassium, or veratridine stimulation (22,23) in a calcium-dependent manner.
5. It produces biological responses in bioassay preparations which can be distinguished from those provoked by other neurotransmitter substances (5).
6. Its application provokes slow synaptic responses in the CNS (27) and PNS (50), which are not suppressed by classical neurotransmitter antagonists.
7. Specific agonists and antagonists to substance P and related tachykinins are being found (see later).

8. Substance P actions are terminated by peptidases (specific?) (30). No reuptake mechanism for substance P has been convincingly demonstrated.

Although these peptides display many "transmitter-like" characteristics, it is important to realize that their "transmitter status" is complicated further for the following aspects:

1. It is becoming apparent that in some cases (probably all) we are not dealing with a single peptide, but rather a family of related peptides which might be present in the same or different neurons.
2. There is growing evidence that more than one of these substances are stored in a single neuron. The idea of "cotransmission" has emerged to support this evidence (for reviews see refs. 3 and 7). The fact that peptides are stored and released along with other transmitters (or transmitter candidates) opens questions on the precise role of sensory peptides.
3. As most synaptic actions of peptides (see above) are relatively slow, there is room for the discovery of yet unknown small molecules produced by sensory neurons which could elicit fast synaptic responses in the manner of the classical neurotransmitter substances.

Currently under way in many laboratories are research efforts addressed to find clues to these important interrogants. But, whatever is the definitive role of these sensory peptides, it is clear that they participate in sensory mechanisms, both in the CNS and PNS. They have also offered rather novel opportunities to investigate sensory subsets, distribution of sensory fibers, and synaptic arrangements involving sensory terminals.

THE TACHYKININ STORY

The so-called "substance P" neurons (immunoreactive, containing, positive) probably belong to a family of related peptides. This has emerged from biochemical studies which demonstrated that important amounts of tachykinins with very similar amino acid sequence to substance P is present in tissue extracts (25,26,34). Although currently there is some confusion as to how many of these peptides are present in various parts in the nervous system and how they should be named, it is becoming clearer that at least three of these tachykinins are important constituents. These are: (a) substance P (SP), which was suspected earlier to be a sensory transmitter (32) and which was chemically identified by Leeman and co-workers (4); (b) substance K, also referred to as neurokinin A (SK, NKA); and (c) neuromedin K, also referred to as neurokinin B (NK, NKB).

Applying molecular biology techniques, Nawa and collaborators (40) have been able to identify two tachykinin precursor molecules in the mammalian brain. They were named α-preprotachykinin, containing an SP sequence, and β-preprotachykinin, containing an SP and SK sequence separated by an intervening peptide sequence. It is still uncertain whether these preprotachykinins are present in different subsets of primary sensory neurons, or whether the precursor peptides are differentially processed in such substrates. From the biochemical information available in the CNS, it seems that there is a good parallelism in the relative concentrations of the active peptides in most brain regions (35). On the other hand, some experimental studies would indicate that NKB might be present in a different neuron, centrally located (42).

It is appealing to think that these various extracted peptides are the natural ligands for multiple tachykinin receptors. Thus, the existence of three tachykinin receptor types has been proposed (29). These receptor types are SP-P where SP and physalaemin are the most potent agonists, and SP-E, where eleidosin and kassinin are the more potent. In addition to these observations, it has been found that the mammalian peptide SK is more potent than eleidosin in the receptor categorized as SP-E, while evidence is accumulating for an additional receptor subtype, where SK would be the most potent agonist (48). A number of peptides with antagonistic actions have been found by amino acid substitution of the tachykinin backbone (16,39,49). They are not, at present, sufficiently specific to differentiate receptor subtypes, in addition they possess agonistic properties in varying degrees.

ORGANIZATION OF TACHYKININ-CONTAINING PRIMARY SENSORY NEURONS

An interesting aspect of the organization of tachykinin-containing primary sensory neurons is their symmetric nature, in that the peptide is present both at central and peripheral ends of primary sensory neurons. This was proposed by Hokfelt and collaborators (21) and demonstrated experimentally in the trigeminal system (10). The idea that the neuroactive tachykinins are present at both ends of primary sensory neurons is in agreement with one of the landmarks of the history of neuronal transmission. As it was expressed by Sir Henry Dale in a letter to Feldberg (44): "There is a good deal of probability that chemical transmission of antidromic vasodilation at the *peripheral* end of a sensory neuron might be expected to use the same substance as transmission of a sensory impulse to a motor cell of a central synapse. It is, of course, merely a guess, but a point of some interest."

As well anticipated by Dale, these peptides, released from sensory neurons, exert actions both in the CNS and PNS. In the CNS, they are somehow involved in pain processing mechanisms, whereas in the periphery they seem to be involved in local sensory responses in a wide variety of target systems.

In the CNS, SP-containing fibers are assumed to participate in the first signal to pain perception. SP applied iontophoretically facilitates transmission in nociceptive-driven neurons of the spinal cord (20); the peptide is absent in the dorsal horn of patients with familial dysautonomia (inability to perceive pain) (46), and its release from trigeminal nucleus tissue slices is inhibited by morphine and endogenous opiates (24). The opiate-mediated inhibition of tachykinin released from primary sensory neurons refreshed the concept of central gating (38) of this information. Jessell et al. (24) proposed for this gating an axo-axonic synaptic mechanism between SP-containing primary sensory neurons and local circuit enkephalinergic cells. The direct, ultrastructural visualization of SP and enkephalin immunoreactive sites would indicate that both peptide-containing systems act on a common dendrite (8).

The presence of tachykinins in peripheral branches of sensory neurons promotes revision of some classical concepts on the significance of neuronal processes. The terminal branching of sensory neurons are in fact "dendritic" processes which were regarded classically as mere sites of sensory transduction, much more so than in the case of small caliber, unmyelinated sensory fibers which terminate as "free endings." It has now been shown that these free endings contain and release neuroactive peptides. These peripheral sensory branches are distributed in many organs in a very specialized fashion. In this chapter we briefly discuss aspects of sensory-peptidergic innervation of the skin and autonomic ganglia.

In the skin, these terminals are related to blood vessels, sweat glands, and hair follicles (10,21). This arrangement is propitious for the engagement of sensory peptides in antidromic neurogenic responses. Thus, it has been seen that the antidromic stimulation of the saphenous nerve (31) or the mental branch (sensory) of the trigeminal nerve (6) leads to vasodilation and plasma extravasation in their corresponding vascular territories, responses which are reduced approximately by half with the application of substance P antagonists.

Some of these tachykinin-induced antidromic, sensory responses are direct, whereas others are mediated by cutaneous mast cells and, possibly, some yet unidentified cholinergic component (6,31). Figure 1 summarizes these interactions in the trigeminal territory.

Sensory peptides in peripheral sensory branches not only can offer a substrate to understand the old enigma of cutaneous antidromic responses, but also provoke new questions. For instance, there are indications that peptides released by peripheral sensory branches might affect immunocompetent cells (45), and also exert thropic actions over cells of the connective tissue

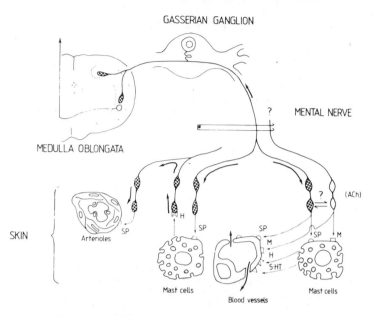

FIG. 1. Antidromically released SP would activate tachykinin receptors (SP) in blood vessels and mast cells. Activated mast cells in turn would release histamine (H) and serotonin (5-HT) which reinforce these peptidergic actions and probably further sensitize sensory fibers. A hypothetical cholinergic involvement is also indicated. ACh, acetyl choline; M, muscarinic receptors. (From ref. 6.)

(41). In a holistic manner, nociceptors would not only transfer information to the CNS, but they could respond, independently, to local injuries.

This concept of independent responses of sensory fibers in the periphery is further stressed by the novel findings of the relation of sensory-peptidergic fibers to autonomic neurons. It is now clear that the network of the substance P immunoreactive fibers originates in sensory neurons (14,36). These sensory terminals (dendritic) establish synaptic contacts with dendrites of autonomic prevertebral ganglia (36,37). Peptides released at this point are able to produce slow, noncholinergic, excitatory postsynaptic potentials (28,50). A sensory-synaptic arrangement of this sort offers further evidence for "reverse" information transfer (9) and offers a framework to explain sensory-autonomic reflexes without the participation of the CNS.

CONCLUSIONS

Peptides and, in particular, tachykinins are strong candidates as neuroactive (neurotransmitter?) substances. They are involved in defined synaptic mechanisms in the CNS and they participate in a number of local responses in the periphery.

REFERENCES

1. Brimijoin, S., Lundberg, J. M., Brodkin, E., Hökfelt, T., and Nilsson, G. (1980): Axonal transport of substance P in the vagus and sciatic nerves of the guinea pig. *Brain Res.*, 191:443–457.
2. Chan-Palay, V., and Palay, S. L. (1977): Ultrastructural identification of SP cells and their processes in rat sensory ganglia and their terminals in the spinal cord by immunocytochemistry. *Proc. Natl. Acad. Sci. USA*, 74:4050–4054.
3. Chan-Palay, V., and Palay, S. (1984): *Coexistence of Neuroactive Substances in Neurons.* Wiley, New York.
4. Chang, M. M., and Leeman, S. E. (1970): Isolation of a sialogogic peptide from bovine hypothalamic tissue and its characterization as substance P. *J. Biol. Chem.*, 245:4784–4790.
5. Couture, R., and Regoli, D. (1982): Smooth-muscle pharmacology of substance P. *Pharmacology*, 24:1–25.
6. Couture, R., and Cuello, A. C. (1984): Studies on the trigeminal antidromic vasodilatation and plasma extravasation in the rat. *J. Physiol.*, 346:273–285.
7. Cuello, A. C. (editor) (1982): *Co-Transmission.* Proceedings of a symposium held at Oxford during the 50th anniversary meeting of the British Pharmacological Society. McMillan, London.
8. Cuello, A. C. (1983): Central distribution of opioid peptides. *Br. Med. Bull.*, 39:11–16.
9. Cuello, A. C. (1983): Dendrites as sites of storage and release of neurotransmitter substances: an extension of Dale's principle. In: *Dale's Principle and Communication Between Neurones*, edited by N. N. Osborne. Pergamon Press, Oxford.
10. Cuello, A. C., Del Fiacco, M., and Paxinos, G. (1978): The central and peripheral ends of the substance P-containing sensory neurones in the rat trigeminal system. *Brain Res.*, 152:499–510.
11. Cuello, A. C., Jessell, T., Kanazawa, I., and Iversen, L. L. (1977): Substance P: localization in synaptic vesicles in rat central nervous system. *J. Neurochem.*, 29:747–751.
12. Cuello, A. C., and Kanazawa, I. (1978): The distribution of substance P immunoreactive fibres in the rat central nervous system. *J. Comp. Neurol.*, 178:129–156.
13. Cuello, A. C., Priestley, J. V., and Matthews, M. R. (1982): Localization of substance P in neuronal pathways. In: *Substance P in the Nervous System*, pp. 55–58. Ciba Foundation Symposium 91. Pitman, London.
14. Dalsgaard, C. J., Hökfelt, T., Elfvin, L. G., Skirboll, L., and Emson, P. (1982): Substance P-containing primary sensory neurons projecting to the inferior mesenteric ganglion: evidence from combined retrograde tracing and immunohistochemistry. *Neuroscience*, 7:647–654.
15. Floor, E., Grad, O., and Leeman, S. E. (1982): Synaptic vesicles containing substance P purified by chromatography on controlled pore glass. *Neuroscience*, 7:1647–1655.
16. Folkers, K., Horig, J., Rampold, G., Lane, P., Rossell, S., and Bjorkroth, U. (1982): Design and synthesis of effective antagonists of substance P. *Acta Chem. Scand.*, 36:389–398.
17. Gamse, R., Lembeck, F., and Cuello, A. C. (1979): Substance P in the vagus nerve. *Naunyn-Schmiedebergs Arch. Pharmacol.*, 306:37–44.
18. Gilbert, R. F. T., and Emson, P. C. (1978): *Neurosci. Lett. (Suppl.)*, 1:218.
19. Harmar, A., Schofield, J. G., and Keen, P. (1980): Cycloheximide-sensitive synthesis of substance P by isolated dorsal root-ganglia. *Nature*, 284:267–269.
20. Henry, J. L. (1980): Substance P and pari-am updating. *Trends Neurosci.*, 3:95–97.
21. Hökfelt, T., Kellerth, J.-O., Nilsson, G., Pernow, B. (1975): Experimental immunohistochemical studies on the localization and distribution of substance P in cat primary sensory neurons. *Brain Res.*, 100:235–252.
22. Iversen, L. L., Jessell, T., and Kanazawa, I. (1976): Release and metabolism of substance P in rat hypothalamus. *Nature*, 264:81–83.
23. Jessell, T. M. (1978): Substance P release from the rat substantia nigra. *Brain Res.*, 151:469–478.
24. Jessell, T. M., Iversen, L. L., and Kanazawa, I. (1977): Opiate analgesics inhibit substance P release from rat trigeminal nucleus. *Nature*, 268:549–551.

25. Kangawa, K., Minamino, N., Fukuda, A., and Matsuo, H. (1983): Neuromedin-K—A novel mammalion tachykinin identified in porcine spinal cord. *Biochem. Biophys. Res. Commun.*, 114:533–540.
26. Kimura, S., Okada, M., Sugita, Y., Kanazawa, I., and Munekato, E. (1983): Novel neuropeptides, neurokinin-alpha, and neurokinin-beta isolated from porcine spinal cord. *Proc. Jpn. Acad. (Ser. B.)*, 59:101–104.
27. Konishi, S., and Otsuka, M. (1974): Excitatory action of hypothalamic substance P on spinal motoneurones of newborn rats. *Nature*, 252:734–735.
28. Konishi, S., Tsunoo, A., and Otsuka, M. (1979): Substance P and noncholinergic excitatory synaptic transmission in guinea-pig sympathetic ganglia. *Proc. Jpn. Acad.*, 55:525–530.
29. Lee, C. M., Iversen, L. L., Hanley, M. R., and Iversen, L. L. (1982): The possible existence of multiple receptors for substance P. *Naunyn-Schmiedebergs Arch. Pharmacol.*, 318:281–287.
30. Lee, C. M., Sandberg, B. E. B., Hanley, M. R., and Iversen, L. L. (1981): Purification and characterisation of a membrane-bound substance P-degrading enzyme from human brain. *Eur. J. Biochem.*, 114:315–327.
31. Lembeck, F., and Holzer, P. (1979): Substance P as neurogenic mediator of antidromic vasodilation and neurogenic plasma extravasation. *Naunyn-Schmiedebergs Arch. Pharmacol.*, 310:175–183.
32. Lembeck, F., and Zetler, G. (1962): Substance P: A polypeptide of possible physiological significance, especially within the nervous system. *Int. Review Neurobiol.*, 4:159–215.
33. Ljungdahl, A., Hökfelt, T., and Nilsson, G. (1978): Distribution of substance P-like immunoreactivity in the central nervous system of the rat. *Neuroscience*, 3:861–943.
34. Maggio, J. E., Sandberg, B. E. B., Bradley, C. V., Iversen, L. L., Santikarn, S., Williams, B. H., Hunter, J. C., and Hanley, M. R. (1983): Substance K: a novel tachykinin in mammalian spinal cord. In: *Substance P-Dublin 1983*, edited by P. Skrabanek and D. Powell, pp. 20–21. Boole Press, Dublin.
35. Maggio, J. E., and Hunter, J. C. (1984): Regional distribution of kassinin-like immunoreactivity in rat central and peripheral tissues and the effect of capsaicin. *Brain Res.*, 307:370–373.
36. Matthews, M. R., and Cuello, A. C. (1982): Substance P-immunoreactive peripheral branches of sensory neurones innervate guinea-pig sympathetic neurones. *Proc. Natl. Acad. Sci. USA*, 79:1668–1672.
37. Matthews, M. R., Connaughton, M., and Cuello, A. C. (1986): Ultrastructure and distribution of substance P-immunoreactive sensory collaterals in the guinea pig prevertebral sympathetic ganglia. *J. Comp. Neurol. (in press)*.
38. Melzack, R., and Wall, P. D. (1965): Pain mechanisms: a new theory. *Science*, 150:971–979.
39. Mizrahi, J., Escher, E., D'Orleans-Juste, P., and Regoli, D. (1982): Substance P antagonists *in vitro* and *in vivo*. *Eur. J. Pharmacol.*, 82:101–105.
40. Nawa, H., Hirose, T., Takashima, H. Inayama, S, and Nakanishi, S. (1983): Nucleotide sequences of cloned CDNAs for two types of bovine brain substance P percursor. *Nature*, 306:32–36.
41. Nilsson, J., v. Euler, A. M., and Dalsgaard, C-J. (1985): Stimulation of connective tissue cell growth by substance P and substance K. *Nature*, 315:61–62.
42. Ogawa, T., Kanazawa, I., and Kimura, S. (1985): Regional distribution of substance P, neurokinin-alpha, and neurokinin-beta in rat spinal cord, nerve roots, and dorsal-root ganglia, and the effects of dorsal-root section or spinal transection. *Brain Res.*, 359:152–157.
43. Otsuka, M., and Konishi, S. (1976): Release of substance P-like immunoreactivity from isolated spinal cord of newborn rat. *Nature*, 264:83–84.
44. Paton, W. D. M. (1976): Sir Henry Dale (1875–1968): some letters and papers. In: *Notes and Records of the Royal Society of London*, 30(2):231–248.
45. Payan, D. G., Levine, J. D., and Goetzl, E. J. (1984): Modulation of immunity and hypersensitivity by sensory neuropeptides. *J. Immunol.*, 132:1601–1604.
46. Pearson, J., Brandeis, L., and Cuello, A. C. (1982): Depletion of substance P-containing axons in substantia gelatinosa of patients with diminished pain sensitivity. *Nature*, 275:61–63.

47. Pickel, V. M., Reis, D. J., and Leeman, S. E. (1977): Ultrastructural localization of substance P in neurons of rat spinal cord. *Brain Res.,* 122:534–540.
48. Quirion, R. (1985): Multiple tachykinin receptors. *Trends Neurosci.,* 8:183–185.
49. Regoli, D., Escher, E., and Mizrahi, J. (1984): Substance P structure activity studies and the development of antagonists. *Pharmacology,* 28:301–320.
50. Tsunoo, A., Konishi, S., and Otsuka, M. (1982): Substance P as an excitatory transmitter of primary afferent neurons in guinea pig sympathetic ganglia. *Neuroscience,* 4:2025–2037.

Advances in Pain Research and Therapy,
Vol. 10. Edited by M. Tiengo et al.
Raven Press, Ltd., New York © 1987.

Endorphins and Substance P in Chronic Pain

Lars Terenius

Department of Pharmacology, University of Uppsala, Uppsala, Sweden

Pain is the most frequent clinical complaint and symptom. Not infrequently are available methods for pain treatment insufficient or inappropriate; persistent pain may become chronic. By definition, chronic pain is a therapeutic failure and a challenge for research. Recently, there has been considerable progress in the mapping of transmitters and pathways of potential importance for pain and pain modulation.

Several peptides have been found in the thin nonmyelinated afferent fibers known to be involved in nociception. These fibers terminate in the most dorsal parts of the dorsal horn of the spinal cord. Approximately 80% of substance P terminals in spinal cord are from these fibers. Based on its distribution and biological actions substance P has been proposed as a transmitter for nociceptive stimuli (e.g., ref. 13.)

Locally in the spinal cord there is also rich representation of pathways with opioid peptides. Substance P nerve terminals overlap with terminals from local enkephalinergic neurons (7). Dynorphin pathways are found locally in the spinal cord with termination mainly in laminae II and IV, areas which receive dense innervation from afferent fibers (5). It is also evident that not only μ(morphine)-type receptors at the spinal level mediate analgesia, but also agents affecting δ- and κ-receptor types. This is an interesting observation since the endogenous opioids have higher affinity for these types, enkephalins for δ-receptors and the dynorphin peptides for κ-receptors (Table 1).

The spinal cord also receives input from fibers in the medulla, some of which have substance P or substance P and serotonin (4,8). Electrical stimulation or morphine microinjection in these areas is known to activate descending systems, some of which may be opioid or activate pathways with an opioid link (18).

It seems pertinent to consider whether this new information about pathways involved in pain and pain modulation and, more explicitly, the alleged role of substance P and opioid peptides in these pathways can be used to

TABLE 1. *Affinities of various opioid peptides for opioid receptor types*[ab]

Endogenous opioid	Relative affinity		
	μ-Receptor	κ-Receptor	δ-Receptor
β-Endorphin	100	2	90
Met-enkephalin	10	1	100
Leu-enkephalin	8	1	100
Dynorphin A	20	100	10

[a]The highest affinity equals 100.
[b]From ref. 14

provide better understanding of chronic pain syndromes. Since chronic pain is an operational term, there is no reason to anticipate that etiology will be uniform. An important goal is, therefore, to provide better diagnostic techniques and improve the taxonomy of chronic pain. The work reviewed in this chapter deals with chronic clinical pain.

Chemical analysis of the cerebrospinal fluid (CSF) content of substance P and opioid peptides has been performed. It has been assumed that the CSF content reflects the activity in CNS pathways. Since CSF is sampled at a lumbar level, contributions may be mainly of local origin, and therefore reflect activity in the spinal cord.

PATIENT SELECTION AND DEFINITIONS

Patients included in these studies had suffered from severe persistent pain for at least 6 months. Patients older than 60 years, who were known abusers of alcohol or drugs, or had been taking narcotic analgesic drugs during the past month were excluded. All patients underwent a thorough neurologic investigation, including X-ray and sensitivity testing, and a psychiatric evaluation during the examination period for approximately one week at a neurologic clinic. Patients with verified organic lesions in the nervous system were termed neurogenic pain patients. When no organic lesion was observed and the patient showed signs of psychiatric disturbance, they were termed psychogenic pain or, lately, idiopathic pain. In this chapter, the term idiopathic pain is used throughout.

During the examination perioid at the hospital, a lumbar puncture was performed in the morning, and CSF (12.5 ml) divided into aliquots of 4 ml and stored frozen at −80°C until analysis.

A control group consisted of healthy volunteers without neurological or psychiatric history.

CHEMICAL ANALYSES

Substance P

Antiserum against substance P was obtained by repeated injections of a substance-P-thyroglobulin conjugate intracutaneously into rabbits. For radioimmunoassay, ^{125}I-labeled Tyr^8-substance P was utilized. The radioimmunoassay procedure has been described in detail elsewhere (15). Briefly, the CSF sample was fractionated on a Sephadex ion exchanger. The fraction containing substance P was saved, lyophilized, and reconstituted in the radioimmunoassay system. Each assay included standard samples.

Opioid Peptides

Opioid peptides were measured by receptor-assay. This type of assay measures opioid activity regardless of structure. It was chosen rather than radioimmunoassay primarily because of the large number of different kinds of opioid peptides that could contribute, and the difficulty in selecting any of them for analysis. The procedure has been described by Terenius and Wahlström (17). Prior to the assay, the CSF sample is fractionated by chromatography on a Sephadex G10 column. The major opioid activity elutes in two fractions, I and II. The former contains opioid peptides of nine to 20 amino acids including dynorphins, the latter enkephalyl peptides with six to eight amino acids. Neither fraction contains β-endorphin or enkephalins (11). This procedure is general in the sense that all opioid activity is measured, and it may be considered similar in scope to the use of naloxone as an antagonist.

SUBSTANCE P MEASUREMENTS

Substance P levels were generally lower in patients than in controls. Patients with the subdiagnosis neurogenic pain had the lowest levels (Table 2). Low CSF levels have also been reported in peripheral neuropathy and

TABLE 2. *Immunoreactive substance P in CSF of healthy volunteers and patients with chronic pain[a]*

Subjects	n	Substance P (fmol/ml CSF)
Healthy volunteers	35	9.6 ± 3.2
Chronic pain, neurogenic	23	6.0 ± 4.2
Chronic pain, idiopathic	37	7.2 ± 5.3

[a]Means ± SD.

autonomic dysfunction (12). However, in patients with arachnoiditis and with strong pain complaints, levels were higher than in controls (9). Several studies have indicated that substance P can be released from the spinal cord by strong somatic stimulation (cf., ref. 13). This may be occurring in arachnoiditis, explaining the elevated levels. Judging from substance P measurements alone, there is no comparable activation of afferents in the chronic neurogenic pain syndrome. Rather there may be a lack of input, i.e., deafferentation.

OPIOID PEPTIDE MEASUREMENTS

Using the radioreceptor assay we observed that patients with chronic pain deviated markedly from the volunteers. In neurogenic pain, levels were very significantly lower than control. In the idiopathic syndromes, levels tended to be higher. Interestingly, higher than control levels were also observed in depressive disorders (Table 3). There was also a co-variation between opioid peptide and serotonin metabolite levels. Thus, the measured indicators of two systems with potential pain modulatory role (*vide infra*) are lower than control in neurogenic pain. Commonalities between chronic idiopathic pain and depressive disorders have been suggested on purely clinical grounds, and it is interesting that they extend to the variables measured here.

Transcutaneous nerve stimulation (TNS) and acupuncture have become important new modalities for treating chronic pain. There is evidence that this treatment is particularly successful in chronic neurogenic pain. There is also direct evidence, using our procedure for chemical measurements and indirect evidence using naloxone injection, that these treatments release opioid peptides. It is, therefore, an attractive hypothesis that electrostimulation and acupuncture treatment is effective via release of opioid peptides (ref. 16, and references cited therein).

There are also data suggesting that TNS treatment with high frequency activates nonopioid mechanisms. However, even this treatment modality has

TABLE 3. *Distribution of cases with regard to opioid peptide levels in CSF measured with radioreceptor assay*[a]

Subjects	Opioid peptides (pmol/ml)[b]		
	<0.6	0.6–1.2	>1.2
Healthy volunteers	3	12	4
Neurogenic pain syndromes	29	2	2
Idiopathic pain syndromes	3	9	10
Depressive disorders	—	3	12

[a]From ref. 1.
[b]Calculated as met-enkephalin equivalents.

TABLE 4. *Levels of opioid peptides in CSF of patients with chronic pain measured in radioreceptor assay[ab]*

Subjects	n	Prior to treatment	Change with treatment
Neurogenic	11	0.21 ± 0.13	0.69 ± 0.15[c]
Nonneurogenic	7	1.04 ± 0.38	0.16 ± 0.24
Responders[d]	5	—	0.71 ± 0.25
Nonresponders	12	—	0.40 ± 0.17

[a]Met-enkephalin equivalents pmol/ml; prior to treatment and 1 week after daily treatments with high-frequency TNS.
[b]From ref. 2.
[c]$p < 0.001$ (Student's *t*-test).
[d]Remaining responders (20–100%) at 3 months.

the best prospects in patients with chronic neurogenic pain and pain mainly located in the extremities. Moreover, the group with the best therapeutic outcome also had the lowest CSF opioid levels (10). A more recent study has again raised the question whether the neurochemical markers discussed here (substance P, opioid peptides, and the serotonin metabolite in CSF) serve as predictors for a therapeutic response to high frequency TNS treatment. In this study (2) patients gave one CSF sample prior to the treatment and a second sample after one week of daily treatment. Treatment was continued and the effect evaluated after 30 days and 3 months. As earlier observed, patients with neurogenic pain had the lowest opioid peptide levels. One week of treatment raised these levels significantly. There was a tendency for higher elevation in long-term responders than in nonresponders (Table 4).

NEUROPEPTIDE AND NEUROENDOCRINE MARKERS IN CHRONIC PAIN

Many CNS functions are sensitive to stress and psychologic discomfort. This includes sensitivity to pain (16). It is not uncommon to observe hyperactivity in the hypothalamus-pituitary-adrenal axis in patients with chronic pain. This is observed as a resistance to cortisol suppression in the dexamethasone suppression test (DST), which examines the hypothalamic response to exogenously given glucocorticosteroid and is used as a neuroendocrine marker for major depressive disorders (3). In a recent study, France and Krishnan (6) reported 14 out of 80 patients with chronic back pain who had an abnormal response. Thirty-five patients satisfied DSM-III criteria for major depression, and all cases with abnormal DST were included among them. In our own studies (L. von Knorring and B. Almay, *unpublished*) eight of nine patients with an abnormal DST were classified as idiopathic.

CONCLUSIONS

The studies reviewed here indicate certain possibilities to categorize chronic pain with chemical markers. Patients with chronic neurogenic pain seem to form a quite distinct category in a state of pronounced central hypoendorphin activity. Several studies indicate that such pain is probably not elicited via activation of substance-P-containing afferents. These patients have normal activity in the hypothalamus-pituitary-adrenal axis. Chronic pain where the psychic components dominate, and there is no apparent organic pathology, is a different clinical reality. This pain, here called idiopathic, is frequently accompanied by supernormal CSF endorphins and abnormal DST, which is also recorded in major depression (with or without pain complaints).

ACKNOWLEDGMENT

This work was supported by the Swedish Medical Research Council grant 5095.

REFERENCES

1. Almay, B. G. L., Johansson, F., von Knorring, L., Terenius, L, and Wahlström, A. (1978): Endorphins in chronic pain. I. Differences in CSF endorphin levels between organic and psychogenic pain syndromes. *Pain*, 5:153–162.
2. Almay, B. G. L., Johansson, F., von Knorring, L., Sakurada, T., and Terenius, L. (1985): Long-term high frequency transcutaneous electrical nerve stimulation (hi-TNS) in chronic pain. Clinical response and effects on CSF-endorphins, monoamine metabolites, substance P-like immunoreactivity (SPLI) and pain measures. *J. Psychosom. Res.*, 29:247–257.
3. Carroll, B. J., Feinberg, M., Greden, T. F., Tarika, J., Albala, A. A., Haskett, R. F., James, N. M., Kronfol, Z., Lohr, N., Steiner, M., de Vigne, J. P., and Young, E. (1981): A specific laboratory test for the diagnosis of melancholia. *Arch. Gen. Psychiatry*, 38:15–22.
4. Chan-Palay, V., Jonsson, G., and Palay, S. L. (1978): Serotonin and substance P coexist in neurons of the rat's central nervous system. *Proc. Natl. Acad. Sci. USA*, 75:1582–1586.
5. Fields, H. L., and Basbaum, A. I. (1984): Endogenous pain control mechanisms. In: *Textbook of Pain*, edited by P. D. Wall and R. Melzack, pp. 142–152. Churchill Livingstone, Edinburgh.
6. France, R. D., and Krishnan, K. R. R. (1985): The dexamethasone suppression test as a biologic marker of depression in chronic pain. *Pain*, 21:49–55.
7. Hökfelt, T., Ljungdahl, A., Terenius, L., Elde, R., and Nilsson, G. (1977): Immunohisto-chemical analysis of peptide pathways possibly related to pain and analgesia. *Proc. Natl. Acad. Sci. USA*, 74:3081–3085.
8. Hökfelt, T., Ljungdahl, A., Steinbusch, H., Verhofstad, A., Nilsson, G., Brodin, E., Pernow, B., and Goldstein, M. (1978): Immunohistochemical evidence of substance P-like immunoreactivity in some 5-hydroxytryptamine-containing neurons in the rat central nervous system. *Neuroscience*, 3:517–538.
9. Hosobuchi, Y., Emson, P. C., and Iversen, L. L. (1982): Elevated cerebrospinal fluid substance P in arachnoiditis is reduced by systemic administration of morphine. *Adv. Biochem. Psychopharmacol.*, 33:497–500.
10. Johansson, F., Almay, B. G. L., von Knorring, L, and Terenius, L. (1980): Predictors for

the outcome of treatment with high frequency transcutaneous electrical nerve stimulation in patients with chronic pain. *Pain,* 9:55–61.

11. Nyberg, F., Nylander, I., and Terenius, L. (1986): Enkephalin-containing polypeptides in human cerebrospinal fluid. *Brain Res.,* 371:278–286.
12. Nutt, J. G., Mroz, E. A., Leeman, S. E., Williams, A. C., Engel, W, K., and Chase, T. N. (1980): Substance P in human cerebrospinal fluid: Reductions in peripheral neuropathy and autonomic dysfunction. *Neurology,* 30:1280–1285.
13. Otsuka, M., and Konishi, S. (1983): Substance P—the first peptide neurotransmitter? *Trends Neurosci.,* 6:317–320.
14. Paterson, S. J., Robson, L. E., and Kosterlitz, H. W. (1983): Classification of opioid receptors. *Br. Med. Bull.,* 39:31–36.
15. Rimón, R., Le Grevés, P., Nyberg, F., Heikkilä, L., Salmela, L., and Terenius, L. (1984): Elevation of substance P-like peptides in the CSF of psychiatric patients. *Biol. Psychiatry,* 19:509–516.
16. Terenius, L. (1981): Endorphins and pain. *Front. Horm. Res.,* 8:162–177.
17. Terenius, L., and Wahlström, A. (1975): Morphine-like ligand for opiate receptors in human CSF. *Life Sci.,* 16:1759–1764.
18. Zorman, G., Belcher, G., Adams, J. E., and Fields, H. L. (1982): Lumbar intrathecal naloxone blocks analgesia produced by microstimulation of the ventromedial medulla in the rat. *Brain Res.,* 236:77–84.

Advances in Pain Research and Therapy,
Vol. 10. Edited by M. Tiengo et al.
Raven Press, Ltd., New York © 1987.

Center Median-Parafascicular Thalamic Complex and Mediodorsal Nucleus Unitary Responses to Noxious Stimuli and Their Conditioning by Limbic and Mesencephalic Stimulations

*M. Mancia, *M. Mariotti, *A. Caraceni, *A. Formenti,
*L. Imeri, and **M. Palestini

*Istituto di Fisiologia Umana II, Università degli Studi, 20133 Milan, Italy; and
**Faculty of Medicine, University of Chile, Santiago, Chile

A role of the thalamus in pain has been postulated since the description of the thalamic syndrome by Dejerine and Roussy (14). In the past, different regions of the thalamus have been subjected to neurolesions as possible "pain centers" (48).

At present the role of spatially recognizing and discriminating nociceptive sensations is attributed to the ventrobasal complex and its projection to the somatosensory cortex, whereas the role of conferring the unpleasant feelings associated with pain and the control of motor responses to nociceptive stimuli is attributed to the intralaminar nuclei (2,7,28,57).

There are different opinions concerning the part played by the posterior complex of the thalamus in the neurological mechanisms of pain (2,12,28,40). Recent anatomical data suggest that the nucleus submedius could have an important function in relation to pain sensation (11,43). Furthermore, it is probable that the n.reticularis of the thalamus is involved in the modulation of nociceptive transmission (39). Already, it appears from this brief review that the relationship between thalamus and pain sensation is complex and uncertain.

The aim of our research was to examine, using electrophysiological methods, the responses of the center median parafascicular thalamic complex (CM-Pf) and mediodorsal nucleus (MD) to nociceptive stimulation. Since these nuclei are involved in aversive and emotional responses to pain, as well as in memory and alerting processes (20,28), the scope of our research was also to study the eventual conditioning influence of limbic and reticular stimulation on the neuronal responses of these nuclei to nociceptive input.

MATERIALS AND METHODS

Two series of experiments were carried out by means of extracellular recordings from CM-Pf and MD nuclei. Forty adult cats were used. The animals were operated on under ether anesthesia maintained with intravenous sodium pentobarbital. The level of anesthesia was checked by electroencephalogram (EEG) synchronization and on the basis of absence of reactions to nociceptive stimulus after the effect of curare had ended. The animals were curarized and artificially ventilated. The temperature was kept constant and the EEG monitored throughout the length of the experiment. Control experiments were carried out on seven animals *encéphale isolé* (spinal sections at C-2). Unit activity was recorded extracellularly using glass micropipettes (resistance 4–5 MΩ) inserted stereotaxically into the CM-Pf complex [anterior (A),6.5–7; lateral (L), 1.2–2.5; high (H), 4–1] or MD nucleus (A, 8–9.5; L, 1–2.5; H, 5–2) (27). The micropipettes were filled with KCl and pontamine skyblue for staining the beginning and the end of each penetration in order to reconstruct the electrode track. Homolateral tooth pulp stimulation (TPS) was applied using monopolar electrodes introduced in the upper canine tooth through a lateral hole (intensity, 100–300 μA; duration, 0.1 msec). The threshold intensity of the nociceptive stimulus was fixed at the start of each experiment at three times the threshold to obtain the jaw-opening reflex. All recorded cells were tested for antidromic identification from cortical areas of projections and from the head of the caudate nucleus in the case of CM-Pf. The antidromic response was evaluated on the basis of latency and frequency of response as well as, in some experiments, using the collision test.

Bipolar stimulation electrodes were inserted stereotaxically in the following structures: mesencephalic reticular formations (MRF): A,3; L,2.5; H,−8), dorsal hippocampus (HIPP)(A,4; L,5; H,7), lateral amygdala (AMY)(A,11.5; L,11; H,−6), septum (SPT)(A,15; L,1; H,2). These structures were stimulated with trains of four stimuli at 300 Hz, 50–60 μA intensity, and 0.1-msec duration. The neuronal response was studied using peri- and poststimulus histograms with a frequency of stimulation of 1 Hz for 100 repeated stimuli, bin width of 1 msec, and with a dot raster displayer. The position of the recording and stimulating electrodes was reconstructed histologically in each experiment.

RESULTS

CM-Pf

Of 199 neurons tested, 25% of the cells were facilitated in their spontaneous discharge by TPS (Table 1). The effect was present with varying latencies (average 12 msec) and the response could be concentrated or dispersed in time (Fig. 1A, 1B). Occasionally TPS produced facilitatory and inhibitory

TABLE 1. *Center median parafascicular thalamic complex responses*

Structures stimulated[a]	Tested	Excited	Inhibited	No effect
NOX (TPS)	199	50	16	133
MRF	131	72	9	50
PAG	131	43	11	77
NGC	131	56	0	75
AMY	57	1	7	49
HIPP	57	2	7	48
SPT	21	4	5	12

[a]NOX (TPS), noxious stimulation, tooth pulp stimulation; MRF, mesencephalic reticular formation; PAG, periaqueductal gray; NGC, nucleus gigantocellularis; AMY, lateral amygdala; HIPP, dorsal hippocampus; SPT, septum.

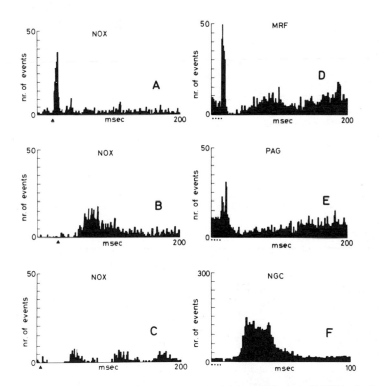

FIG. 1. Poststimulus histograms (100 repeated trials) of different CM-Pf units following single-shock TPS (**A,B,C**) and high-frequency (4 impulses at 300 Hz) stimulation of mesencephalic reticular formation (**D**), periacqueductal gray (**E**), and nucleus gigantocellularis (**F**). *Solid triangles* and *dots* indicate stimuli.

discharge sequences (Fig. 1C). Inhibition was observed in 8% of the cases, with latency of 20 msec and average duration of 50 msec.

High frequency MRF stimulation had a facilitatory effect on 56% of the tested neurons. Inhibition was limited to 6.8%. High frequency stimulation of nucleus gigantocellularis (NGC) and periaqueductal gray (PAG) also produced facilitation of spontaneous neuronal discharge in 43% and 33%, respectively. PAG produced inhibition in 8.3% of neurons. Figure 1D to 1F shows the intensity, latency, and duration of the effects following high frequency MRF, PAG, and NGC stimulation.

High frequency stimulation of both AMY and HIPP, studied in 57 neurons, produced inhibitory effects in 12% neurons (Table 1) with a mean latency of 12 msec (Fig. 2A, 2B). Out of 21 tested neurons, SPT stimulation gave rise to five inhibitions (Table 1; Fig. 2C), while four cells showed facilitation followed by inhibition. Convergence of TPS and HIPP stimulation was observed in only five out of 55 tested neurons.

Stimulation of the somatosensory cortex and caudate nucleus never produced antidromic activation of those thalamic neurons that responded to TPS.

MD

Out of 222 MD tested neurons, 18% were facilitated in their spontaneous discharge by TPS (Table 2) with latencies, in general, between 5 and 10 msec. The effect could be concentrated or spaced in time (Fig. 3A, 3B).

TABLE 2. *Mediodorsal nucleus responses*

Structures stimulated[a]	Tested	Excited	Inhibited	No effect
NOX (TPS)	222	40	5	177
AMY	63	23	0	40
HIPP	137	30	5	102
SPT	38	6	3	29
MRF	20	4	0	16
TPS conditioning				
HIPP + NOX	49	11	3	35
AMY + NOX	15	4	1	10
SPT + NOX	7	2	0	5
MRF + NOX	10	4	0	6

[a]NOX (TPS), noxious stimulation, tooth pulp stimulation; AMY, lateral amygdala; HIPP, dorsal hippocampus; SPT, septum; MRF, mesencephalic reticular formation.

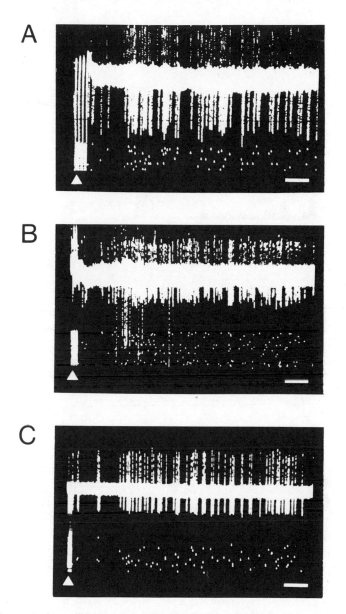

FIG. 2. Three different CM-Pf units inhibited in their spontaneous discharge by high-frequency (4 impulses at 300 Hz) lateral amygdala (**A**), dorsal hippocampus (**B**), and septum (**C**) stimulation. *Triangles* indicate beginning of the train. Time: A, 20 msec/division; **B** and **C**, 40 msec/division.

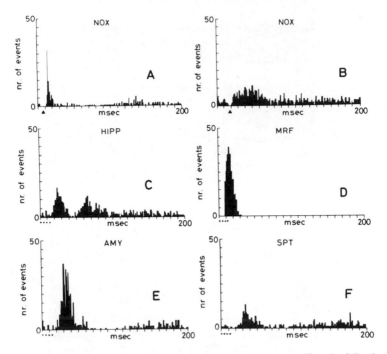

FIG. 3. Poststimulus histograms (100 repeated trials) of different MD units following single-shock TPS (**A,B**) and high-frequency (4 impulses at 300 Hz) stimulation of dorsal hippocampus (**C**), mesencephalic reticular formation (**D**), lateral amygdala (**E**), and septum (**F**). *Solid triangles* and *dots* indicate stimuli.

High-frequency stimulation of the HIPP had an excitatory effect in ~22% of the tested units. The same facilitatory effect followed high-frequency stimulation of the AMY (36%), SPT (15%), and MRF (20%) (Table 2). Generally, these effects were observed with a latency between 20 and 50 msec for limbic structures, and 10 and 20 msec for MRF (Fig. 3C–3F).

Convergence on the same cells was seen by nociceptive, limbic, and mesencephalic impulses (Table 2). High-frequency conditioning stimulation of these central structures could produce a marked increase of neuronal responses to TPS (Figs. 4, 5). The maximum effect was observed with HIPP stimulation (22% of tested neurons) (Table 2) with an interval between conditioning and test stimulus of 30 to 40 msec (Fig. 4A–4C). Conditioning stimulation of HIPP, MRF, AMY, and SPT was often capable of making evident a nociceptive response of neurons that do not otherwise respond to a noxious stimulus alone (Fig. 4D–4F, Fig. 5A–5F).

The MD cells facilitated by TPS were never fired by antidromic stimulation of the prefrontal cortex.

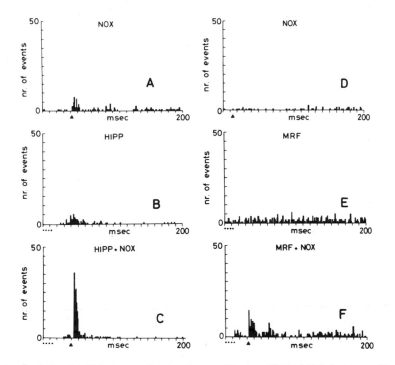

FIG. 4. Poststimulus histograms showing the conditioning effect of high-frequency (4 stimuli at 300 Hz) hippocampal (**A, B, C**) and mesencephalic (**D, E, F**) stimulation on noxious response of two different MD units. *Solid triangles* indicate noxious stimuli and *solid dots* hippocampal and mesencephalic stimuli. Note the potentiation of noxious response following hippocampal conditioning in **C** and its facilitation by mesencephalic conditioning in **F**.

DISCUSSION

General Remarks

In discussing the results presented in this chapter we wish to underline that dental pulp stimulation may be considered a model of nociceptive activation (32), although this type of stimulation might involve fibers other than pain afferents (15,32). As to the functional characteristics of the recorded cells, since additional studies of the effect of low threshold somatic stimulation were not carried out, we are unable, at present, to confirm whether we are dealing with specific nociceptive or multireceptive neurons.

The percentage of cells facilitated by nociceptive stimulation both in CM-Pf and MD appears modest, although this may be explained by the fact that the receptive field we used for stimulation was very much reduced. Using the same type of activation (TPS) in CM-Pf, data similar to ours have been obtained (58). None of the neurons facilitated by nociceptive input in CM-Pf

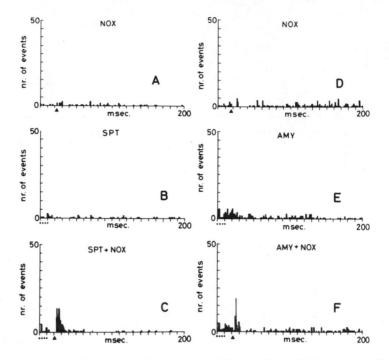

FIG. 5. Poststimulus histograms showing the conditioning effect of high frequency (4 stimuli at 300 Hz) septal (**A, B, C**) and amygdaloid (**D, E, F**) stimulation on noxious response of two different MD units. *Solid triangles* indicate noxious stimuli and *solid dots* septal and amygdaloid stimuli. Note the clear facilitation of noxious responses following septal and amygdaloid conditioning.

and MD seem to project to the cerebral cortex. We must, therefore, think that the intralaminar and MD neurons involved in nociception are either interneurons or neurons with intrathalamic or subcortical projections. Furthermore, it must be remembered that the percentage of CM-Pf and MD cells activated by cortical stimulation by other authors (1,8,16,54) was also very low.

No substantial difference was found in the CM-Pf and MD unitary responses to TPS and central stimulations comparing the results obtained in anesthetized and *encéphale isolé* animals. However, the percentage of responding neurons was slightly higher in the latter preparations than in anesthetized animals.

CM-Pf Responses

Various data of clinical and experimental nature suggest that the CM-Pf plays a central role in the elaboration of nociceptive input. CM nucleus has been a target of neurosurgical lesions carried out for alleviation of pain (56).

Lesions of Pf nucleus raise the nociceptive threshold both in humans (49) and in animals (13), and a bilateral lesion of CM-Pf abolishes the escape reaction induced by stimulation of dental pulp in the cat (35). Moreover, it has been revealed that the intralaminar nuclei (together with MD) are the thalamic areas with the highest concentrations of opiate receptors (38,45).

Electrophysiological experiments demonstrated that neurons of CM-Pf complex respond to stimulation of both dental pulp (58) and wide receptive fields (3,51). Nociceptive responses of this type have also been recorded in CM-Pf in humans, during neurosurgical operations (26).

CM-Pf neurons respond to nociceptive stimulation in various ways, with facilitation and inhibition. Others (57) also found this type of response in CM-Pf both in specific nociceptive and multireceptive neurons. These cells could be part of the spinothalamic system, since neurons in this system can be activated antidromically from the CM-Pf (22). Nociceptive input can, in any case, also reach these nuclei by means of the spinoreticular system through the nucleus reticularis gigantocellularis (9,29,30).

Anatomical and physiological data allow one to consider CM-Pf complex as an area of interaction between nociception and motor control, on one hand, and nociception and electrocortical alerting system on the other. In fact, the CM-Pf receives an input from the motor cortex (33) and the entopeduncolar nucleus (36,37). Other afferents reach CM-Pf complex from the cerebellar nuclei (4), the substantia nigra (33), and other structures related with postural functions and space orientation, such as the superior collicolus and vestibular nuclei (33). On the efferent side, the CM-Pf sends fibers to the striatum (see ref. 28 for review) and the sensorimotor cortex (6,47). Therefore, these nuclei seem to be involved in the elaboration of motor responses to noxious stimuli. On the other hand, since the CM-Pf complex participates in the processes of EEG desynchronization (28), it may represent an area of interaction between nociception and cortical alerting mechanisms. These considerations may indirectly explain the analgesic effect of the lesions of these nuclei (57).

Our results agree with those reported in the literature, and confirm the participation of CM-Pf in the integration of nociceptive afferent input. The limbic system appears to have an inhibitory effect on the CM-Pf, but its capacity to condition the nociceptive responses seems to be limited by lack of convergence.

MD Responses

The mediodorsal nucleus is the main thalamic nucleus projecting to the prefrontal cortex (20). It is often associated with higher functions such as memory and attention (21,31,53). Surgical lesions of MD give rise to a prefrontal syndrome (46) and relieve intractable pain (23).

Afferents to MD arising from the limbic structures have been demonstrated by anatomical studies. In particular the projections from the amygdala are well documented in the monkey (41). There are projections to MD from septal areas, hypothalamus (25; I. Gritti et al., *unpublished observations*), cingulate cortex (5), periacqueductal gray, raphe nuclei, reticular formation, superior colliculus, and sensorimotor cortical areas (25, 52; I. Gritti et al., *unpublished observations*). Afferents reach the MD from the olfactory cortex and olfactory tubercle (42). Moreover, it has been recently suggested that the olfactory tubercle-MD-prefrontal cortex circuit can be considered analogous to the striatal-cortical one. On the basis of these data, a function of MD in linking limbic structures to motor systems has been postulated (24,54,55).

Neurophysiological experiments demonstrated MD responses to peripheral stimuli (10,18,19), some described as painful (10,19), and to stimulation of limbic structures such as the amygdala, septum, and hippocampus (16,17,44).

Our results clearly confirm a nociceptive facilitatory input to MD. Noteworthy are those MD neurons that respond to nociceptive input and which are strongly facilitated by conditioning high-frequency stimulation of central structures, such as HIPP, AMY, SPT, and MRF. The conditioning stimulus is often capable of making evident a nociceptive response of neurons that do not otherwise respond to a noxious stimulus alone. Among these structures the hippocampus appears to have the maximum conditioning effect.

The conditioning effect generally occurs with a 20 to 40-msec interval between conditioning and test stimuli, thus suggesting a long polysynaptic pathway. It also appears worthwhile emphasizing the specificity of the facilitatory effect on MD neurons by stimulation of limbic structures. The same structures in fact are inhibitory on CM-Pf, as observed also by other authors (34,50).

Finally, one is tempted to speculate on a possible role of the limbic system, functionally linked to the MD, both in the process of emotional elaboration of nociceptive input, and in the mechanism of memorization of painful experiences.

REFERENCES

1. Albe-Fessard, D., Cesaro, P., and Hamon, B. (1983): Effect of striatal stimulation on cellular activities of medial thalamic neurons studied in rat. *Exp. Brain Res.,* 50:34–44.
2. Albe-Fessard, D., Berkley, K. J., Kruger, L., Ralston, H. J., and Willis, W. D., Jr. (1985): Diencephalic mechanisms of pain sensation. *Brain Res. Rev.,* 9:217–296.
3. Albe-Fessard, D., and Kruger, L. (1962): Duality of unit discharges from cat centrum medianum in response to natural and electrical stimulation. *J. Neurophysiol.,* 25:3–20.
4. Asanuma, C., Thach, W. T., and Jones, E. G. (1983): Anatomical evidence for segregated focal groupings of efferent cells and their terminal ramifications in the cerebellothalamic pathway of the monkey. *Brain Res. Rev.,* 5:267–297.

5. Balaydier, C., and Maguiere, F. (1980): The duality of the cingulate gyrus in the monkey. Neuroanatomical study and functional hypothesis. *Brain,* 103;525–554.
6. Bentivoglio, M., Molinari, M., Minciacchi, D., and Macchi, G. (1983): Organization of the cortical projections of the posterior complex and intralaminar nuclei of the thalamus as studied by means of retrograde tracers. In: *Somatosensory Integration in the Thalamus,* edited by G. Macchi, A. Rustioni, and R. Spreafico, p. 337–364. Elsevier, Amsterdam.
7. Besson, J. M., Guilbaud, G., Abdelmoumene, M., and Chauch, A. (1982): Phisiologie de la nociception. *J. Physiol. (Paris),* 78:7–107.
8. Bowsher, D. (1974): Thalamic convergence and divergence of information generated by noxious stimulation. In: *Advances in Neurology, Vol.4,* edited by J. J. Bonica, pp.223–232. Raven Press, New York.
9. Bowsher, D., Mallart, A., Petit, D., and Albe-Fessard, D. (1968): A bulbar relay to the CM. *J. Neurophysiol.,* 31:288–300.
10. Casey, K. L. (1966): Unit analysis of nociceptive mechanisms in the thalamus of the awake squirrel monkey. *J. Neurophysiol.,* 29:727–750.
11. Craig, A. D., and Burton, H. (1981): Spinal and medullary lamina I projection to nucleus submedius in medial thalamus: a possible pain center. *J. Neurophysiol.,* 45:443–466.
12. Curry, M. J. (1972): The exteroceptive properties of neurones in the somatic part of the posterior group (PO). *Brain Res.,* 44:439–462.
13. Dafny, N., and Gildenberg, P. (1984): Morphine effects on spontaneous, nociceptive, antinociceptive and sensory evoked responses of parafasciculus thalami units in morphine naive and morphine dependent rats. *Brain Res.,* 323:11–20.
14. Dejerine, J., and Roussy, G. (1906): Le syndrome talamique. *Rev. Neurol.,* 14:521–532.
15. Dong, W. K., and Chudler, E. H. (1984): Origin of tooth pulp evoked far-field and early nearfield potentials in the cat. *J. Neurophysiol.,* 51:859–889.
16. Edinger, H., Siegel, A., and Troiano, R. (1975): Effect of stimulation of prefrontal cortex and amygdala on diencephalic neurons. *Brain Res.,* 97:17–31.
17. Encabo, H., and Bekermann, A. J. (1971): Responses evoked in MD by subcortical stimulation. A microelectrode study. *Brain Res.,* 28:35–46.
18. Encabo, H., and Volkind, R. (1968): Evoked somatic activity in nucleus medialis dorsalis; a microelectrode study. *Electroencephalogr. Clin. Neurophysiol.,* 25:252–258.
19. Feltz, P., Krauthamer, G., and Albe-Fessard, D. (1967): Neurons of the medial diencephalon. I. Somatosensory responses and caudate inhibition. *J. Neurophysiol.,* 30:55–80.
20. Fuster, J. H. (1980): *The Prefrontal Cortex,* Raven Press, New York.
21. Fuster, J. H., and Alexander, G. E. (1973): Firing changes in cells of the nucleus medialis dorsalis associated with delayed response behavior. *Brain Res.,* 61:79–91.
22. Giesler, G. J., Yezierski, R. P., Gerhart, K. D., and Willis, W. D. (1981): Spinothalamic tract neurons that project to medial and/or lateral thalamic nuclei: evidence for a physiologically novel population of spinal cord neurons. *J. Neurophysiol.,* 46:1285–1308.
23. Hecaen, H., Talairach, J., David, M., and Dell, M. B. (1949): Coagulations limitées du thalamus dans l'algie du syndrome thalamique. Resultats therapeutiques et physiologiques. *Rev. Neurol.,* 81:917–931.
24. Heimer, L., Switzer, R. D., and Vantbesen, G. W. (1982): Ventral striatum and ventral pallidum. Components of the motor system? *Trends Neurosci.,* 5:83–87.
25. Irle, E., Markowitsch, H. J., and Streicher, M. (1984): Cortical and subcortical including sensory-related afferents to the thalamic mediodorsal nucleus of the cat. *J. Hirnforsch.,* 25:29–51.
26. Ishijima, B., Yoshimasu, N., Fukushima, T., Hori, T., Sekino, H., and Samo, K. (1975): Nociceptive neurons in the human thalamus. *Confin. Neurol. (Basel),* 37:99–106.
27. Jasper, H. H., and Ajmone-Marsan, C. (1954): *A Stereotaxic Atlas of the Diencephalon of the Cat.* National Research Council of Canada, Ottawa.
28. Jones, E. G. (1985). *The Thalamus.* Plenum Press, New York.
29. Levante, A., Cesaro, P., and Albe-Fessard, D. (1983): Electrophysiological and anatomical demonstration of a bulbar relayed pathway toward the medial thalamus in the cat. *Neurosci. Lett.,* 38:139–144.
30. Mancia, M., Margnelli, M., Mariotti, M., Spreafico, R., and Broggi, G. (1974): Brain stem thalamus reciprocal influences in the cat. *Brain Res.,* 69:297–314.
31. Markowitsch, H. J. (1982): The thalamic mediodorsal nucleus and memory: a critical evaluation of studies in animal and man. *Neurosci. Biobehav. Rev.,* 6:351–380.

32. Mason, P., Strassman, A., and Maciewicz, R. (1985): Is the jaw opening reflex a valid model of pain? *Brain Res. Rev.*, 10:137–146.
33. McGuinness, C. M., and Krauthamer, G. M. (1980): The afferent projections to the centrum medianum of the cat as demonstrated by retrograde transport of horseradish peroxidase. *Brain Res.*, 184:255–269.
34. McKenzie, J. S., and Rogers, D. K. (1973): Hippocampal suppression of intralaminar thalamic unit responses in cats and comparison with suppression evoked from the caudate nucleus. *Brain Res.*, 64:1–15.
35. Mitchell, C. L., and Kaelber, W. W. (1966): Effect of medial thalamic lesions on responses elicited by tooth pulp stimulation. *Am. J. Physiol.*, 210:263–269.
36. Nauta, W. J. H., and Mehler, W. R. (1966): Projections of the lentiform nucleus in the monkey. *Brain Res.*, 1:3–42.
37. Parent, A., and De Bellefeuille, L. (1983): The pallidointralaminar and pallidonigral projections in primate as studied by retrograde double-labeling method. *Brain Res.*, 278:11–28.
38. Pert, C. B., Kumar, M. J., and Snyder, S. H. (1976): Autoradiographic localization of opiate receptors in the rat brain. *Proc. Natl. Acad. Sci. USA*, 73:3729–3733.
39. Peschanski, M., Guilbaud, G, and Gautron, M. (1980): Neuronal responses to cutaneous electrical and noxious mechanical stimuli in the nucleus reticularis thalami of the rat. *Neurosci. Lett.*, 20:165–170.
40. Poggio, G. F., and Mountcastle, V. B. (1960): A study on the functional contributions of the lemniscal and spinothalamic systems to somatic sensibility: Central nervous mechanisms in pain. *Bull. Johns Hopkins Hosp.*, 106:266–316.
41. Porrino, L. J., Grane, A. M., and Goldman-Rakic, P. S. (1981): Direct·and indirect pathways from the amygdala to the frontal lobe in the rhesus monkey. *J. Comp. Neurol.*, 198:121–136.
42. Price, J. L., and Slotnick, B. M. (1983) Dual olfactory representation in the rat thalamus: an anatomical and electrophysiological study. *J. Comp. Neurol.*, 215:63–77.
43. Ralston, H. J. (1984): Synaptic organization of spinothalamic tract projections to the thalamus, with special reference to pain. In: *Advances in Pain Research and Therapy, Vol. 6*, edited by L. Kruger and J. C. Liebeskind, pp. 183–195. Raven Press, New York.
44. Sager, O., and Butkhuzi, S. (1962): Electrographical study of the relationship between the dorsomedian nucleus of the thalamus and the rhinencephalon (hippocampus and amygdala). *Electroencephalogr. Clin. Neurophysiol.*, 14:835–846.
45. Sar, M. Stumpf, W. E., Miller, R. J., Chang, K. J., and Cuatrecasas, P. (1978): Immunohistochemical localization of enkephalin in rat brain and spinal cord. *J. Comp. Neurol.*, 182:17–38.
46. Spiegel, E. A., Wycis, H. T., Freed, H., and Orchinik, C. (1952): The central mechanism of emotions (experience with circumscribed thalamic lesions). *Am. J. Psychiatry*, 108:426–432.
47. Strick, P. L. (1975): Multiple sources of thalamic input to the primate moter cortex. *Brain Res.*, 88:372–377.
48. Sweet, W. H. (1980): Central mechanism of chronic pain (neuralgias and certain other neurogenic pain). In: *Pain*, edited by J. J. Bonica, pp. 287–303. Raven Press, New York.
49. Sweet, W. H. (1981): Cerebral localization of pain. In: *New Perspectives in Cerebral Localization*, edited by R. A. Thompson, pp. 205–240. Raven Press, New York.
50. Urabe, M., and Ito, H. (1968): Inhibitory effects of the limbic system on the nucleus CM of the thalamus. *Physiol. Behav.*, 3:695–702.
51. Urabe, M., Tsubokawa, T., and Watanabe, Y: (1966): Alteration of activity of single neurons in the nucleus centrum medianum following stimulation of peripheral nerve and application of noxious stimuli. *Jpn. J. Physiol.*, 16:421–435.
52. Velayos, J. Z., and Reinoso-Suarez, F. (1982): Topographic organization of the brainstem afferents to the mediodorsal thalamic nucleus. *J. Comp. Neurol.*, 206:17–27.
53. Victor, M., Adams, R. D., and Collins, G. H. (1971): *The Wernicke-Korsakoff Syndrome: a Clinical and Pathological Study of 245 Patients, 82 with Post-Mortem Examinations.* Davis, Philadelphia.
54. Vives, F., and Mogenson, G. J. (1985): Electrophysiological evidence that the mediodorsal nucleus of the thalamus is a relay between the ventral pallidum and the medial prefrontal cortex in the rat. *Brain Res.*, 344:329–337.

55. Young, W. S., III, Alheid, G. F., and Heimer, H. (1984): The ventral pallidal projection to the mediodorsal thalamus: a study with fluorescent retrograde tracers and immunohisto-fluorescence. *J. Neurosci.,* 4:1626–1638.
56. White, J. C., and Sweet, W. H. (1969): *Pain and Neurosurgeon.* Thomas, Springfield.
57. Willis, W. D. (1985). *The Pain System.* Karger, Basel.
58. Woda, A., Azerad, J., Guilbaud, G., and Besson, J. M. (1975). Etude microphysiologique des projections thalamiques de la pulpe dentaire chez le chat. *Brain Res.,* 89:193–213.

Advances in Pain Research and Therapy,
Vol. 10. Edited by M. Tiengo et al.
Raven Press, Ltd., New York © 1987.

Pain, Motility, Neuropeptides, and the Human Skin: Immunohistochemical Observations

Olle Johansson

Department of Histology, Karolinska Institute, S-104 01 Stockholm, Sweden

During the last three decades histochemistry has played an increasingly important role in our attempts to understand the function of the nervous system. Starting with acetylcholinesterase staining at the end of the 1940s, followed by the formaldehyde-induced fluorescence method for visualization of monoamines, also employing techniques such as routine electron microscopy and autoradiography, and finally exploiting the enormous potential of immunohistochemistry, this extensive work has led to profound knowledge of the distribution of various transmitters and neuroactive compounds in the central and peripheral nervous system. Retrograde tracing studies and analysis at the ultrastructural level have provided information on the connectivity between these systems and on possible mechanisms underlying chemical transmission. The high resolution of the histochemical techniques has allowed the demonstration of more than one transmitter candidate in a neuron, suggesting that chemical transmission may represent a more complex phenomenon than was hitherto thought. New techniques are currently being introduced, for instance, hybrid histochemistry; and it may also be predicted that, during the coming decade, histochemistry will remain a valuable tool in our attempts to understand the nervous system.

The last few years we have witnessed extensive research to elucidate the role of neuropeptides at the brain and spinal cord level, particularly with regard to involvement in pain and motility mechanisms. This work has shown great complexity with regard to the number of peptides present and to their localization. Briefly, in the spinal cord peptides of different kinds may not be found only in primary afferent fibers originating in dorsal root ganglia, but also in local neurons as well as in supraspinal descending systems. There are also peptide-containing preganglionic efferent neurons with cell bodies in the sympathetic and parasympathetic intermediolateral columns. In some cases the peptide occurs with a "classical" transmitter in the same neurons and, in other cases, more than one peptide can be seen in a neuron. Thus, a high degree of complexity exists with regard to the distribution and possible functions of peptides in the spinal cord [for further results, see A. Cuello (Chap. 1) and Hökfelt et al. (26,27)].

The present chapter focuses on the peripheral parts of these systems as exemplified by the occurrence of peptide-containing nerves and cells in normal human skin, as visualized by the use of indirect immunohistochemistry. Recently, several studies have indicated the presence of certain peptides in different structures of normal as well as pathological skin. Using radioimmunoassay and/or immunohistochemistry, e.g., substance P (SP), neurokinin A (NKA), calcitonin gene-related peptide (CGRP), γ-melanocyte stimulating hormone (γ-MSH), prodynorphin–opioid peptides, somatostatin, vasoactive intestinal polypeptide (VIP), peptide histidine isoleucine amide (PHI), or neuropeptide tyrosine (NPY) immunoreactive nerves (5,6,13,22,25,28–30,32,34,36,39,47,49,52,56,58,61,67,70,71), VIP-containing mast cells (12), somatostatin immunoreactive dendritic cells (40), and methionine-enkephalin or VIP-containing Merkel cells (21,23) have been observed in experimental animals as well as in man. Specific peptide patterns have also been found within human skin cellular elements of various skin diseases such as symptomatic cutaneous mastocytoma (72), acanthosis nigricans (4), urticaria pigmentosa (28,34), diabetic lipodystrophy (37), lichen sclerosus et atrophicus (36), and bullous pemphigoid, as well as factitious and cold urticaria (68,69); however, up till now not in, e.g., psoriasis (35,38) or angioma (O. Johansson, K. Nordlind, and S. Lidén, *unpublished observations*).

METHODOLOGY

The structural characterization of peptides offers possibilities to raise more or less specific antisera to these compounds; these antisera can then be used for radioimmunological or immunohistochemical analyses of systems containing these peptides. The latter technique was introduced by Coons (11) more than 40 years ago and was originally based on principles of fluorescence, i.e., the markers used for detection were fluorescent compounds conjugated to the antibodies. Subsequently, other markers have been introduced, for example, the enzyme horseradish peroxidase, which can be used for studies both at the light and electron microscopic level (2,55). More recent modifications include the peroxidase-antiperoxidase (PAP) technique of Sternberger (59).

The main virtue of all immunohistochemical techniques are their general applicability. Thus, any substance against which an antiserum can be raised may be traced in tissue sections, provided that it is retained at its endogenous storage site during the immunohistochemical procedure. In order to obtain this, it is mostly necessary to fix the tissues. Fixation is also necessary to obtain an acceptable morphology. Since fixation frequently destroys antigenicity, the preparation of the tissues for immunohistochemistry is often a balance between a good (or at least acceptable) morphology and retention, on one hand, and a tolerable degree of antigenicity destruction on the other. It is important to note that the immunohistochemical techniques do not provide absolute specificity. It is possible that the antibody raised to a certain antigen also reacts with antigens with a similar structure, so-called cross-reactivity. Therefore, terms such as "NPY-like immunoreactivity" have been considered appropriate in the text. A procedure for tissue processing and indirect immunohistochemistry, which has turned out to be suitable for many antigens present in the skin, has been developed (A. Ljungberg and O. Johansson, *in preparation*) and is summarized below.

Healthy adult volunteers without any history or heredity of skin diseases were used. Punch biopsies (3 mm) were surgically excised under local anesthesia. After immersion for 2 to 4 hr in an ice-cold picric acid/formalin or para-benzoquinone (PBQ)/formalin solution, the tissue pieces were rinsed for at least 24 hr in ice-cold phosphate buffer, sectioned perpendicularly at 14 μm on a cryostat, and processed for indirect immunohistochemistry according to Coons and collaborators (see ref. 11). The sections were incubated with the antisera or control sera, respectively, diluted in 0.01 M phosphate buffered saline (PBS), kept overnight at +4°C in a humid atmosphere, rinsed in PBS for 10 min with three changes, then incubated for 30 min at +37°C with fluorescein-isothiocyanate (FITC)- or tetramethylrhodamine-isothiocyanate isomer R (TRITC)-labeled antiserum, rinsed as before and mounted. As an additional control, certain sections were only incubated with the second antiserum. The sections were studied and photographed in a Zeiss fluorescence microscope. After photography, the cover slips were removed and, after rinsing, certain sections were stained with hematoxylin-eosin for routine histology. For further methodological details, the reader is referred to Johansson and Nordlind (34) and Johansson (29,30).

RESULTS

The present chapter focuses on the occurrence of peptide-containing nerves and cells in normal human skin as investigated by the use of an indirect immunohistochemical technique. Utilizing this, it was possible to describe in detail a network of peptide immunoreactive nerve fibers in the epidermis and dermis as well as certain types of positive dermal cells. The results are briefly summarized below.

SP

Immunoreactivity for the peptide SP could be seen in the upper dermis, in or around Meissner's corpuscles, and close to as well as within the epidermis as single free nerve endings. However, SP-like immunoreactivity was also observed in nerve fiber bundles in the deeper parts of the dermis as well as innervating hair follicles, eccrine sweat glands, and blood vessels.

NKA

NKA positive nerve endings were localized both in the epidermis and the dermis, especially in the stratum papillare. Furthermore, NKA-like immunoreactivity was found within nerves of the stratum reticulare and, finally, also single positive nerve fibers could be observed close to blood vessels, sweat glands, and hair follicles.

CGRP

The immunoreactivity pattern for this peptide paralleled that found for SP, thus CGRP positive nerve fibers could be seen in the dermis and close to, as well as within, the epidermis as single free nerve endings. Also, the Meissner's corpuscles contained immunoreactive nerve fibers. Furthermore, CGRP-like immunoreactivity was observed in nerve fiber bundles in more deeply located parts of the dermis as well as, to some extent, innervating blood vessels, sweat glands, and hair follicles.

γ-MSH

Immunoreactivity for γ-MSH was observed within nerve fibers of the dermis, both in the apical as well as the deeper parts, and of the epidermis. Strong evidence for a preferential localization of γ-MSH-like immunoreactivity to sensory nerves was seen. Smooth and/or varicose fibers were frequently found in the stratum papillare close to the epidermis (the fibers were smooth and running perpendicular to the surface in the papillae, and at the basal parts of the epithelial crypts they were varicose and running parallel to the basal membrane; this latter localization pointed to a possible innervation of the Merkel cells since sometimes single, varicose fibers were seen to enter the most basal parts of the stratum basale), entering the epidermal-dermal junctional zone as well as penetrating into the basal layer of the proper epidermis as free nerve endings. The Meissner's corpuscles were densely innervated. The more deeply located γ-MSH immunoreactive fibers were seen running in the connective tissue matrix either in nerve fiber bundles or as smooth, single preterminal axons, however, showing a plexus of varicosities when approaching their terminal fields. Single fibers could be found in association with blood vessels (mostly arteries), sweat glands (not with the eccrine, although the apocrine has some few fibers between the acini), hair follicles (having a dense plexus at their base), however, rarely around sebaceous glandular acini, and so far not observed to innervate the erector pili muscles. It should be noted that it was difficult to draw any definite conclusions with regard to these structures being directly *innervated* or the fibers being *en passage* on their way to *other* structures. Finally, single strongly immunoreactive neutrophilic granulocytes were seen in the upper part of the dermis.

Somatostatin

Following immunohistochemistry, somatostatin immunoreactive nerve fibers could be seen in the dermis, both in the upper as well as in more deeply located parts. The fibers sometimes formed free nerve endings, especially close to the epidermis. The somatostatin positive networks were generally sparse and only single fibers could be seen close to, e.g., hair follicles. Fibers were rarely found intermingled with the Meissner's corpuscles of the stratum papillare of the dermis. Also, immunoreactive dendritic cells were observed in the dermis (Fig. 1A).

VIP

After incubation with VIP antiserum, single VIP immunoreactive nerve endings could be seen in the apical parts of the dermis (stratum papillare) situated closely to the epidermal-dermal junctional zone as free nerve endings. In the deeper parts of the dermis, as well as of the subcutis, VIP immunoreactive nerve fibers could be found within fiber bundles, terminating with a medium dense-dense network innervating sweat glands, hair follicles (especially the hair papillae) (Fig. 1C), sebaceous glands, and blood vessels. Single fibers were observed close to the erector pili smooth muscles.

PHI

Incubation with PHI antiserum resulted in fluorescent nerve fibers that were observed in the dermis, mainly in the deeper parts and in the subcutis. The PHI fibers were mainly seen close to and around blood vessels (both arteries and veins) and sweat glands (both eccrine and apocrine), and were of a fine-caliber type with smooth preterminal axons and a sparse plexus of varicosities at their terminal field. Furthermore, they were observed around hair follicles and also the hair papillae, however, more rarely around sebaceous glands. Single PHI immunoreactive fibers could be seen in close vicinity to the erector pili muscles. Finally, also single (somatic?) immunoreactive nerve fibers were found in the apical parts of the dermis, close to the epidermal-dermal junctional zone, as free nerve endings.

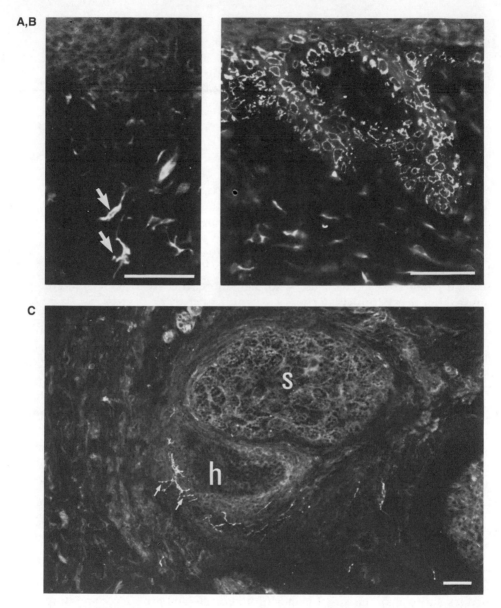

FIG. 1. Immunofluorescence micrographs of the skin after incubation with antiserum to somatostatin (**A**), NPY (**B**), and VIP (**C**). In **A**, immunoreactive dendritic cells (*arrows*) are seen in the upper dermis close to the epidermis. In **B**, NPY positive basal cells of the epidermis are shown. Note the granular appearance. In **C**, VIP immunoreactivity is observed within nerve fibers around a hair follicle (h). The nerve terminals are readily visible (*arrows*); s = sebaceous gland. *Bars* indicate 50 μm.

NPY

After incubation with NPY antibodies, fluorescent nerve fibers were observed in the dermis, mainly in the deeper parts and in the subcutis. Only rarely were the fibers found in the stratum papillare close to the epidermis, without ever entering the epidermal-dermal junctional zone or the proper epidermis as free nerve endings. The NPY immunoreactive fibers were of a fine-caliber type and were seen running in the connective tissue matrix either in nerve fiber bundles or as smooth, single preterminal axons. They showed a medium dense-dense plexus of varicosities when approaching their terminal fields where they could be found close to and around blood vessels (arteries, but not with certainty associated with veins), and eccrine sweat glands with very few in association with the apocrine glands and with sparse amounts around sebaceous glandular acini/hair follicles. It may be noted that this is in contrast to Tainio et al. (61) who were unable to observe any NPY immunoreactive nerves in the nerve plexuses around the human axillary eccrine or apocrine sweat glands. No evidence for a localization of NPY-like immunoreactivity to sensory nerves was seen. Finally, a weak-strong staining in the cytoplasm of the stratum basale cells (Fig. 1B) as well as in the cells of the outer root sheath of hair follicles could be observed. The immunoreactive material in these cells seemed to be of granular nature; however, only future electron microscopic investigations can reveal the true character of these presumable granules.

None of the fluorescent structures described above could be observed after incubation with control serum (antiserum adsorbed with the respective corresponding peptide) or only with the second, FITC- or TRITC-labeled, antiserum. However, after incubation with blocked antiserum or only with the second antiserum some diffuse general "background staining" of a low intensity was seen in the connective tissue fiber network.

FUNCTIONAL SIGNIFICANCE

The skin is far more than an inert wrapping for the body. It is a large multifaceted organ with a complex structure, capable of rapid regeneration. It is responsible for many of the body's reactions to the environment, providing sensory information, protection, and temperature control. The skin's tough flexibility allows us to perform delicate tasks, use subtle expressions, and still be capable of rough manual labor.

The body interprets external stimuli as heat, cold, pain, light touch, pressure, itch, and even tickle. Heat and cold perception trigger a variety of temperature control measures. Pain, pressure, and touch usually lead to direct avoidance. Itch, or pruritus, is a response to weak but persistent stimulation, perhaps of pain or pressure nerve fibers; it can be overridden by painful stimuli or steady pressure, as well as by the usual responses of rubbing and scratching. Tickle is caused by persistent light movements, as when a fly lands on the skin or when someone purposely tickles a child. The response is usually minor avoidance behavior, such as a flick of the hand or jerking away.

The distribution of nerve fibers in the skin has earlier been described by the use of different light and electron microscopic techniques (e.g., see ref. 54). The cutaneous innervation is divided into a sensory and an autonomic portion. The sensory nerve fibers are found in the epidermis and dermis as free or specialized nerve endings, around blood vessels, sweat glands, and hair follicles. Autonomic fibers are found innervating blood and lymphatic vessels, sweat glands, hair papillae, sebaceous glands, and in erector pili muscles associated with hair follicles.

Due to space limitations, it is impossible to discusss all the functional implications of the findings described above. However, some recent observations regarding the physiology and pharmacology of these neuropeptides may be mentioned and for further details, the reader is referred to the literature.

One of the first peptides to be shown to be functionally important in the skin was SP. Its high content in spinal dorsal roots prompted Lembeck (42) to suggest that SP may act as a transmitter in primary sensory neurons. After the structural characterization, the transmitter role of SP was strengthened by the elegant biochemical and electrophysiological studies by Otsuka and collaborators (41,62,63,66), demonstrating a marked excitatory action of SP on spinal motoneurons. Parallel electrophysiological investigations on the dorsal horn suggested a possible relation between pain transmission and SP (24). SP has not only been associated with pain and itch sensations but also with events such as neurogenic inflammation, where SP-mediated vasodilation and plasma extravasation occurs after antidromic stimulation of sensory nerves (43). These mechanisms have been suggested to take part via axon collaterals of SP containing primary sensory neurons (43,54; see also ref. 13). After intradermal injection of peptides (such as SP) cutaneous mast cells, blood vessels, and neurons are stimulated leading to histamine release, vasodilation/edema, and pain/itch (see refs. 19,20). SP is believed to activate dermal mast cells to release histamine which stimulates either two separate populations of "pain" and "itch" nerves, or one type of neuron conveying both pain and itch. By antidromic stimulation, dilation of blood vessels, i.e., the flare response, is produced via release of SP and possibly other peptides. SP released from the nerve terminals acts directly on the blood vessels and also on adjacent mast cells to cause secretion of histamine that, in turn, causes vasodilation and activation of other sensory nerves, leading to an extension of the flare reaction. Also, other peptides have histamine-releasing properties, such as VIP, neurotensin (NT), and dynorphin. Somatostatin, which is an inhibitor of many secretory processes, also induces histamine release. Recently, it has been shown that CGRP, apart from inducing histamine release, produces a delayed erythema in human skin lasting more than 3 hr after injection. Furthermore, the novel peptide CGRP has been shown to have a number of other biological activities including contraction of the guinea pig ileum (65), stimulation of sympathetic outflow (17), and vasodilation (8). Enkephalins and other opioids that are known to inhibit pain have the opposite effect on itch and enhance histamine-induced flare and itch responses in human skin. The mechanism responsible for this effect is not known; however, it is not due to histamine or prostaglandin release (data from refs. 7,8,18–20,57).

Regarding γ-MSH, there are excellent morphological conditions for a local sensory influence of γ-MSH, or a γ-MSH-like peptide, at the human skin level. The peptide may be involved in transmitter events related to nociception. On the other hand, γ-MSH released from these nerve endings and/or neutrophilic granulocytes may also exert a direct effect on connective tissue cell types, such as mast cells or granulocytes, thus participating in neurogenic inflammatory responses, pruritus, etc. This possibility should also be kept in mind when discussing other neuropeptides present in the skin.

In several studies it has been demonstrated that intra-arterial VIP causes vasodilation (44,45). Preliminary observations have suggested the presence of PHI-like immunoreactivity in peripheral autonomic neurons with a similar distribution to that of VIP (10). PHI has 13 amino acids in identical positions to VIP and PHI, although with a somewhat lower potency, shares many of the biological effects of VIP (3,9,14,60). However, it may be noted that in the cat submandibular gland preparation PHI could not be proven to have the powerful vasodilating action of VIP (50). Lundberg and collaborators (46) have demonstrated that in their experimental model systemic administration of PHI and VIP induced hypotension, probably due to peripheral vasodilation in both guinea pig and cat. Furthermore, both PHI and VIP caused an inhibition of the vagally induced increase in respiratory insufflation pressure in guinea pig. In this study, VIP was approximately five to ten times more potent than PHI with regard to hypotensive effects and two-to-threefold, considering respiratory smooth muscle relaxant effects in the guinea pig. Furthermore, in the cat VIP was 50-fold more potent in inducing hypotension.

Regarding the peptide NPY, Lundberg and collaborators (52) found that it exerts effects similar to the sympathetic nervous response. Thus, NPY induces local vasoconstriction in the cat submandibular salivary gland in addition to systemic hypertension (51,53). Furthermore, NPY inhibits the electrically induced contraction of the rat (53) and mouse (1) vas deferens. Since NPY does not seem to inhibit the contractile response to exogenous norepinephrine (1,53), NPY probably inhibits norepinephrine release via a presynaptic action. NPY may, therefore, have several actions in the sympathetic vascular and smooth muscle responses, resulting in both stimulatory and inhibitory effects on sympathetic function.

The above described innervation patterns point to possible dual functional origins for, e.g., PHI, VIP, and SP immunoreactive fibers, i.e., some fibers belong to the somatic nervous system whereas others belong to the autonomic nervous system. Furthermore, the different neuropeptides are also frequently found coexisting with each other or with "classical" transmitters. For instance, CGRP and substance P-like immunoreactivity have been shown to coexist in dorsal root ganglion cells and the spinal cord (16,64) as well as in the human skin (C.-J. Dalsgaard et al., *in preparation*), and a coexistence of prodynorphin-opioid peptides and leucine-enkephalin with SP in a major population of trigeminal and dorsal root ganglion cells has been proposed (70). Although no further attempts were made to show coexistence between SP, γ-MSH, NKA, and VIP, respectively, in the fibers of the human skin, it is tempting to suggest, based on the above-mentioned studies (13,29,30), that these neuropeptides may, at certain levels, serve together as co-transmitters or co-modulators of sensory function. Coexistence of VIP and PHI at the cellular level is a situation commonly encountered in many different tissues and species (15,46), however, it was not possible with the present technique to unequivocally establish it. Furthermore, some of the PHI and VIP immunoreactive nerves found in the present investigation may also contain acetylcholine (cf. refs. 33,44,47–49). Some peripheral neurons may thus contain at least two peptides, VIP and PHI, together with the "classical" transmitter acetylcholine. Such a situation has been demonstrated earlier, for example, in central 5-hydroxytryptamine neurons which also contain TRH- and SP-like immunoreactivities (31). Finally, coexistence of NPY and norepinephrine at the cellular level is a situation commonly encountered in many different tissues and species (52,53).

In summary, peptides are apparent in sensory and autonomic nerve terminals and fibers of the human skin. Thus, certain neuropeptides should also be considered when examining the role of different peripheral neurotransmitter candidates. Furthermore, peptides and "classical" transmitters may, at this level, serve together as co-transmitters or co-modulators of sensory and/or autonomic function. From these preliminary data, it is clear that future work in the field of human skin and peptides in physiology and pathophysiology of, for instance, pain and motility is of considerable importance.

ACKNOWLEDGMENTS

This research was supported by grants from the Swedish Medical Research Council (14X-07162, 12P-6965), Magnus Bergvalls Stiftelse, Sven och Ebba-Christina Hagbergs Stiftelse, The Swedish Society of Medicine, Stiftelsen Lars Hiertas Minne, Edvard Welanders Stiftelse, Åke Wibergs Stiftelse, and the Karolinska Institute Research Funds. For a generous·supply of antisera the author is grateful to Drs. E. Brodin, Stockholm; A.C. Cuello, Montreal; R.P. Elde, Minneapolis; J. Fahrenkrug, Copenhagen; J.A. Fischer, Zurich; L. Terenius, Uppsala; and E. Theodorsson-Norheim, Stockholm, respectively. For skillful technical assistance I thank Ms. A.-C. Andersson, Dr. A. Enhamre, Ms. W. Hiort, Ms. S. Nilsson, Ms. A. Peters, Ms. S. Soltesz-Mattisson, and Ms. K. Åman.

REFERENCES

1. Allen, J. M., Tatemoto, K., Polak, J. M., Hughes, J., and Bloom, S. R. (1982): Two novel related peptides, neuropeptide Y (NPY) and peptide YY (PYY) inhibit the contraction of the electrically stimulated mouse vas deferens. *Neuropeptides,* 3:71–77.
2. Avrameas, S. (1969): Coupling of enzymes to proteins with glutaraldehyde. Use of conjugates for the detection of antigens and antibodies. *Immunochemistry,* 6:43–47.
3. Bataille, D., Gespach, C., Laburthe, M., Amiranoff, B., Tatemoto, K., Vauclin, N., Mutt, V., and Rosselin, G. (1980): Peptide having N-terminal histidine and C-terminal isoleucineamide (PHI). Vasoactive intestinal peptide (VIP) and secretin-like effects in different tissues from the rat. *FEBS Lett.,* 114:240–242.
4. Bernstein, J. E., Rothstein, J., Soltani, K., and Levine, L. E. (1983): Neuropeptides in the pathogenesis of obesity-associated benign acanthosis nigricans. *J. Invest. Dermatol.,* 80:7–9.
5. Björklund, H., Dalsgaard, C.-J., Jonsson, C.-E., and Hermansson, A. (1986): Sensory and autonomic innervation of non-hairy and hairy human skin. An immunohistochemical study. *Cell Tissue Res.,* 243:51–57.
6. Bloom, S.R., and Polak, J.M. (1983): Regulatory peptides and the skin. *Clin. Exp. Dermatol.,* 8:3–18.
7. Brain, S. D., and Williams, T. J. (1986): The potent vasodilator properties of human calcitonin gene-related peptide (CGRP) in human skin. In: *Cellular Pharmacology of the Skin, Third Annual Symposium of the Skin Pharmacology Society* (Abstr.), p. 25. Stockholm.
8. Brain, S. D., Williams, T. J., Morris, H. R., and MacIntyre, I. (1985): Calcitonin gene-related peptide is a potent vasodilator. *Nature,* 313:54–56.
9. Brennan, L. J., Mc Longhlin, T. A., Mutt, V., Tatemoto, K., and Wood, J. R. (1982): Effects of PHI, a newly isolated peptide, in gall bladder function in the guinea-pig. *J. Physiol. (Lond.),* 329:71–72.
10. Christofides, N. D., Yiangai, Y., Blank, M. A., Tatemoto, K., Polak, J. M., and Bloom, S. R. (1982): Are peptide histidine isoleucine and vasoactive intestinal peptide co-synthesized in the same prohormone? *Lancet,* 2:1398.
11. Coons, A. H. (1958): Fluorescent antibody methods. In: *General Cytochemical Methods, Vol. 1,* edited by J. F. Danielli, pp. 399–422. Academic Press, New York.
12. Cutz, E., Chan, W., Track, N.S., Goth, A., and Said, S. I. (1978): Release of vasoactive intestinal polypeptide in mast cells by histamine liberators. *Nature,* 275:661–662.
13. Dalsgaard, C. -J., Jonsson, C. -E., Hökfelt, T., and Cuello, A. C. (1983): Localization of substance P-immunoreactive nerve fibers in the human digital skin. *Experientia,* 39:1018–1020.
14. Dimaline, R., and Dockray, G. J. (1980): Actions of a new peptide from porcine intestine (PHI) on pancreatic secretion in the rat and turkey. *Life Sci.* 27:1947–1951.
15. Fahrenkrug, J., Bek, T., Lundberg, J. M., and Hökfelt, T. (1985): VIP and PHI in cat neurons: co-localization but variable tissue content possible due to differential processing. *Reg. Peptides,* 12:21–34.
16. Fischer, J., Forssmann, W. G., Hökfelt, T., Lundberg, J. M., Reinecke, M., Tschopp, F. A., and Wiesenfeld-Hallin, Z. (1985): Immunoreactive calcitonin gene-related peptide and substance P: coexistence in sensory neurones and behavioural interaction after intrathecal administration in the rat. *J. Physiol.,* 362:29P.
17. Fisher, L. A., Kikkawa, D. O., Rivier, J. E., Amara, S. G., Evans R. J., Rosenfeld, M.

G., Vale, W. W., and Brown, M. R. (1983): Stimulation of noradrenergic sympathetic outflow by calcitonin gene-related peptide. *Nature,* 305:534–536.

18. Foreman, J. C. (1986): Substance P and calcitonin gene-related peptide: Pharmacology in human skin. In: *Cellular Pharmacology of the Skin, Third Annual Symposium of the Skin Pharmacology Society* (Abstr.), p. 23. Stockholm.

19. Hägermark, Ö. (1986): Skin as a response organ for neuropeptides. In: *Cellular Pharmacology of the Skin, Third Annual Symposium of the Skin Pharmacology Society* (Abstr.), p. 11. Stockholm.

20. Hägermark, Ö., Hökfelt, T., and Pernow, B. (1978): Flare and itch induced by substance P in human skin. *J. Invest. Dermatol.,* 71:233–235.

21. Hartschuh, W., Weihe, E., Büchler, M., Helmstaedter, V., Feurle, G. E., and Forssmann, W. G. (1979): Met-enkephalin-like immunoreactivity in Merkel cells. *Cell Tissue Res.,* 201:343–348.

22. Hartschuh, W., Weihe, E., and Reinecke, M. (1983): Peptidergic (neurotensin, VIP, substance P) nerve fibers in the skin. Immunohistochemical evidence of an involvement of neuropeptides in nociception, pruritus and inflammation. *Br. J. Dermatol.,* (Suppl. 25) 109:14–17.

23. Hartschuh, W., Weihe, E., Yanaihara, N., and Reinecke, M. (1983): Immunohistochemical localization of vasoactive intestinal polypeptide (VIP) in Merkel cells of various mammals: Evidence for a neuromodulator function of the Merkel cell. *J. Invest. Dermatol.,* 81:361–364.

24. Henry, J. L. (1976): Effects of substance P on functionally identified units in cat spinal cord. *Brain Res.,* 114:439–451.

25. Hökfelt, T., Johansson, O., Kellerth, J. -O., Ljungdahl, Å., Nilsson, G., Nygårds, A., and Pernow, B. (1977): Immunohistochemical distribution of substance P. In: *Substance P,* edited by U.S. von Euler and B. Pernow, pp. 117–145. Raven Press, New York.

26. Hökfelt, T., Skirboll, L., Dalsgaard, C. -J., Johansson, O., Lundberg, J. M., Norell, G., and Jancsó, G. (1982): Peptide neurons in the spinal cord with special reference to descending systems. In: *Brain Stem Control of Spinal Mechanisms,* edited by B. Sjölund, and A. Björklund, pp. 89–117. Elsevier, Amsterdam.

27. Hökfelt, T., Skirboll, L., Lundberg, J. M., Dalsgaard, C. -J., Johansson, O., Pernow, B., and Jancsó, G. (1983): Neuropeptides and pain pathways. In: *Advances in Pain Research and Therapy, Vol. 5,* edited by J. J. Bonica, U. Lindblom, and A. Iggo, pp. 227–246. Raven Press, New York.

28. Johansson, O. (1985): Morphological characterization of the somatostatin-immunoreactive dendritic skin cells in urticaria pigmentosa patients by computerized image analysis. *Scand. J. Immunol.,* 21:431–439.

29. Johansson, O. (1986): Evidence for PHI-immunoreactive nerve fibers in the human skin: Coexistence with VIP?. *Med. Biol.* 64:67–73.

30. Johansson, O. (1986): A detailed account of NPY-immunoreactive nerves and cells of the human skin. Comparison with VIP-, substance P- and PHI-containing structures. *Acta Physiol. Scand.,* 128:147–153.

31. Johansson, O., Hökfelt, T., Pernow, B., Jeffcoate, S. L., White, N., Steinbusch, H. W. M., Verhofstad, A. A. J., Emson, P. C., and Spindel, E. (1981): Immunohistochemical support for three putative transmitters in one neuron: Coexistence of 5-hydroxytryptamine, substance P- and thyrotropin releasing hormone-like immunoreactivity in medullary neurons projecting to the spinal cord. *Neuroscience,* 6:1857–1881.

32. Johansson, O., Ljungberg, A., and Vaalasti, A. S. (1987): Evidence for γ-MSH containing nerves and neutrophilic granulocytes in the human skin using indirect immunofluorescence. *J. Invest. Dermatol. (in press).*

33. Johansson, O., and Lundberg, J. M. (1981): Ultrastructural localization of VIP-like immunoreactivity in large dense-core vesicles of 'cholinergic-type' nerve terminals in cat exocrine glands. *Neuroscience,* 6:847–862.

34. Johansson, O., and Nordlind, K. (1984): Immunohistochemical localization of somatostatin-like immunoreactivity in skin lesions of *urticaria pigmentosa* patients. *Virchows Arch.* (*Cell. Pathol.*), 46:155–164.

35. Johansson, O., and Nordlind, K. (1985): Immunohistochemical screening of psoriasis. *Arch. Dermatol. Res.,* 277:156.

36. Johansson, O., and Nordlind, K. (1986): Immunoreactivity to material like vasoactive intestinal polypeptide in epidermal cells of lichen sclerosus et atrophicus. *Am. J. Dermatopathol.,* 8:105–108.
37. Johansson, O., Nordlind, K., Efendić, S., and Lidén, S. (1985): The immunohistochemical observation of somatostatin-like and avian pancreatic polypeptide-like immunoreactivity in certain cellular elements of diabetic lipodystrophic skin. *Dermatologica,* 171:233–237.
38. Johansson, O., Olsson, A., Enhamre, A., Hammar, H., and Goldstein, M. (1987): Phenylethanolamine *N*-methyltransferase-like immunoreactivity in psoriasis: An immunohistochemical study on catecholamine synthesizing enzymes and neuropeptides of the skin. *Acta. Derm. Venereol.* (Stockh.) 67:1–7.
39. Johansson, O., and Vaalasti, A. (1987): Immunohistochemical evidence for the presence of somatostatin-containing sensory nerve fibers in the human skin. *Neurosci. Lett.,* 73:225–230.
40. Johansson, O., Vaalasti, A., and Ljungberg, A. (1987): Somatostatin-like immunoreactivity is also found in normal human dermal dendritic skin cells. *Nature (in press).*
41. Konishi, S., and Otsuka, M. (1974): Excitatory action of hypothalamic substance P on spinal motoneurones of newborn rats. *Nature,* 252:734–735.
42. Lembeck, F. (1953): Zur Frage der zentralen Übertragung afferenter Impulse. III. Mitteilung. Das Vorkommen und die Bedeutung der Substanz P in den dorsalen Wurzeln des Rückenmarks. *Naunyn-Schmiedebergs Arch. Pharmacol.,* 219:197–213.
43. Lembeck, F., and Holzer, P. (1979): Substance P as neurogenic mediator of antidromic vasodilation and neurogenic plasma extravasation. *Naunyn-Schmiedebergs Arch. Pharmacol.,* 310:175–183.
44. Lundberg, J. M. (1981): Evidence for coexistence of vasoactive intestinal polypeptide (VIP) and acetylcholine in neurons of cat exocrine glands. Morphological, biochemical and functional studies. *Acta Physiol. Scand.,* (Supp. 496) 1–57, *Doctoral Dissertation,* Stockholm.
45. Lundberg, J. M., Änggård, A., Fahrenkrug, J., Hökfelt, T., and Mutt, V. (1980): Vasoactive intestinal polypeptide in cholinergic neurons of exocrine glands: Functional significance of coexisting transmitters for vasodilation and secretion. *Proc. Natl. Acad. Sci. USA,* 77:1651–1655.
46. Lundberg, J. M., Fahrenkrug, J., Hökfelt, T., Martling, C. -R., Larsson, O., Tatemoto, K., and Änggård, A. (1984): Co-existence of peptide HI (PHI) and VIP in nerves regulating blood flow and bronchial smooth muscle tone in various mammals including man. *Peptides,* 5:593–606.
47. Lundberg, J. M., Hedlund, B., Änggård, A., Fahrenkrug, J., Hökfelt, T., Tatemoto, K., and Bartfai, T. (1982): Costorage of peptides and classical transmitters in neurons. In: *Systemic Role of Regulatory Peptides,* edited by S. R. Bloom, J. M. Polak, and E. Lindenlaub, pp. 93–119. Schattauer Verlag, Stuttgart.
48. Lundberg, J. M., and Hökfelt, T. (1983): Coexistence of peptides and classical transmitters. *TINS,* 6:325–332.
49. Lundberg, J. M., Hökfelt, T., Schultzberg, M., Uvnäs-Wallensten, K., Köhler, C., and Said, S. I. (1979): Occurrence of vasoactive intestinal polypeptide (VIP)-like immunoreactivity in certain cholinergic neurons of the cat: Evidence from combined immunohistochemistry and acetylcholinesterase staining. *Neuroscience,* 4:1539–1559.
50. Lundberg, J. M., and Tatemoto, K. (1982): Vascular effects of the peptides PYY and PHI: Comparison with APP and VIP. *Eur. J. Pharmacol.,* 83:143–146.
51. Lundberg, J. M., and Tatemoto, K. (1982): Pancreatic polypeptide family (APP, BPP, NPY and PYY) in relation to sympathetic vasoconstriction resistant to α-adrenoceptor blockade. *Acta. Physiol. Scand.,* 116:393–402.
52. Lundberg, J. M., Terenius, L., Hökfelt, T., and Goldstein, M. (1983): High levels of neuropeptide Y in peripheral noradrenergic neurons in various mammals including man. *Neurosci. Lett.,* 42:167–172.
53. Lundberg, J. M., Terenius, L., Hökfelt, T., Martling, C. R., Tatemoto, K., Mutt, V., Polak, J., Bloom, S. R., and Goldstein, M. (1982): Neuropeptide Y (NPY)-like immunoreactivity in peripheral noradrenergic neurons and effects of NPY on sympathetic function. *Acta Physiol. Scand.,* 116:477–480.
54. Miller, M. R., Ralston H. J., III, and Kasahara, M. (1958): The pattern of cutaneous innervation of the human hand. *Am. J. Anat.,* 102:183–218.

55. Nakane, P. K., and Pierce, G. B. (1967): Enzyme-labelled antibodies for the light and electronmicroscopic localization of tissue antigens and antibodies. *J. Cell. Biol.*, 33:307–311.

56. O'Shaughnessy, D. J., McGregor, G. P., Ghatei, M. A., Blank, M. A., Springall, D. R., Gu, J., Polak, J. M., and Bloom, S. R. (1983): Distribution of bombesin, somatostatin, substance-P and vasoactive intestinal polypeptide in feline and porcine skin. *Life Sci.*, 32:2827–2836.

57. Piotrowski, W., and Foreman, J. C. (1986): Some effects of calcitonin gene-related peptide in human skin and on histamine release. *Br. J. Dermatol.*, 114:37–46.

58. Polak, J. M., and Bloom, S. R. (1981): The peripheral substance P-ergic system. *Peptides*, (Suppl. 2) 2:133–148.

59. Sternberger, L. A. (1979): *Immunocytochemistry, 2nd ed.* Wiley, New York.

60. Szecowka, J., Tatemoto, K., Mutt, V., and Efendić, S. (1980): Interaction of a newly isolated intestinal polypeptide (PHI) with glucose and arginine to affect the secretion of insulin and glucagon. *Life Sci.*, 26:435–438.

61. Tainio, H., Vaalasti, A., and Rechardt, L. (1986): The distribution of sympathetic adrenergic, tyrosine hydroxylase- and neuropeptide Y-immunoreactive nerves in human axillary sweat glands. *Histochemistry*, 85:117–120.

62. Takahashi, T., Konishi, S., Powell, D., Leeman, S. E., and Otsuka, M. (1974): Identification of the motoneuron-depolarizing peptide in the bovine dorsal root as hypothalamic substance P. *Brain Res.*, 73:59–69.

63. Takahashi, T., and Otsuka, M. (1975): Regional distribution of substance P in the spinal cord and nerve roots of the cat and the effect of dorsal root section. *Brain Res.*, 87:1–11.

64. Terenghi, G., Gibson, S. J., McGregor, G. P., Ghatei, M. A., Mulderry, P. K., Bloom, S. R., and Polak, J. M. (1985): Co-localisation of substance P and calcitonin gene-related peptide immunoreactivity in primary sensory neurones. In: *Substance P. Metabolism and Biological Actions*, edited by C. C. Jordan and P. Oehme. Taylor and Francis, London (*in press*).

65. Tippins, J. R., Morris, H. R., Panico, M., Etienne, T., Bens, P., Girgis, S., MacIntyre, I., Azria, M., and Attinger, M. (1984): The myotropic and plasma-calcium modulating effects of calcitonin gene-related peptide (CGRP). *Neuropeptides*, 4:425–434.

66. Tsunoo, A., Konishi, S., and Otsuka, M. (1982): Substance P as an excitatory transmitter of primary afferent neurons in guinea-pig sympathetic ganglia. *Neuroscience*, 7:2025–2037.

67. Vaalasti, A., Tainio, H., and Rechardt, L. (1985): Vasoactive intestinal polypeptide (VIP)-like immunoreactivity in the nerves of human axillary sweat glands. *J. Invest. Dermatol.*, 85:246–248.

68. Wallengren, J., Ekman, R., and Möller, H. (1986): Substance P and vasoactive intestinal peptide in bullous and inflammatory skin disease. *Acta Derm. Venereol.*, 66:23–28.

69. Wallengren, J., Möller, H., and Ekman, R. (1986): Release of substance P (SP) and vasoactive intestinal peptide (VIP) in physical urticaria. In: *Cellular Pharmacology of the Skin, Third Annual Symposium of the Skin Pharmacology Society*, (Abstr.) p. 26. Stockholm.

70. Weihe, E., Hartschuh, W., and Nohr, D. (1986): Co-existence of opioid peptides and substance P in sensory afferents. In: *Cellular Pharmacology of the Skin, Third Annual Symposium of the Skin Pharmacology Society*, (Abstr.) p. 26. Stockholm.

71. Weihe, E., Hartschuh, W., and Weber, E. (1985): Prodynorphin opioid peptides in small somatosensory primary afferents of guinea pig. *Neurosci. Lett.*, 58:347–352.

72. Wesley, J. R., Vinik, A. I., O'Dorisio, T. M., Glaser, B., and Fink, A. (1982): A new syndrome of symptomatic cutaneous mastocytoma producing vasoactive intestinal polypeptide. *Gastroenterology*, 82:963–967.

Advances in Pain Research and Therapy,
Vol. 10. Edited by M. Tiengo et al.
Raven Press, Ltd., New York © 1987.

Psychological Treatment: The Importance of Objective Behavioral Goals in Pain Management

Eldon Tunks

Chedoke-McMaster Hospital, Hamilton, Ontario L8N 325, Canada

The importance of the psychological dimension in chronic pain has long been recognized. Of the various forms of psychological treatment used, some emphasize emotional relief or the development of insight, and others focus on various aspects of overt behavior and behavioral management. Most pain clinics provide access to at least one form of psychological treatment, and many multidisciplinary clinics depend on well developed psychologically based treatment programs. Since the late 1960s, behavioral methods, such as operant conditioning, biofeedback, or cognitive-behavioral therapy have shown promise in the management of chronic pain. The hallmark of behavioral methods of treatment is the clinical focus on objective, rather than subjective, therapeutic goals. This chapter concerns itself with the importance of objective behavioral goals as an essential ingredient for successful outcome, both in the therapies that are explicitly "behavioral" and also in the therapies such as psychodynamic or cognitive therapy which deal with subjective data and conversations with the patient.

CHARACTERISTICS OF THE CHRONIC PAIN PATIENT

Crook et al. (11) carried out an epidemiological survey to discover the prevalence and characteristics of acute pain and chronic pain problems in the community. Comparisons were then made between chronic pain sufferers in the community who for the most part had not been referred to specialty clinics, and chronic pain patients who had been referred to a university hospital pain clinic (12). These two groups did not seem to differ in the duration of their pain problems, nor in the bodily locations of their pains, nor in demographic variables such as age, sex, marital status, original occupation, or social class. Clear differences did however emerge in several psychosocial and behavioral variables. The patients who attended the chronic pain specialty clinic reported more difficulties in activities of daily living, and more pain on activity. They were more frequent users of the health-care system, and often experienced complications of job loss, litigation, alcohol and drug abuse. They endorsed more somatic symptoms and more depression, and admitted more frequently to social withdrawal in response to pain. More than half of the pain clinic patients blamed the onset of their pain on an accident, often at work, and they were very frequently unemployed (12). These findings suggest that patients who are likely to be referred to specialty pain clinics may not be typical of pain sufferers in general. It is likely that it is not the pain diagnosis alone, but also a loading on behavioral and psychosocial variables, that causes certain patients to be referred to specialists. Treatment of such patients in a pain clinic should emphasize the need for behavioral change.

PSYCHOLOGICAL TREATMENT

Up to 1968, psychological treatment for chronic pain was formulated mainly in psychodynamic terms, either through psychoanalytic theories, as illustrated by the work of Engel (15), or through some variation of psychosomatic theory that considered individual responses and the effects of stress. Psychological treatment likely would be long, expensive, and possibly ineffective.

A marked departure from the traditional subjective viewpoint came from Fordyce et al. (20) in their publication in 1968 of a case report of the use of operant conditioning methods for treatment of three chronic pain patients. They followed this up in 1973 with a study of 36 such patients, noting that on follow-up, patients reported less pain, improved medication use and activity levels (21). This caused a great deal of excitement, and stimulated the application of the operant conditioning method in many other pain clinics, usually as part of a multidisciplinary approach, and generally with favorable results. These have been fully reviewed by several authors (3,9,47,49). Consequently, there is a recognition that psychological methods are effective in pain management. In addition, behavioral approaches have built-in objective clinical goals which can serve as measures which are valuable both for program evaluation and also for research.

GOALS OF OPERANT BEHAVIORAL INTERVENTION

The various reports of operant behavioral treatment programs have been reviewed in detail elsewhere (3,9,46,47,49,50). With regard to the importance of objective behavioral goals in chronic pain management, a few studies are of particular interest.

Intuitively, one might assume that pain ought to be aggravated proportionately to the degree of exercise, and relieved by rest. An operant learning model of pain would postulate the opposite; a chronic pain problem is reinforced by rest, whereas reinforcement of activity while withholding reinforcement of pain behavior leads to reduction in pain behavior and increase in activity. Fordyce et al. (22) reported a study in which physiotherapists observed 25 patients, studying their tolerance during specific exercises over a period of several sessions. Observations were made of the number of repetitions of each exercise performed in any given session; of the kinds of pain behavior during the same session; of verbal complaints, guarding, or gestures indicating pain; and of moaning or statements implying inability or difficulty to continue due to pain. There was a strikingly significant negative correlation between exercise performed per session and pain behavior in the same session. That is, as the amount of exercise rose, the verbal and the nonverbal indicators of pain fell in frequency. This suggests that the illness behavior associated with chronic pain is more subject to environmental reinforcement than to nociception. It would follow from this that when treating chronic pain patients, the treatment goal would be primarily to change the pain behavior, rather than to limit the expectations of treatment according to the patient's complaints.

The role of the spouse as a possible reinforcer of illness behavior, was examined in a study by Block et al. (6). A taped structured interview was given to 20 married chronic pain patients, who were required to report their pain levels in two different conditions; on one occasion the spouse was present, whereas on the other occasion the ward clerk who acted as a neutral observer was present. Patients who had indicated that their spouses were relatively nonsolicitous in response to their pain behavior reported significantly lower pain levels in the spouse-observed condition. On the contrary, patients who reported that their spouses were relatively solicitous in responding to pain behavior reported higher pain levels in the spouse-observed condition. In keeping with the awareness that family dynamics may reinforce illness behavior, an important ingredient in many pain management programs is some form of family intervention directed to the goal of teaching family members to modify their responses in such a way as to cease reinforcement of illness behavior, and instead to reinforce active and well behavior.

Considering the above, it is important to know what sort of reinforcement is apt to be effective in achieving the therapeutic goal. Cairns and Pasino (8) studied nine patients with chronic low back pain in three conditions. In the "verbal reinforcement condition," therapists observed the patients while exercising on bicycle or walking. Beginning with the ninth session, the therapists began to praise the patient and to converse with him only if exercise levels increased. In the "graph" and the "verbal reinforcement plus graph condition," daily performance levels of one of the exercises were plotted on a graph prominently over the patient's bed for six sessions. Over the next six sessions, while continuing the graph, the therapists also verbally praised any increase in performance on that exercise, while other exercise still remained under base-line (unreinforced) conditions. In the "control condition," patients were instructed to walk or to use the exercise bicycle, while observing therapists made no specific response. Only during the times of verbal reinforcement, with or without a graph, did exercise behavior increase. The graph did not significantly increase the exercise behavior. In the condition in which only one exercise was being verbally reinforced, the unreinforced activity actually decreased. This study points out the specific reinforcing value of verbal communication, with the added suggestion that therapeutic goals that are selected for reinforcement should be carefully chosen, since generalization of the treatment effect to all illness behavior will not necessarily occur. Very similar findings were reported by Doleys et al. (13).

Observations such as those in the research described above have reaffirmed the suspicion that many behaviorally oriented therapists have of psychological therapies that depend primarily on conversations with the patient. Indeed, verbalizations about pain can even be considered a form of illness behavior. It is possible that such verbalizations may not even be trusted for factual data; for example, Linton and Melin (30) showed that memory for reported pain is faulty after a few weeks. The behaviorists' preference for action rather than words has led sometimes to the accusation that behavioral therapies neglect the essential empathy to aid chronic pain sufferers, and this has been the subject of increasing debate in the literature (18,19,33–35,38,41).

Notwithstanding the demonstrated effectiveness of operant conditioning methods, in practically all pain-management programs that use operant conditioning methods, multiple other interventions, including "supportive psychotherapy," are also simultaneously used, so that it would be difficult to attribute success of the programs to the operant conditioning alone (3,42,48). Moreover, other studies have demonstrated that, apart from operant conditioning, there are also other kinds of psychological treatment that may be combined with multimodal treatment programs with equally satisfactory results: biofeedback, cognitive-behavioral, or psychodynamic psychotherapy (23,33,39).

GOALS OF BIOFEEDBACK THERAPY

Biofeedback therapy involves objective behavioral goals; these are to learn to demonstrate control of certain bodily functions which are monitored instrumentally. The assumptions underlying biofeedback therapy are that the illness to be treated depends on abnormal activity in an organ system that is controlled by the nervous system, but not within the individual's awareness: By instrumentation, it is possible to monitor that organ system; feedback from the instrumentation to the individual will allow the patient to become aware of and to learn to voluntarily modify those responses, leading to improvement in the illness. Depending on the illness, different sorts of instrumental feedback may be used. On the surface one might be tempted to conclude that the success of biofeedback therapy depends primarily on the ability to objectify and then to modify a previously involuntary and unconscious physiological process. As most of the recent reviews point out, it is doubtful that such clear specificity exists. Although supporting the impression that biofeedback treatment of various types seems to produce beneficial results, these reviews note that, for the most part, biofeedback is about as effective as structured relaxation training, (with which the biofeedback procedure is often also admixed) (9,26,29,46–48,50,51).

Most of the electromyographic (EMG) biofeedback research is confined to studies of tension headache subjects, although some involves other problems such as chronic back pain (46) or myofascial-pain dysfunction syndrome (40). It is often assumed that the pain of tension headache is due to sustained and abnormal muscle contraction. Zitman (51) notes that the published studies do seem to show that during pain-free periods, tension headache patients have higher resting EMG levels than controls, but EMG levels during attacks correlate more poorly with the headache episodes. For example, Gray et al. (24) compared biofeedback treatment of muscles near the source of pain, biofeedback from an area remote from the pain, and relaxation only. Although pain improved for all groups, the EMG levels did not significantly change. Furthermore, EMG levels recorded from subjects during headaches were not different from nonheadache values. Holroyd et al. (25) compared EMG biofeedback with a credible pseudotherapy (patients trained to meditate, with the expectation that improvement would occur automatically), and with a symptom-monitoring control group. They found that only the biofeedback group had pain improvement, even though subjects rated the experimental conditions as equally credible. The authors suggested that cognitive rather than physiological factors were mainly responsible for the treatment effect. In another study, Andrasik and Holroyd (1) used an ingenious method to train tension headache subjects either to decrease, to maintain, or to increase forehead tension levels. All three groups improved, compared to a no-treatment control group.

Skin temperature biofeedback has been applied mostly to treatment of migraines. The assumptions behind this are that migraine is associated with an abnormality of sympathetic tone. This tone can be corrected by biofeedback if the hands can be warmed, thereby reducing the sympathetic tone. Initial uncontrolled reports appeared to support these assumptions, but later reviews noted that there was not a clear relationship between the specific goal of hand-warming and the desired clinical effect (9,26,48,51). Jessup et al. (26) noted that hand-warming, hand-cooling, or no treatment all produced similar improvement. Zitman (51) criticized the basic assumptions underlying this biofeedback approach, concluding that there is insufficient evidence to assume that migraine is related to a general vasomotor dysfunction, that the published studies do not support the idea that changes in finger temperature can produce changes in the vasomotor response of cranial vessels, that temperature changes that can be produced are usually of small magnitude, and that the degree of increase of temperature change does not seem to be related to the relief of symptoms.

Increasingly sophisticated studies such as described above are gradually pointing to the conclusion that the efficacy of biofeedback depends on changing the patient's sense of control and interpretation of his disorder. In this way, attention is turning to cognitive factors as the major mediators in the success of biofeedback, rather than physiological conditioning alone (1,16,32,47). The objective behavioral goal of acquiring control over a particular bodily function serves the purpose of increasing self-awareness, increasing the belief in self-control, and providing a structured therapeutic experience in which the subject may mobilize coping strategies which can be effectively generalized to pain management. The therapeutic goal should not be restricted to modification of a physiological process alone, but rather to provide a task through which the patient may develop an awareness of bodily control, while learning to employ effective coping strategies (47). In this way, the focus on objective goals (such as learning to control biofeedback output) continues to be essential, but for reasons of promoting changes in coping behavior rather than because of specific "autonomic response-disease" connections.

GOALS OF COGNITIVE THERAPY

Cognitive therapy, or cognitive-behavioral therapy, is actually a group of therapeutic methods which may be applied in various combinations. At the core of the approach is the assumption that thoughts often mediate actions, that maladaptive behaviors are often tied to problems in style of thinking or to lack of effective available cognitive coping methods, and that these problems can be corrected by an approach which combines overt goal-oriented tasks (such as self-monitoring, stress inoculation and practice of specific coping strategies, or biofeedback) with cognitive training (reappraisal of stress, studying possible cognitive coping alternatives, or analysis of maladaptive thoughts). What is common to all of these methods is that some objective measurement, usually some form of self-monitoring, is built into the treatment, and that the patient is engaged in a structured therapeutic experience which is designed to enhance his or her sense of mastery. Often, cognitive coping methods are explicitly discussed and practiced, with the assumption that the patient's strategies are absent or deficient.

Considering the wide variation in types of cognitive therapy, it is difficult to evaluate or compare them. Certainly they are becoming popular and seem to be effective. The most comprehensive reviews of the field note that laboratory studies of individual cognitive coping methods have often failed to demonstrate superiority, or even efficacy, of these methods in volunteers. The reason for this finding may be that many subjects may already have their own well developed coping strategies which are preferable and more versatile. Furthermore, laboratory studies of normal volunteers may not be comparable to clinical situations (44,47). Cognitive therapies represent a compromise between behavior therapies which focus primarily on objective goals, and insight-oriented psychotherapies which concentrate primarily on talking and subjective states. The strength of cognitive-behavioral therapy is the use of objective behavioral goals around which the patient can orient his task of learning to cope.

GOALS OF DYNAMIC PSYCHOTHERAPY

Psychotherapy aims at using the patient-therapist relationship to develop insight, through the means of explanations and interpretations of unconscious processes. The insight is believed to permit the patient to rearrange his coping in a more economical and comfortable way. Although many pain clinics have endorsed operant conditioning or other psychological methods as their main therapeutic endeavor, supportive psychotherapy usually remains. Karasu et al. (2), in the largest review of the psychotherapy and behavior therapy literature, came to the conclusions that little or no difference can be shown in the effectiveness of one form of psychotherapy or behavior therapy in comparison to another, except that when behavior therapies tended to focus on more narrow therapeutic goals (such as bed-wetting or phobias), the results were better, and that therapy of some type is generally better than control or no therapy. Luborsky et al. (31) used a box score method to compare all published studies of psychotherapy. Six studies showed that behavior therapy was better than psychotherapy, whereas thirteen showed that there was no difference. However, the behavior therapy studies mostly involved desensitization procedures, and the studies that showed behavior therapies superior usually involved specific behavioral conditions which are rarely ever treated by psychotherapy. In his review of psychotherapies for psychosomatic disorders, including pain, Kellner (27) found that the combination of psychological treatment methods with other methods was more effective than solitary treatments. Likewise, Draspa (14) and Sarno (39) both showed that psychotherapy can be combined with multimodal treatment approaches, with good results. It should be noted that multimodal programs usually include counseling and advice about objective issues, such as vocational counseling or physical fitness, for example. Although in theory psychotherapy is based on subjective experiences and goals, in the context of a multimodal approach the psychotherapeutic intervention takes on a focus on objective goals, not dissimilar to the goals of behavioral therapies.

Bellissimo and Tunks (5) argued that it is fully compatible with any psychotherapy to establish with the patient objective behavioral goals in addition to those that are more subjective. Such behavioral goals, which might be used in the context of a "treatment contract," help to increase the perceived relevance of the therapy for the pain problem, serve as benchmarks against which to measure progress or lack of it, allow for development of a sense of mastery, improve the participation of patients who lack psychological sophistication, reduce the time period required for a successful outcome, and provide an effective and realistic focus to keep the patient actively engaged in therapy.

GOALS OF MULTIDISCIPLINARY APPROACHES

Many pain clinics provide multidisciplinary treatment for chronic pain. Group education and discussion, relaxation training, vocational counseling, exercise, transcutaneous electrical nerve stimulation (TENS), medication reduction, and other methods are combined in the treatment package; thus, there are multiple goals of a psychological, biological, and social nature. Despite many anecdotal reports supporting the usefulness of these eclectic programs, there are many problems in their evaluation. The use of multiple outcome measures raises the statistical probability that some treatment effects will occur just by chance. There are problems in (a) measurement of treatment effect, (b) standardization of measures to be used, (c) follow-up methodologies, (d) designing adequate controls, (e) dealing with contamination effects, and (f) comparing studies that have different intake procedures and criteria, and serve different populations. These problems are discussed in other reviews (3,29,42,46,47,49). Many of these programs include physical or medical therapies, such as prescription of antidepressants, TENS, and exercise.

Antidepressants may be given because of the assumption that chronic pain often represents a "masked depression" (7), but Pilowsky et al. (37) reported in a controlled study that amitriptyline had no appreciable effect in a mixed group of chronic pain patients.

TENS is favored by many clinics because it may provide an alternative to medications which can be abused, is noninvasive, and can be self-applied. However, Thorsteinsson et al. (45), in a double-blind cross-over study, found the efficacy of TENS scarcely better than placebo.

In a review of physiotherapy methods for low back pain, Nachemson (36) raised doubts that most methods were of any real use, apart from maintaining good muscle tone, education regarding good posture, and a reasonable amount of activity. In a more recent review, Flor and Turk (17) reviewed available physical treatments such as medication, orthopedic or neurosurgical procedures, steroid injections or nerve blocks, chemonucleolysis, manipulation, traction, braces, TENS, and physiotherapy for back pain. Whereas there is some evidence that improvement may result from medical or surgical treatment of some cases of acute back pain associated with progressive neurological lesions, these treatments are usually disappointing in chronic back pain (17). Flor et al. (16) did a study comparing EMG biofeedback, pseudotherapy (false feedback), and conventional physiotherapy of exercises, massage, ultrasound, heat, and medication. Only the biofeedback group improved significantly, measured by pain duration, intensity, and quality, EMG levels, reduction in negative self-statements (cognitive improvements), and impairment reported at follow-up.

The above evidence suggests that the goals of physical therapy may, for the most part, be insufficient to the management of chronic pain. However, it may yet be that psychological or behavioral therapies are more effective when combined with certain physically oriented therapies, especially when the latter emphasize education and exercise (14). Such exercise and education programs generally include systems to increase activity in the patients, often by use of quotas. In this case, the physical therapy may support the cognitive and behavioral change in conjunction with the psychological treatment (16).

Lest it should sound as if only multidisciplinary programs are valid for chronic pain management, it should be noted that there are many physicians who have a particular commitment to the management of pain, but who do not have access to a multidisciplinary program. Yet, their results may be quite good. Although they are not psychotherapists or behaviorists by training, successful clinicians are usually individuals who demonstrate an attitude of empathy, and who motivate the patient to actively participate in treatment. If one observes them in their work, one can see that the medical, surgical, or anesthesiological treatment they offer is well integrated into a broader understanding of the chronic pain problem, engendering hope and motivation for change in their patients.

In summary, multidisciplinary units alter the patient's orientation to the pain problem by means of multiple therapeutic experiences, the majority of which involve objective behavioral goals.

IMPORTANCE OF SETTING SPECIFIC GOALS

Outside the field of pain studies, Kolb and Boyatzis (28) studied Master's degree students in the Management course at Massachusetts Institute of Technology. These students participated in groups in which each individual was encouraged to reflect on his own behavior and to select a limited and well defined goal that he would like to achieve. He then was to keep an objective record of his performance in the form of a graph which measured progress day to day. There were two factors that predicted success in changing: the individual's commitment to his change goal, and the amount of feedback he received from other group members. Expectation of success and self-monitoring were also found to be significant factors in success.

In the chronic pain literature, despite the apparent diversity in approaches represented by operant behavior therapy, cognitive-behavioral therapy, and traditional psychotherapy, goal-setting is presented as an essential element in treatment (5,29,47). For example, in a multidisciplinary pain management unit, Catchlove and Cohen (10) compared 20 patients who were treated but given no specific instruction about return to work, with 27 patients who received the same treatment but who were instructed at the outset of treatment that they would be expected to return to work on a specific day. Twenty-five percent of the no-instruction group returned to work, compared to 59% of the instruction group—a statistically significant difference.

The Chedoke-McMaster Pain Program in Hamilton, Canada (4; E. Tunks and S. Banerjee, *unpublished observations*) is a multidisciplinary pain program that includes an inpatient unit which was initially established in 1972 as an operant conditioning program, following the method described by Fordyce. The program was subsequently altered, making use of groups, and introducing "milieu therapy"; in this condition, patients were expected to help each other to learn more adaptive ways to manage their pain, but it was left up to each individual to work toward his/her own goals. After 2 years, the program was altered again, still retaining the emphasis on groups and the therapeutic milieu, but adding a requirement that all patients were to negotiate with the staff each week measurable objective goals, such as increases in exercise quotas or decreases in medication. Forty-four consecutive patients were included in the operant conditioning cohort, 77 consecutive patients in the group/milieu therapy condition, and 44 consecutive patients in the group/milieu therapy plus objective goals condition. Outcomes were assessed by examinations or observations by the attending physician, nurse, occupational therapist, and physiotherapist at the time of admission, discharge, 6 weeks follow-up, and 6-months follow-up. Patients who could not be traced were counted as treatment failures.

Activity levels were rated as improved if significant improvements in uptime, participation in work placements, and exercise were observed during hospitalization; there was no significant difference between groups in activity level noted at the time of discharge; 75% of the patients in the "operant conditioning" and in the "group/milieu plus goals" condition, and 83% of those in the group/milieu condition showed substantial increase in activity.

Intake of sedatives, psychotropic drugs, analgesic drugs, laxatives, and other drugs was reduced in 59% of the patients in the operant conditioning, and in 77% of the patients in the groups/milieu plus goals conditions, compared to 35% in the group/milieu therapy condition. Twenty-eight percent of the patients in the operant conditioning, and 50% of the patients in the groups/milieu plus goals conditions completely discontinued their analgesics, compared to only 9% in the groups/milieu therapy condition. All of these differences were statistically significant.

At the time of admission to the program, almost all patients were disabled with respect to vocational, avocational, and social roles. At 6-months follow-up after treatment, approximately 40 to 50% in all three treatment conditions were employed, in training or school, or actively seeking work. However, if one considered only those patients who on admission were unemployed and without potential jobs—not retired, not housewives, and not students, the majority of whom were in receipt of pensions or compensation or were engaged in litigation—change in status to employed by the time of discharge or 6-months follow-up favored those who were treated with methods emphasizing objective goals. Thirty-two percent of such patients in the operant conditioning, 21% of those in groups/milieu plus goals condition, and 15% of those in the groups/milieu condition found work. Although change of employment figures were not statistically different, the distinct impression was that functional outcome was greatly improved by treatment programs that demanded contractual goal-setting, whether the program followed the model of operant conditioning or milieu and group therapies.

CONCLUSIONS

As noted by Sternbach (43), there are not enough data to support a conclusion that one type of psychological therapy is better than another in cases of chronic pain, or that one kind of therapy is better suited for a specific kind of patient. However, regardless of the brand of therapy, a specific goal orientation increases the probability of success.

Treatment goals based only on treatment of presumed biological causes of pain are less likely to produce change when treating chronic pain than are goals related to changing behavior and manner of coping.

When dealing with chronic pain, especially when the patients suffer psychological and social complications, multidisciplinary treatment may be better than the component methods taken by themselves. In such multimodal programs, the physical therapy components that emphasize education and active exercise may influence cognitive and behavioral change.

Verbal encouragement may be one of the most important factors in facilitating goal attainment and behavioral change.

Specific goal-setting as part of the treatment process is compatible with all psychologically based therapies. The more specific and measurable the goal, the greater the likelihood of reaching the desired goal of pain control.

REFERENCES

1. Andrasik, F., and Holroyd, K. A. (1980): A test of specific and nonspecific effects in the biofeedback treatment of tension headache. *J. Consult. Clin. Psychol.,* 48:575–586.
2. APA Commission on Psychotherapies (1982): *Psychotherapy Research: Methodological and Efficacy Issues.* American Psychiatric Association, Washington, D.C.
3. Aronoff, G. M., Evans, W. O., and Enders, P. L. (1983): A review of followup studies of multidisciplinary pain units. *Pain,* 16:1–11.
4. Banerjee, S. N., and Tunks, E. (1981): Inpatient pain program—behavior modification vs. therapeutic community. *58th Annual Session of American Congress of Rehabilitation Medicine,* San Diego.
5. Bellissimo, A, and Tunks, E. (1984): *Chronic Pain: the Psychotherapeutic Spectrum.* Praeger, New York.
6. Block, A. R., Kremer, E. F., and Gaylor, M. (1980): Behavioral treatment of chronic pain: the spouse as a discriminative cue for pain behavior. *Pain* 9:243–252.
7. Blumer, D., and Heilbronn, M. (1982): Chronic pain as a variant of depressive disease: the pain-prone disorder. *J. Nerv. Ment. Dis.,* 170:381–406.
8. Cairns, D., and Pasino, J. A. (1977): Comparison of verbal reinforcement and feedback in the operant treatment of disability due to chronic low back pain. *Behav. Ther.,* 8:621–630.
9. Cameron, R. (1982): Behavior and cognitive therapies. In: *Chronic Pain: Psychosocial Factors in Rehabilitation,* edited by R. Roy and E. Tunks, pp. 79–103. Williams & Wilkins, Baltimore.
10. Catchlove, R., and Cohen, K. (1983): Directive approach with Workmen's Compensation patients. In: *Advances in Pain Research and Therapy, Vol. 5.,* edited by J. J. Bonica, U. Lindblom, and A. Iggo, pp. 913–918. Raven Press, New York.
11. Crook, J., Rideout, E., and Browne, G. (1984): The prevalence of pain complaints in a general population. *Pain,* 18:299–314.
12. Crook, J., and Tunks, E. (1985): Defining the "chronic pain syndrome": an epidemiological method. In: *Advances in Pain Research and Therapy, Vol. 9,* edited by H. L. Fields, R. Dubner, and F. Cervero, pp. 871–877. Raven Press, New York.
13. Doleys, D. M., Crocker, M., and Patton, D. (1982): Response of patients with chronic pain to exercise quotas. *Phys. Ther.* 62:1111–1114.
14. Draspa, L. J. (1959): Psychological factors in muscular pain. *Br. J. Med. Psychol.* 32:106–116.
15. Engel, G. L. (1959): Psychogenic pain and the pain-prone patient. *Am. J. Med.,* 26:899–918.
16. Flor, H., Haag, G., Turk, D. C., and Koehler, H. (1983): Efficacy of EMG biofeedback, pseudotherapy, and conventional medical treatment for chronic rheumatic back pain. *Pain,* 17:21–31.
17. Flor, H., and Turk, D. C. (1984): Etiological theories and treatments for chronic back pain. I, Somatic models and interventions. *Pain,* 19:105–121.
18. Fordyce, W. E. (1983): Behavior is behavior is . . . *Contemp. Psychol.,* 28:730.
19. Fordyce, W. E. (1983): Behaviorism strikes back. *Contemp. Psychol.,* 28:888.
20. Fordyce, W. E., Fowler, R., Lehmann, J., and De Lateur, B. (1968): Some implications of learning in problems of chronic pain. *J. Chron. Dis.,* 21:179–190.
21. Fordyce, W. E., Fowler, R. S., Lehmann, J. F., De Lateur, B. J., Sand, P. L., and Trieschmann, R. B. (1973): Operant conditioning in the treatment of chronic pain. *Arch. Phys. Med. Rehab.,* 54:399–408.
22. Fordyce, W. E., McMahon, R., Rainwater, G., Jackins, S., Questad, K, Murphy, T, and De Lateur, B. (1981): Pain complaint-exercise performance relationship in chronic pain. *Pain,* 10:311–321.
23. Gottlieb, H. J., Koller, R., and Alperson, B. L. (1982): Low back pain comprehensive rehabilitation program: a followup study. *Arch. Phys. Med. Rehab.,* 63:458–461.
24. Gray, C. L., Lyle, R. C., McGuire, R. J., and Peck, D. F. (1980): Electrode placement, EMG feedback, and relaxation for tension headaches. *Behav. Res. Ther.,* 18:19–23.
25. Holroyd, K. A., Andrasik, F., and Noble, J. (1980): A comparison of EMG biofeedback and a credible pseudotherapy in treating tension headache. *J. Behav. Med.,* 3:29–39.

26. Jessup, B. A., Neufeld, R. W. J., and Merskey, H. (1979): Biofeedback therapy for headache and other pains; an evaluative review. *Pain,* 7:225–270.
27. Kellner, R. (1975): Psychotherapy in psychosomatic disorders. *Arch. Gen. Psychiatry,* 32:1021–1028.
28. Kolb, D. A., and Boyatzis, R. E. (1970): Goal setting and selfdirected behavior change. *Hum. Rel.,* 23:439–457.
29. Linton, S. J. (1986): Behavioral remediation of chronic pain: a status report. *Pain,* 24:125–141.
30. Linton, S. J., and Melin, L. (1982): The accuracy of remembering chronic pain. *Pain,* 13:281–285.
31. Luborsky, L, Singer, B., and Luborsky, L. (1975): Comparative studies of psychotherapies. Is it true that "Everyone has won and all must have prizes"? *Arch. Gen. Psychiatr.,* 32:995–1008.
32. Meichenbaum, D. (1976): Cognitive factors in biofeedback therapy. *Biofeedback Self Regul.* 1:201–216.
33. Merskey, H. (1982): Pain and behavior therapy. *Contemp. Psychol.,* 27:1006.
34. Merskey, H. (1983): Multimodal does not just mean behavioral. *Contemp. Psychol.,* 28:730–731.
35. Merskey, H. (1983): Psychiatric doubts not assuaged? *Contemp. Psychol.,* 28:888.
36. Nachemson, A. (1969): Physiotherapy for low back pain patients. *Scand. J. Rehab. Med.,* 1:85–90.
37. Pilowsky, I., Hallett, E. C., Bassett, D. L., Thomas, P. G., and Penhall, R. K. (1982): A controlled study of amitriptyline in the treatment of chronic pain. *Pain,* 14:169–179.
38. Rachlin, H., et al. (1985): Pain and behavior. *Behav. Brain Sci.,* 8:43–83.
39. Sarno, J. E. (1976): Chronic back pain and psychic conflict. *Scand. J. Rehab. Med.,* 8:143–153.
40. Scott, D. S., and Gregg, J. M. (1980): Myofascial pain of the temporomandibular joint: a review of the behavioral-relaxation therapies. *Pain,* 9:231–241.
41. Steger, J. C. (1981): Pain: interface between the physiological and psychological. *Contemp. Psychol.,* 26:943–944.
42. Sternbach, R. A. (1983): Fundamentals of psychological methods in chronic pain. In: *Advances in Pain Research and Therapy. Vol. 5,* edited by J. J. Bonica, U. Lindblom, and A. Iggo, pp. 777–780. Raven Press, New York.
43. Sternbach, R. A. (1984): Recent advances in psychologic pain therapy. In: *Advances in Pain Research and Therapy, Vol. 7,* edited by C. Benedetti, C. R. Chapman, and G. Moricca, pp. 251–255. Raven Press, New York.
44. Tan, S-Y. (1982): Cognitive and cognitive-behavioral methods for pain control: a selective review. *Pain,* 12:201–228.
45. Thorsteinsson, G., Stonnington, H. H., Stillwell, G. K., and Elveback, L. R. (1978): The placebo effect of transcutaneous electrical stimulation. *Pain,* 5:31–41.
46. Turk, D. C., and Flor, H. (1984): Etiological theories and treatments for chronic back pain. II. Psychological models and interventions. *Pain,* 19:209–233.
47. Turk, D. C., Meichenbaum, D., and Genest, M. (1983): *Pain and Behavioral Medicine: a Cognitive-Behavioral Perspective.* Guilford, New York.
48. Turner, J. A., and Chapman, C. R. (1982): Psychological interventions for chronic pain: a critical review. II. Relaxation training and biofeedback. *Pain,* 12:1–21.
49. Turner, J. A., and Chapman, C. R. (1982): Psychological interventions for chronic pain: a critical review. I. Operant conditioning, hypnosis, and cognitive-behavioral therapy. *Pain,* 12:23–46.
50. Turner, J. A., and Romano, J. M. (1984): Evaluating psychologic interventions for chronic pain: Issues and recent developments. In: *Advances in Pain Research and Therapy, Vol. 7,* edited by C. Benedetti, C. R. Chapman, and G. Moricca, pp. 257–296. Raven Press, New York.
51. Zitman, F. G. (1983): Biofeedback and chronic pain. In: *Advances in Pain Research and Therapy, Vol. 5,* edited by J. J. Bonica, U. Lindblom, and A. Iggo, pp. 795–808. Raven Press, New York.

Advances in Pain Research and Therapy,
Vol. 10. Edited by M. Tiengo et al.
Raven Press, Ltd., New York © 1987.

Analogies Existing Between the Primary Trigeminal Afferent Fibers Running Within the Oculomotor Nerve and the Ventral Root Primary Afferent Fibers

*R. Bortolami ,*M.L. Lucchi ,*E. Callegari ,**L. Calzà,
+V.E. Pettorossi, and +E. Manni

*Institute of Veterinary Anatomy, University of Bologna, 40100 Bologna, Italy;
**Department of Pathophysiology and Pain Therapy, University of Milan, 20100
Milan, Italy; and +Institute of Human Physiology, Catholic University Medical
School, 00168 Rome, Italy.

A great number of studies have underlined the problem of entry of primary afferents into the spinal cord. In particular, there has been a great deal of interest in the nociceptive afferents and the mechanism that such afferents utilize in the transmission of nociceptive impulses to higher centers (for review see ref. 4). In all these studies, however, the hypothesis that primary afferents could modulate other primary afferents directly, i.e., forming axoaxonic synapses, has never been taken into account.

We have been able to demonstrate that trigeminal primary afferents entering the brainstem through the oculomotor nerve could synapse, at the level of substantia gelatinosa (SG) layer of the nucleus caudalis trigemini (NCT), on other trigeminal primary afferents entering the pons as root fibers of the V nerve (1).

In fact after section of either the ophthalmic branch just near its origin or the oculomotor nerve between its emergence from the interpeduncular fossa and its passage through the dura mater, degenerating fibers could be traced caudally up to the level of NCT. In the SG glomeruli of this nucleus the degenerating axonal terminals were presynaptic to the central axonal endings which, as it is known (6,7), represent the classical V nerve endings.

Since axoaxonic synapses are considered to be the morphological basis of presynaptic inhibition (5,9,18), primary afferents such as the trigeminal fibers running within the oculomotor nerve could modulate directly other trigeminal primary afferents.

Since in the cat it has been evidenced that thin primary afferent fibers can reach the SG of the spinal cord entering from the ventral roots (13), we have also investigated whether these fibers could have the same synaptic

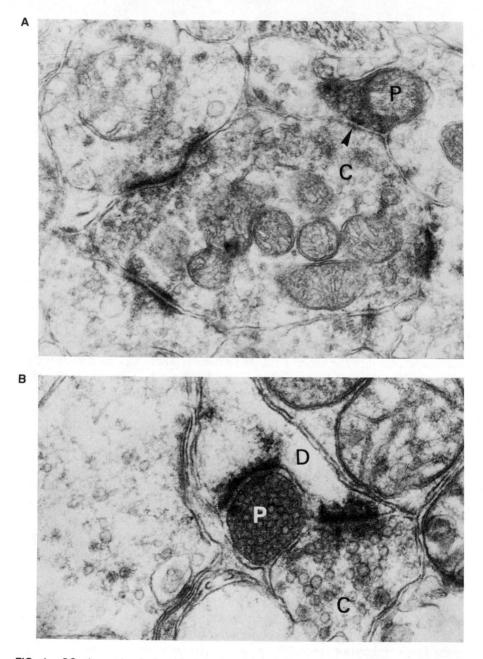

FIG. 1. SG glomerulus in L_5 spinal cord segment ipsilaterally to the section of the corresponding ventral root. **A:** Peripheral degenerating terminal (P) presynaptic (*arrow*) to the central axonal ending (C) (×36,100). **B:** Peripheral degenerating terminal (P) synapsing on a dendritic spine (D) which in turn synapses with the central axonal ending (C). (×48,450).)

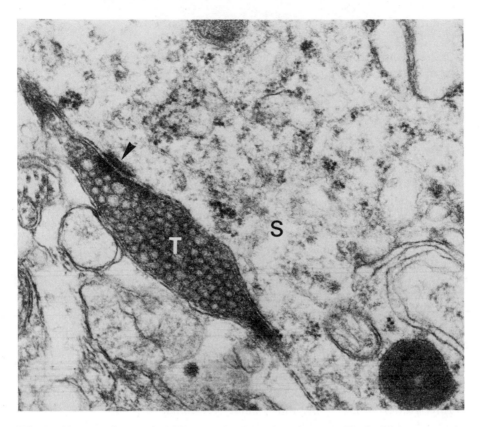

FIG. 2. Degenerating terminal (T) synapsing (*arrow*) on the soma (S) of a SG interneuron in L_5 spinal cord segment ipsilaterally to the section of the corresponding ventral root. (×41,800.)

organization of the trigeminal primary fibers that reach the SG layer of the NCT through the oculomotor nerve.

MATERIALS AND METHODS

In three deeply anesthetized (50 mg/kg i.m. of ketamine plus 0.4 mg/kg i.m. of diazepam) adult cats a laminectomy was done to expose and cut the L_5 ventral root. The animals were allowed to survive for 48 hr after the operation and then, under deep anesthesia, an intracardiac perfusion with buffered aldehydes was performed, as previously described (14). The L_5–L_4 segments of the spinal cord were removed and cut in transverse slices, 100 μm in thickness, with the Vibratome; from each tenth slice the dorsal horn ipsilateral to the rhizotomy was trimmed and processed for electron microscopic observation of the SG Rolandi.

OBSERVATIONS AND DISCUSSION

After ventral rhizotomy, degenerating axonal endings were present within the ipsilateral lamina II of L_5–L_4 spinal segments. The majority of these degenerating endings have been identified within the SG glomeruli. They never represented a central axonal ending which is known to represent the terminal of the dorsal root axon (2,3,8,10–12,15–17), but they were peripheral terminals presynaptic often to the central axonal endings or sometimes to dendritic spines or dendritic shafts, which were in turn synapsing with the central axonal ending (Fig. 1 A,B). Some degenerating endings were also observed synapsing on the soma of SG interneurons (Fig. 2).

From our observations, the ventral root primary afferent fibers can be considered from a synaptologic point of view the equivalent of the trigeminal primary afferents running within the oculomotor nerve. In the SG glomeruli of both the spinal cord and NCT, primary afferents synapse on each other directly.

Since the lamina II of the spinal cord and the SG layer of NCT contain the terminals of thermal and nociceptive afferents, we can assume that quite probably the primary afferents synapsing each other convey impulses of the same type.

On the basis of our data and of the functional role related to the axoaxonic junctions, the presynaptic primary afferents reaching the SG central axonal endings through the ventral roots or through the oculomotor nerve represent an anatomically well defined inhibitory or modulatory pathway of primary afferent fibers on other primary afferents.

ACKNOWLEDGMENTS

This research was supported by grants from CNR and Ministero Pubblica Istruzione.

REFERENCES

1. Bortolami, R., Veggetti, A., Callegari, E., Lucchi, M. L., and Palmieri, G. (1977): Afferent fibers and sensory ganglion cells within the oculomotor nerve in some mammals and man. *Arch. Ital. Biol,* 115:355–385.
2. Coimbra, A., Sodré-Borges, B. P., and Magalhães, M. M. (1974): The substantia gelatinosa Rolandi of the rat. Fine structure, cytochemistry (acid phosphatase) and changes after dorsal root section. *J. Neurocytol.,* 3:199–217.
3. Coimbra, A., Ribeiro-da-Silva, A., and Pignatelli, D. (1984): Effects of dorsal rhizotomy on the several types of primary afferent terminals in lamina I–III of the rat spinal cord. An electron microscope study. *Anat. Embryol.,* 170:279–287.
4. Dubner, R., and Bennett, G. J. (1983): Spinal and trigeminal mechanisms of nociception. *Ann. Rev. Neurosci.,* 6:381–418.
5. Eccles, J. C., Kostyuk, P. G., and Schmidt, R. F. (1962): Presynaptic inhibition of the central actions of flexor reflex afferents. *J. Physiol. (Lond.),* 161:258–281.

6. Gobel, S. (1974): Synaptic organization of the substantia gelatinosa glomeruli in the spinal trigeminal nucleus of adult cat. *J. Neurocytol.*, 3:219–243.
7. Gobel, S., and Binck, J. M. (1977): Degenerative changes in primary trigeminal axons and in neurons in nucleus caudalis following tooth pulp extirpations in the cat. *Brain Res.*, 132:347–354.
8. Gobel, S., and Falls, W. M. (1979): Anatomical observations of horseradish peroxidase-filled terminal primary axonal arborizations in layer II of the substantia gelatinosa of Rolando. *Brain Res.*, 175:335–340.
9. Gray, E.G. (1962): A morphological basis for pre-synaptic inhibition? *Nature*, 193:82–83.
10. Knyihar, E., and Csillik, B. (1976) Effect of peripheral axotomy on the fine structure and histochemistry of the Rolando substance: degenerative atrophy of central processes of pseudounipolar cells. *Exp. Brain Res.*, 26:73–87.
11. Knyihar-Csillik, E., Csillik, B., and Rakic, P. (1982): Ultrastructure of normal and degenerating glomerular terminals of dorsal root axons in the substantia gelatinosa of the rhesus monkey. *J. Comp. Neurol.*, 210:357–375.
12. Knyihar-Csillik, E., Csillik, B., and Rakic, P. (1982): Periterminal synaptology of dorsal root glomerular terminals in the substantia gelatinosa of the spinal cord in the rhesus monkey. *J. Comp. Neurol.*, 210:376–399.
13. Light, A.R., and Metz, C.B. (1978): The morphology of the spinal cord efferent and afferent neurons contributing to the ventral roots of the cat. *J. Comp. Neurol.*, 179:501–516.
14. Lucchi, M. L., Bortolami, R., and Callegari, E. (1972): Ultrastructural features of mesencephalic trigeminal nucleus in cat, rabbit and pig. *J. Submicrosc. Cytol.*, 4:7–18.
15. Murray, M., Battisti, W., and Goldberger, M. E. (1983): Synaptic replacement in deafferented dorsal horn (lamina II) of cat. *Neurosci. Abstr.*, 9:987.
16. Ribeiro-da-Silva, A., and Coimbra, A. (1984): Capsaicin causes selective damage to type I synaptic glomeruli in rat substantia gelatinosa. *Brain Res.*, 290:380–383.
17. Ribeiro-da-Silva, A., Pignatelli, D., and Coimbra, A. (1985): Synaptic architecture of glomeruli in superficial dorsal horn of rat spinal cord, as shown in serial reconstructions. *J. Neurocytol.*, 14:203–220.
18. Walberg, F. (1965): Axoaxonic contacts in the cuneate nucleus, probable basis for presynaptic depolarization. *Exp. Neurol.*, 13:218–231.

Advances in Pain Research and Therapy,
Vol. 10. Edited by M. Tiengo et al.
Raven Press, Ltd., New York © 1987.

Monoamines and Peptides Involved in the Central Control of Pain and Locomotion: Their Alteration in Different Physiopathological Conditions

L. Calzà, L. Giardino, M. Zanni, M. Rigoli, and M. Tiengo

Department of Pathophysiology and Pain Therapy, University of Milan, 20125 Milan, Italy

During the last 10 years there has been a dramatic development of our knowledge of the neurochemical organization of the central nervous system (CNS). One of the important concepts resulting from this study has been that of "peptidergic transmission." Its role in the central control of different functions has been investigated with particular regard to classical transmitter/neuropeptide interactions. This interaction could be carried out both in the case of coexistence of classical transmitters and peptides in the same neuron (4,7) and at local circuit level, through a synaptic contact or in the parasynaptic mode. This means the diffusion of the neuroactive substances in the extracellular fluid of the local circuit microenvironment (30).

These new concepts are based on the anatomical and functional re-examination of various regions of CNS, such as the basal ganglia and spinal cord. For example, it has been shown in the striatum that its heterogeneous neurochemical organization matches with a functional subdivision (13). Further, the dorsal horn of the spinal cord is characterized by an extremely complex neurochemical and anatomical substrate in which the parasynaptic mode of interactions among neurotransmitters is a salient phenomenon (7).

The control of functions, such as pain and locomotion, is due to the interactions among different neuroactive substances present in the neural networks. In this study, the action of same transmitters can be pre-eminent, but not exclusive. The understanding of the central control of a function and its alteration in physiopathological conditions is obviously based on the knowledge of these interactions.

BASAL GANGLIA

Three subcortical nuclei—the caudate nucleus, the putamen, and the pallidum—are collectively called the basal ganglia. Physiological evidence indi-

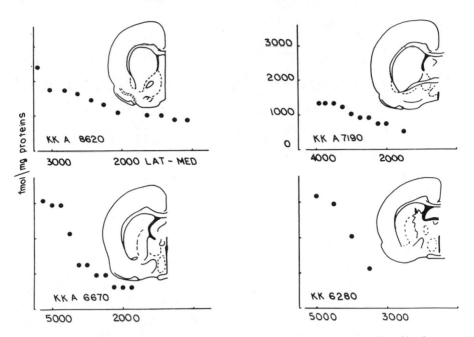

FIG. 1. Rostrocaudal and mediolateral distribution of D2 receptors labeled by 3H-spiperone. The results are obtained by means of quantitative receptor autoradiography. Briefly, the sections are incubated with 3H-spiperone (3 nM in Tris buffer, 50 mM; pH 7.4), 60 min at room temperature, washing buffer: Tris, 50 mM; NaCl, 120 mM; NaCl, 120 mM; KCl, 5 mM; MgCl^2, 1 mM; CaCl$_2$, 2 mM. The unspecific binding has been determined by incubation of the adjacent section with 3H-spiperone (3 nM) + butaclamol (1 μM). The sections are exposed to 3H-Ultrofilm (LKB). Quantitation has been obtained by means of microdensitometrical procedures, using the image analyzer Tesak VDC 501/Computer Digital PDP 11.

cates that the basal ganglia play an important role in the initiation and control of movement. Their chemoarchitecture is extremely rich compared with many other parts of the brain; Graybiel recently listed 110 neuroactive compounds and related substances in the striatum (13,14). Dopamine (DA) was the first neurotransmitter found in the striatum and many data indicate its involvement in the extrapyramidal control of movement. Since 1958, when Carlsson demonstrated that DA was present in the brain, many data have been published on the organization of the DA-ergic innervation of the striatum (3), and a particular effort has been devoted to the study of its heterogeneity. The "dopamine islands" represent the early developing DA system, whereas the "diffuse" DA innervation develops later (22). The islandic system has a lower rate of DA turnover, and it is probably related to other neurochemically defined compartments in the striatum (13). The striatal DA content in adult rats shows a rostrocaudal gradient, whereas no differences are present in the coronal plane (11). Other transmitters are also distributed in such a gradient way. The highest choline acetyltransferase

(ChAT) activity has been detected in the rostral striatum, and it is higher laterally than medially (26); glutamate decarboxylase activity (GAD) and substance P (SP) levels are higher in the caudal rat striatum (29). At present, a similar distribution is under study for several peptides (33). Receptor autoradiography is a very important tool in understanding the neurochemical organization of the CNS. Using this technique, several authors and this laboratory (Fig. 1) demonstrated an increasing mediolateral gradient in the D2-receptor distribution, labeled with 3H-spiperone (cold: (+) butaclamol). This result confirmed previous homogenate binding studies (18,19,31). We also observed a rostrocaudal gradient in D2-receptor distribution, with the highest level in the caudal portion. The autoradiographic study of D1-receptor distribution, performed with 3H-flupentixol, indicates their preferential localization in the periventricular region which is the portion of striatum where the DA islands are still present even during the adulthood (Fig. 2) (10,28). The medial striatum receives afferences from the ventral tegmental area, prefrontal cortex, and amygdala. Here many enkephalinergic (ENK)-positive neurons are located (Fig. 2). The distribution of opioid-like structures in striatum, especially ENK-positive neurons and opioid receptors, is not homogeneous (Fig. 2); many ENK-positive neurons are located in the medial caudatus and clustered in the ventral striatum (nucleus accumbens and olfactory tubercle).

The opioid receptors have two types of distribution (Fig. 3): diffuse and clustered. The first is due to δ-receptors, whereas the clusters are due to μ- and ε-receptors. As can be seen in Fig. 3, the clustered opioid receptors

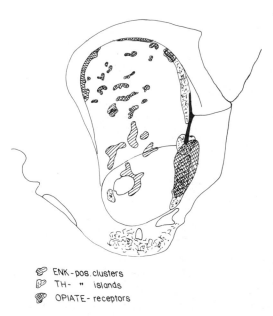

ENK - pos. clusters
TH - " islands
OPIATE - receptors

FIG. 2. Schematic drawing of the distribution of ENK, tyrosine-hydroxylase, and opiate receptors in a coronal section of the rat striatum.

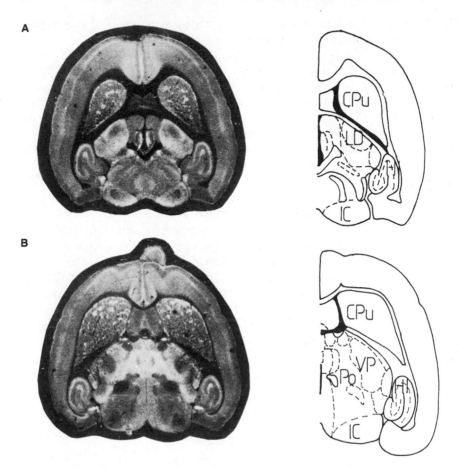

FIG. 3. Distribution of opiate receptors in two horizontal planes of the rat brain. Ligand: 3H-naloxone. Briefly, the sections are incubated with 3H-naloxone (3 nM) in Tris-HCl buffer 50 mM, pH 7.4, 60 min at 0°C, washing buffer Tris HCl 50 mM, pH 7.4. The unspecific binding has been determined by incubation of adjacent sections with 3H-naloxone + cold naloxone (1 mM). **A:** PX=5.9 mm. **B:**PX=5.1 mm. Abbreviations: CPu, caudatoputamen; LD, dorsolateral nucleus of the thalamus; IC, inferior colliculus; HI, hippocampus; VP, ventroposterior nucleus of the thalamus; Po, posterior nucleus of the thalamus.

system shows a preferential rostral distribution particularly in the ventral portion of caudatus. A high-density receptor strip is well defined in its rostrolateral portion. Particular attention has been devoted to DA-ENK interactions in the central control of locomotion and pain. Low opioid doses activate the locomotor system and high doses produce catatonic or cataleptic effects (23). These actions are similar to those obtained by the activation or inhibition of the basal ganglia dopaminergic system. Morphine and endogenous opioids increase DA turnover, whereas enkephalin stimulates the release of DA (21,32). Moreover, striatal DA fibers contain approximately one-third of all the opioid receptors present in the basal ganglia (5,24). The morphine injection in striatum, such as its electrical stimulation, produces a potent analgesia, whereas lesions of the dopaminergic nigrostriatal pathway reduce morphine antinociception (21). The ultrastructural analysis of DA-ENK interaction does not demonstrate axoaxonic synapses involving ENK-ergic elements. Therefore, every interaction between ENK- and DA-ergic neurons is likely to be a nonsynaptic or parasynaptic interaction (6).

DORSAL HORN OF THE SPINAL CORD

The neural circuits first activated by noxious or painful stimulation of peripheral nerves are located in the dorsal horn of the spinal cord and in the nucleus of spinal tract of the trigeminal nerve, particularly in the most

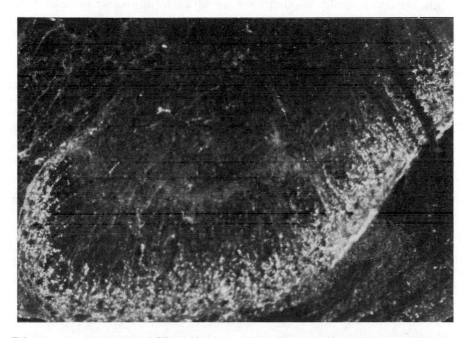

FIG. 4. Microphotograph of SP-positive innervation of the dorsal horn of the rat spinal cord. Indirect immunofluorescence procedures. Briefly, the animals are perfused with paraformaldehyde 4% in PBS, the spinal cord is postfixed by immersion in the same fixative and washed in sucrose 5% in PBS. The sections (14 μm, cryostat Kryostat 1720 Leitz) are incubated with the primary antiserum (Immunonuclear Corporation, 1:500), washed in PBS, incubated with the FITC-conjugate antiserum (Dako, 1:10), washed, cover-slipped, and photographed using the Zeiss photomicroscope (XBO 100, BP 485, FT 510, LP 520 filters, Tri-X pan Kodak film).

superficial layers which include the substantia gelatinosa. The region consists of three major components: (a) the central terminals of primary afferent neurons innervating cutaneous and deep tissues, (b) intrinsic neurons including local interneurons and long projection or output neurons, and (c) the terminal axons of extrinsic neurons originating mainly from descending brainstem pathways.

These structures provide the anatomical basis of the spinal control of pain threshold, through the interactions of associated neurotransmitters and neuropeptides. Particular attention has been devoted to the study of the interaction of SP, ENK, and serotonin (5-HT). SP (Fig. 4) is associated with the primary afferences (8,16); its iontophoretic application in the dorsal horn causes the discharge of nociceptive neurons in lamina V (25). ENK is associated with the pain inhibition at spinal cord level (2,12,15) and probably acts at local circuit level through the intrinsic interneurons of the dorsal horn. The ENK-immunoreactivity in the superficial layers is not affected by sensory denervation, while many immunoreactive cell bodies are revealed after colchicine treatment. 5-HT has a potent inhibitory action when iontophoretically applied near spinal dorsal horn interneurons (15). Its action has been associated with the inhibitory effect on spinal pain transmission neurons produced by the raphe magnus stimulation (9). 5-HT is also involved in morphine analgesia. A great effort has been devoted to the understanding of the ultrastructural basis of SP-ENK-5-HT interaction, but the technical problems associated with double-labeling ultrastructural procedures has not allowed the final picture of this interaction pattern to be defined. The nonsynaptic interaction between SP and ENK seems to be a well-established point. In fact, the explanation of the inhibitory effect of ENK on SP release in the dorsal inhibition is complicated by the presence of many other substances in the primary afferents, in the local interneurons, and in the descending fibers. The coexistence of several peptides, such as SP, ENK, and thyrotropin-releasing hormone (TRH) (17), in the 5-HT spinal projecting neurons further complicates the neurochemical organization of the region. According to the most recent concepts regarding coexistence, the intraneuronal balance of these substances is not stable (4) and not defined during all times of life and in all functional situations of the network.

AGING

The aging process is characterized by impairment of different functions. Coordinate locomotion is frequently lacking, and pain perception, another integrative function, is unbalanced. Besides the morphological modification of the old brain (neuronal loss, increased glia and white matter), several neurochemical changes have been described in the old CNS. None of these

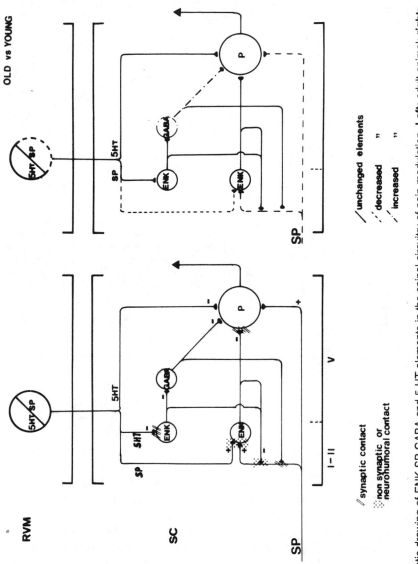

FIG. 5. Schematic drawing of ENK-SP-GABA and 5-HT elements in the spinal circuitry of pain modulation. **Left:** adult animal; **right:** old animal. Abbreviations: I-II-V, I,II,V laminae of the spinal cord; sc, spinal cord; nvm, rostroventral medulla; P, projecting neurons.

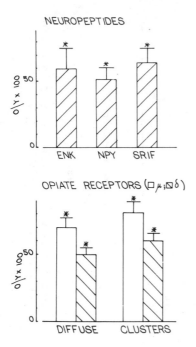

FIG. 6. Effect of aging some peptidergic elements of the striatum in rats: 24 vs. 3 months. The results for neuropeptides are obtained by counting the immunoreactive neurons at the same rostrocaudal level in the striatum of three animals for age. The μ-receptors are visualized using 3H-naloxone; δ-receptors are visualized using 3H-D-ala-D-leu-enkephalin. The quantitation has been performed by means of computerized densitometry (image analyzer Tesak VDC 501/Computer Digital PDP 11). Abbreviations: NPY, neuropeptide Y; SRIF, somatostatin.

phenomena seems to be a "marker" of aging. The ascending dopaminergic neurons and their postsynaptic receptors progressively degenerate with age (1,27), and the number of cholecystokinin (CCK)-positive neurons decrease in the nigrostriatal pathway (1).

Brain opiate receptors and enkephalin-like immunoreactivity disappear during aging (27), the striatal levels of ChAT decrease, whereas benzodiazepine receptors increase with old age (20). We observe in the striatum (Fig. 6) an evident and significant decrease of peptidergic neurons, and also an important decrease of opiate receptors, mainly the δ-type.

In the spinal cord (L. Calzá et al., *in preparation*) we observe a decrease of SP-positive terminals (Fig. 5) [the semiquantitative evaluation has been performed by means of the image analyzer Tesak VDC 501/Computer Digital PDP 11 (see Fig. 7 legend for further information)], while ENK, 5-HT-positive, and GABA-ergic elements are unchanged. These results seem to indicate an imbalance between the transmission of the nociceptive stimulus and its modulation. The SP, involved in the primary afferences, clearly decreases, while the opiatergic system and the serotoninergic descending system, involved in pain inhibition, seem to be less affected. However, discussing the neurochemical modification associated with old age, it is crucial to remember the high individuality of the aging process and the influence of individual experiences (from tooth loss and orofacial trauma, to the memory

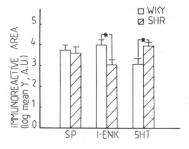

FIG. 7. Semiquantitative evaluation of ENK, SP, and 5-HT immunoreactivity in the dorsal horn of the spinal cord of hypertensive [spontaneously hypertensive (SHR)] rats vs. normotensive [Wistar Kyoto (WKY)] rats. The quantitation is performed as follows: the SP, ENK, and 5-HT terminals are stained by indirect immunofluorescence (antisera from Immunonuclear Corporation) using a dilution curve of the primary antibodies on ten adjacent sections. The sections are photographed using a standard exposure time. The negatives are analyzed using the image analyzer Tesak VDC 501 equipped with the host computer Digital PDP 11. After the standardization of the images according to a dark and a light standard, the area covered by the gray tones included between two thresholds (dark and light) is automatically evaluated. The best interpolating curve of the 10 values of the immunoreactive area is calculated, and the ED_{50} values are used for the statistical analysis.

of a previous experience of pain) on the neuroanatomical and neurochemical organization of the neuronal networks.

HYPERTENSION

Recent studies demonstrated that pain perception and blood pressure regulation may be physiologically related (34,35). Neuroanatomical, electrophysiological, microinjection, and lesion studies provide evidence for a possible relationship between pain regulation and blood pressure control systems (34,35). Many transmitters and peptides associated with pain modulation, as SP, ENK, and 5-HT, are present in the medullary regions of blood pressure control. The semiquantitative analysis of ENK, SP, and 5-HT immunoreactivity in the dorsal horn of the spinal cord of WKY and SHR rats (Fig. 7) indicates: (a) an unchanged amount (quantity) of SP, (b) an evident decrease of ENK (that confirms the results of other authors obtained with different approaches), and (c) an increase of 5-HT in SHR animals. In this case the serotoninergic signal seems to be prominent with respect to the ENK-ergic signal in the inhibition of pain transmission (Fig. 8).

COMMENT

A great ability of the CNS is the adjustment of the circulating information in a network with relation to environmental stimuli. The result is a constant homeostasis. In several pathological conditions, a functional deficit appears when this adjustment capability is depleted. At this moment, the neuro-

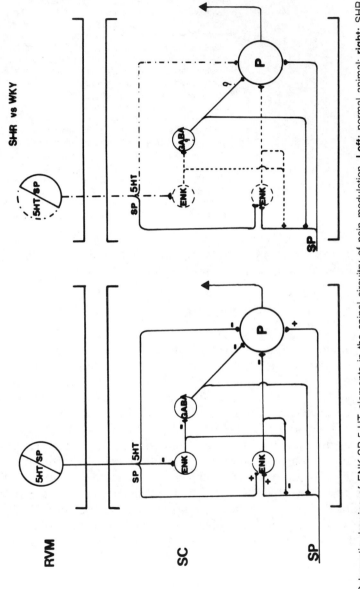
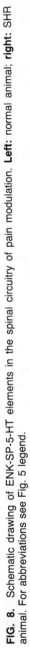

FIG. 8. Schematic drawing of ENK-SP-5-HT elements in the spinal circuitry of pain modulation. **Left:** normal animal; **right:** SHR animal. For abbreviations see Fig. 5 legend.

chemical study of the CNS indicates both the primary deficit and the compensation attempt. This refers to the demand to follow the different stages of the life until old age, the development of hypertension, and so on. In this context our results are to be considered the first step of a wider experimental project.

REFERENCES

1. Agnati, L. F., Fuxe, K., Giardino, L., Calzá, L., Zoli, M., Battistini, N., Benfenati, F., Vanderhaeghen, J. J., Guidolin, D., Ruggeri, M., and Goldstein, M. (1985): Evidence for cholecystokinin-dopamine-receptor interactions in the central nervous system of the adult and old rat. In: *Neuronal Cholecystokinin,* edited by J. J. Vanderhaeghen and I. N. Crawley, pp. 315–333. Annals of the New York Academy of Science, New York.
2. Basbaum, A. I., and Fields, H. L. (1984): Endogenous pain control systems: brainstem spinal pathways and endorphin circuitry. *Ann. Rev. Neurosci.,* 7:309–338.
3. Bjorklund, A., and Lindvall, O. (1984): Dopamine-containing systems in the CNS. In: *Classical Transmitters in the CNS,* edited by A. Bjorklund and T. Hokfelt, pp. 55–111. Elsevier, Amsterdam.
4. Chan Palay, V., and Palay, S (editors) (1984): *Coexistence of Neuroactive Substances.* Raven Press, New York.
5. Chesselet, M. F., and Graybiel, A. M. (1983): Met-enkephalin-like and dinorphyn-like immunoreactivities of the basal ganglia of the cat. *Life Sci.,* 33:37–40.
6. Cuello, A. C. (1983): Central distribution of opioid peptides. *Br. Med. Bull.,* 39:11–16.
7. Cuello, A. C, (editor) (1983): *Cotransmission,* Mac Millan, New York.
8. Cuello, A. C., Del Fiacco, M., and Paxinos, G. (1978): The central and peripheral ends of the substance P-containing sensory neurons in the rat trigeminal system. *Brain Res.,* 152:499–510.
9. Dubner, R., and Bennett, G. J. (1983): Spinal and trigeminal mechanisms of nociception. *Annu. Rev. Neurosci.,* 6:381–418.
10. Dubois, A., Savasta, M., Curet, O., and Scatton, B. (1986): Autoradiographic distribution of the D1 agonist 3H-SKF38393, in the rat brain and spinal cord. Comparison with the distribution of D2 dopamine receptors. *Neuroscience,* 19:125–137.
11. Flint Beal, M., and Martin, J. B. (1985): Topographical dopamine and serotonin distribution and turnover in rat striatum. *Brain Res.,* 358:10–15.
12. Glazer, E. J., and Basbaum, A. I. (1983): Opioid neurons and pain modulation: an ultrastructural analysis of enkephalin in cat superficial dorsal horn. *Neuroscience,* 10:357–376.
13. Graybiel, A. M., Ragsdale, C. W., Yoneoka, E. S., and Elde, R. P. (1981): An immunohistochemical study of enkephalins and other neuropeptides in the striatum of the cat with evidence that the opiate peptides are arranged to form mosaic patterns in register with the striosomal compartments visible by acetylcholinesterase staining. *Neuroscience,* 6:377–397.
14. Graybiel, A. M. (1984): Correspondence between the dopamine islands and striosomes of the mammalian striatum. *Neuroscience,* 13:1157–1187.
15. Hentall, I. D., and Fields, H. L. (1983): Actions of opiates, substance P, and serotonin on the excitability of primary afferent terminals and observations on interneuronal activity in the neonatal rat's dorsal horn *in vitro. Neuroscience,* 9:521–528.
16. Hokfelt, T., Kellertm, J. O., Nilsson, G., and Pernow, B. (1975): Experimental immunohistochemical studies on the localization and distribution of substance P in cat primary sensory neurons. *Brain Res.,* 100:235–252.
17. Johansson, O., Hokfelt, T., Pernow, B., Jeffcoate, S. L., White, N., Steinbush, H. W. M., Verhofstad, A. A. J., Emson, P. C., and Spindel, E. (1981): Immunohistochemical support for three putative transmitters in one neuron: coexistence of 5-hydroxytryptamine, substance P, and thyrotropin releasing hormone-like immunoreactivity in medullary neurons projecting to the spinal cord. *Neuroscience,* 6:1857–1881.

18. Joyce, J. N., Loeschen, S. K., and Marshall, J. F. (1985): Dopamine D2 receptors in rat caudate-putamen: the lateral to medial gradient does not correspond to dopaminergic innervation. *Brain Res.*, 338:209–218.
19. Joyce, J. N., and Marshall, J. F. (1985): Striatal topography of D2 receptors correlates with indexes of cholinergic neuron localization. *Neurosci. Lett.*, 53:127–131.
20. Kendall, D. A., Strong, R., and Enna, S. J. (1982): Modifications in rat brain GABA receptor binding as a function of age. In: *The Aging Brain: Cellular and Molecular Mechanisms of Aging in the Nervous System*, edited by E. Giacobini et al. Raven Press, New York.
21. Lineberry, C. G., and Vierck, C. J. (1975): Attenuation of pain reactivity by caudate nucleus stimulation in monkeys. *Brain Res.*, 98:110–134.
22. Olson, L., Seiger, A., and Fuxe, K. (1972): Heterogeneity of striatal and limbic dopamine innervation: highly fluorescent islands in developing and adult rats. *Brain Res.*, 44:283–288.
23. Pert, A. (1983): In: *Characteristics and Functions of Opioids*, pp. 389–401. Elsevier/North-Holland, Amsterdam.
24. Pollard, H., Llorens-Cortes, C., and Schwartz, J. C. (1977): Enkephalin receptors on dopaminergic neurons in rat striatum. *Nature*, 268:745–747.
25. Randic, M., and Miletic, U. (1977): Effect of substance P in cat dorsal horn neurons activated by noxious stimuli. *Brain Res.*, 128:164–169.
26. Rea, M. A., and Simon, J. R. (1981): Regional distribution of cholinergic parameters within the rat striatum. *Brain Res.*, 219:317–326.
27. Roth, G. S. (1983): Brain dopaminergic and opiate receptors and responsiveness during aging. In: *Aging Brain and Ergot Alkaloids, Aging, Vol. 23*, edited by A. Agnoli et al., pp. 53–60. Raven Press, New York.
28. Savasta, M., Dubois, A., and Scatton, B. (1986): Autoradiographic localization of D1 dopamine receptors in the rat brain with 3HSCH23390. *Brain Res.*, 375:291–301.
29. Scally, M. C., Ulus, I. H., Wurtman, R. J., and Pettibone, D. J. (1978): Regional distribution of neurotransmitter-synthesizing enzymes and substances P within the rat corpus striatum. *Brain Res.*, 143:556–560.
30. Schmitt, F. O. (1984): Molecular regulators of brain function: a new view. *Neuroscience*, 13:991–1001.
31. Tassin, J. P., Cheramy, A., Blanc, G., Thierry, A. M., and Glowinski, J. (1976): Topographical distribution of dopaminergic receptors in the rat striatum. 1. Microestimation of 3H-dopamine and dopamine content in microdiscs. *Brain Res.*, 197:291–301.
32. Tulunary, F. C., Yano, I., and Takemori, A. E. (1976): The effect of biogenic amine modifiers on morphine analgesia and its antagonism by naloxone. *Eur. J. Pharmacol.*, 35:285–292.
33. Zaborszky, L., Alheid, G. F., Beinfeld, M. C., Eiden, L. E., Heimer, L., and Palkovits, M. (1985): Cholecystokinin innervation of the ventral striatum: a morphological and radioimmunological study. *Neuroscience*, 14:427–453.
34. Zamir, N., Simantov, R., and Segal, M. (1980): Pain sensitivity and opioid activity in genetically and experimentally hypertensive rats. *Brain Res.*, 184:299–310.
35. Zamir, N., and Shuber, E. (1980): Altered pain perception in hypertensive humans. *Brain Res.*, 201:471–474.

Advances in Pain Research and Therapy,
Vol. 10. Edited by M. Tiengo et al.
Raven Press, Ltd., New York © 1987.

Flexion Withdrawal Reflex: A Link Between Pain and Motility

*Roberto Casale and **Mario Tiengo

*Foundation "Clinica del Lavoro", Pavia, Rehabilitation Medical Center of
Montescano, Service of Neurophysiology, 27040 Montescano, Italy; and
**Department of Pathophysiology and Pain Therapy, University of Milan, 20122
Milan, Italy

Exteroceptive reflexes are commonly defined as an organized and stereo-typed motor reaction, often complex, and activated by cutaneous and subcutaneous stimuli. From exteroceptive reflexes come the so-called nociceptive or defensive ones, because they are provoked by stimuli that in animals produce pain (20). From a neurophysiological point of view the simplest level of interaction between nociceptive input and motor response and that which in laboratory tests can be most easily isolated from the network is the flexion withdrawal reflex of the lower limb.

FLEXION WITHDRAWAL REFLEX AND MOTOR ORGANIZATION STUDIES

The first to study exteroceptive reflexes, at the beginning of the century, were some of the most important authors of neurological science such as Babinski (1), Sherrington (29), Wernicke (31), and Lloyd (23). Their interest was to study the physiopathology of movement and the influences that exteroceptive inputs place on the motoneuronal spinal pool. Lloyd (23) observed how the muscular reflex discharge, due to the stimulation of the sensitive nerve in the cat, has two electromyographic components at different onset latencies, showing the involvement of two types of fibers at different rates of conduction. Fundamental works on physiopathological mechanisms of the flexion reflex are those of Hagbarth (13) and of Kugelberg et al. (21) which affirm that "there is little doubt that. . . . .the nervous reflexes elicited from the foot. . . .represent the adequate withdrawal movement" of the human lower limb to exteroceptive stimuli. Pinelli and Valle (27) were among the first to include the study of polysynaptic flexion reflexes in the evaluation of spasticity in man in both the lower and upper limbs. Pinelli observed a flexion reflex similar to that of Babinski. More recently, Dimitrijevic and Nathan (10,11) applied it to the study of human spinal spasticity, evaluating phenomena such as habituation and dishabituation.

FLEXION WITHDRAWAL REFLEX AND NOCICEPTION STUDIES

In the 1960s we gradually witnessed a change in the researcher's interests from the motor component of the reflex to its nociceptive aspect. Certainly, one of the scientific events that led to this gradual change of interests was the publication of the spinal gate control theory (25). As Lloyd (23) had experimented on cats, Hugon (18), in the light of this theory, experimented on man underlining the nociceptive aspect of the theory and extending to a "significant degree the Malzack-Wall approach to the human subject."

Stimulating the sural nerve in its retromalleolar course with a random pulse consisting of a train of 8 to 10 shocks at 300 cps we can register from the biceps femoris (caput brevis) muscle two reflex components at different times of onset produced by a stimulus of increasing intensity:

1. Early response of short latency (40–60 msec.) and low threshold provoked by tactile nonpainful stimulation, corresponding to a reflex functionally integrated in the postural control of the foot (28), and called Ra II since it involves group II afferents.
2. Delayed response of longer latency (80–150 msec.) and higher threshold provoked by a more intense stimulus corresponding to Sherrington's (29) nociceptive reflex. This response was called Ra III since it involves group III afferents. In the early experiment carried out by Hugon (17) the painful nature of stimulation able to provoke the Ra III reflex was confirmed in the verbal report of subjects who underwent the stimulation.

The relationship between flexion withdrawal reflex and the pain level was studied by Willer (33) who related the Ra III threshold (expressed in mA) and the pain provoked using a visual analogic scale.

The liminal pain in those experiences, was described by the subjects "as a sharp sensation, like a pin-prick localized at the point of stimulation" (18), while the intensity of the stimulus ready to provoke the reflex was approximately 10 to 13 mA (33). Further works have provided experimental evidence of the excitatory and/or inhibitory influences acting on spinal neuronal activity.

Stress, attention, anxiety, as well as both painful and nonpainful stimuli such as electrical and vibratory stimulation seem to modify the threshold of the reflex (2,4,5,16,32,34).

VIBRATION INFLUENCES BOTH PAIN AND MOTILITY

The study of vibration is of particular interest, inasmuch as it has followed the concerns of clinical neurophysiology, earlier being dedicated to motility and its disorders, and then, in recent years, to pain.

Vibration was used in clinical neurophysiology because it induces a discharge imitating the static fusimotor activation of the primary ending Ia

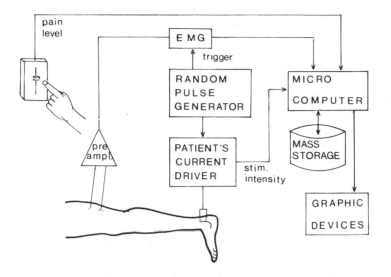

FIG. 1. Schematic representation of the experimental set: A random generator triggers both a current driver, connected with the subject, and an electromyograph for the registration of the reflex response. Pain level is measured by a lever connected with a linear potentiometer and handled by the subject. Stimulation intensity (mA), pain level (in arbitrary units) and EMG signals are acquired on line by a microcomputer providing data storage and analysis, as well as graphic display.

fiber units that normally occurs under isometric contraction (15). Vibration activates not only the latter, but also receptive units such as Pacinian corpuscles and rapidly adapting receptors functionally linked with large-diameter fibers (19). For some years it has been used with the aim of pain control because of this activation and the consequent possibility of modulating nociceptive input at the spinal level (18). Vibration can inhibit monosynaptic reflexes H and T (8,22), as well as influencing polysynaptic reflexes (19); but data on lower limb flexion reflex are not so homogeneous as for H and T reflexes.

Confirming an observation of Delwaide (9), Ertekin and Ackali (12) showed an increase in amplitude and duration of Ra III during vibration. They also observed a facilitatory effect lasting 20 min after vibration ceased. In our laboratory, using a computer-aided system, we are carrying out studies on the effect of vibration on Ra III, and recently we published some data in contrast to Ertekin's observation (5) (Fig. 1). In this research we examined a group of lumbosciatalgic patients without neurophysiological signs of peripheral nerve impairment (sural nerve latency, H reflex latency, and amplitude were normal and statistically not different from those of a control group). Harmless, cramping pain was referred at medium intensity in the leg. Vibration stimulus of 100 Hz was applied for approximately 20 to 25 min to the Achilles tendon after having reached the reflex threshold, and after its amplitude had been stabilized. We measured the pain level with a

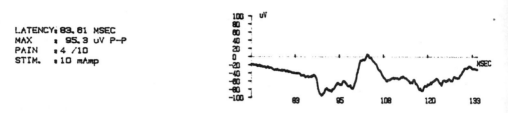

CENTRO MEDICO DI RIABILITAZIONE – MONTESCANO –
SERVIZIO DI NEUROFISIOLOGIA

F. CAMP. : 7935 HERTZ
NAME : O. E. ' 3-2B   DELAY : 70 MSEC.
NERVE : SURAL DX
STIMULATION : RANDOM TRAINS (8-9 SHOCKS) AT 300 C/SEC.
COMMENTS : VIBRATION PROJ. (NORM./BASAL)

LATENCY: 83.61 MSEC
MAX   : 95.3 uV P-P
PAIN   : 4 /10
STIM. : 10 mAmp

FIG. 2. Sample of graphic display. **Upper:** General data, such as stimulation parameter and technical data, are plotted. **Lower left:** Different wave parameters, such as latency and maximal amplitude; stimulation intensity (mA) and the relative subjective pain intensity (arbitrary units) are shown as well. **Lower right:** Ra III wave is plotted. Sampling frequency and acquisition delay are plotted in the upper general part.

modified representation of graphic self-pain estimate consisting of a lever attached to a linear potentiometer. Both pain level and stimulation intensity were registered and displayed on the computer's screen with the elicited reflex response, and then plotted (Fig. 2).

The application reduced the pain level by 60 to 70% with almost an immediate effect, and inhibited the Ra III up to its disappearance, increasing the reflex threshold (Fig. 3). Nevertheless, such barrage seemed to be unstable as we registered Ra-III-like randomly high amplitude potentials after this almost total inhibition (6).

The discrepancy between Ertekin's data and ours could be explained, as suggested by Wall and Cronly-Dillon (30), since vibration reduced the effects of low-intensity painful stimulation, whereas it increased that of high intensity. During Ertekin's experiments, many subjects reported an increase in pain provoked by electrical stimulation during vibration. This leads us to think that the electrical stimulus used by this author was of higher intensity than our "threshold" stimulus which was just sufficient to provoke a stable reflex. In the first case, vibration could not interfere with nociceptive input but, on the contrary, could be added to them, clinically increasing the pain and instrumentally increasing the amplitude and length of the reflex. In the second case, vibration could create a barrage, even if incomplete, and would stop provoking an incomplete barrage only at high frequencies (14), while

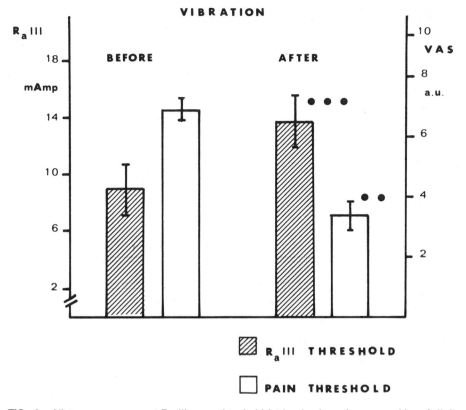

FIG. 3. Histograms represent Ra III wave threshold (*striped columns*) expressed in mA (*left scale*), and subjective pain intensity (*empty columns*) expressed in arbitrary units (*right scale*) before and after a 20-min 100-Hz vibration treatment in lumbosciatalgic patients. *Black dots* represent statistical significance.

for those approximate or inferior to 100 Hz such a blockage would result as ineffective or at least unstable.

This hypothesis could also be clinically supported by the positive results obtained by some authors (5,24,26) in certain pathologies, and by the poor effectiveness we have observed during 1985 in the treatment of certain types of pain in paraplegics and in patients with intense pain (R. Casale and A. Arrigo, *unpublished data*).

To add to this, Ottoson (24) himself had signaled the increase of pain level in the treatment of cephalic pain when the vibration was placed far from the painful area. In such conditions, factors such as the intensity of the conditioned stimulus and the intensity of spontaneous pain seem to be relevant (3). Sites, parameters, and time of application of vibration as well as electrical stimulation can be of further relevance.

Finally we must not forget that the vibratory stimulus at 100 Hz provokes changes in sympathetic tone (4). Experiments carried out in our laboratory forced us to maintain whichever exteroceptive stimulus that can produce, at least in the initial phase of application, a sympathomimetic "phasic" response. This sympathomimetic response in some clinically healthy subjects is of huge intensity altering measurements of nociceptive reflex as well as threshold.

ACKNOWLEDGMENTS

The author wishes to thank Prof. Paolo Pinelli for his helpful comments; Dr. M. Buonocore and Dr. A. Modica for their assistance; and Ms. J. McKay for her linguistic help.

REFERENCES

1. Babinski, J. (1898): Du phenomene des orteils et sa valeur semiologique. *Semaine Med.,* 18:321–322.
2. Bathien, N. (1971): Reflexes spinaux chez l'homme et niveaux d'attention. *Electroencephalogr. and Clin. Neurophysiol.,* 30:32–37.
3. Bini, G., Cruccu, G., Hagbarth, K. E., Shady, W., and Torebjork, E. (1984): Analgesic effect of vibration and cooling on pain induced by intraneuronal electrical stimulation. *Pain,* 18:239–248.
4. Boureau, F., Willer, J. C., and Dehen, H. (1977): L'action de l'acupuncture sur le doleur. Basis physiologiques. *Nouv. Presse Med.,* 6:1871–1874.
5. Casale, R., Buonocore, M., Bozzi, M., and Bodini, G. C. (1986): Variazioni pletismografiche indotte dalla applicazione di uno stimolo vibratorio a 100 Hz nel normale Boll. Soc. Ital. Bid. Sper. (*in press*).
6. Casale, R., Giordano, A., and Tiengo, M. (1985): Risposte riflesse nocicettive spinali. Variazione della risposta riflessa nocicettiva RaIII e del dolore lomosciatalgico indotte da TENS e vibrazione. *Minerva Anestesiol.,* 51:217–229.
7. Casale, R., and Tiengo, M. (1984): Neurophysiological effects of the administration of a vibratory antalgic stimuli in healthy and lumbosciatalgic patients. *Pain, (Suppl.),* 2:57.
8. Delwaide, P. J. (1969): Approche de la physiopathologie de la spasticite¹: Reflexe de Hoffmann et vibration appliquees sur le tendon d' Achille. *Rev. Neurol.,* 121:72–74.
9. Delwaide, P.J. (1973): Human monosynaptic reflexes and presynaptic inhibition. An interpretation of spastic hyperreflexia. In: *New Development in Electromyography and Clinical Neurophysiology, Vol. 3,* edited by J.E. Desmedt, pp. 509–527. Karger, Basel.
10. Dimitrijevic, M. R., and Nathan, P. W. (1970): Studies of spasticity in man. 4: Changes in flexion reflex with repetitive cutaneous stimulation in spinal man. *Brain,* 93:743–768.
11. Dimitrijevic, M. R., and Nathan, P. W. (1971): Studies of spasticity in man. 5: Dishabituation of the flexion reflex in spinal man. *Brain,* 94:77–90.
12. Ertekin, C., and Ackali, D. (1978): Effect of continuous vibration on nociceptive flexor reflexes. *J. Neurol. Neurosurg. Psychiatry,* 41:532–537.
13. Hagbarth, K. E. (1960): Spinal withdrawal reflex in the human lower limbs. *J. Neurol. Neurosurg. Psychiatry,* 23:222–227.
14. Hagbarth, K. E. (1973): Effects of muscle vibration in normal man and in patients with motor disease. In: *New Development in Electromyography and Clinical Neurophysiology, Vol. 3,* edited by J.E. Desmedt, pp. 428–443. Karger, Basel.
15. Hagbarth, K. E., and Eklund, G. (1966): Motor effects of vibratory stimuli in man. In: *Granit Nobel Symposium 1, Muscular Afferent and Motor Control,* edited by Alquist and Wikseel, pp. 171–196, Stockholm.

16. Handewerker, H. O., Iggo, A., and Zimmermann, M. (1975): Segmental and supraseg-mental actions on dorsal horn neurons responding to noxious and non-noxious skin stimuli. *Pain,* 1:147–165.
17. Hugon, M. (1967): Reflexes polysynaptiques cutaneé et commandes volontaires. Thèse Science, Phis., Paris.
18. Hugon, M. (1973): Exteroceptive reflexes to stimulation of the sural nerve in normal man. In: *New Developments in Electromyography and Clinical Neurophysiology, Vol. 3,* edited by J. E. Desmedt, pp. 713–729. Karger, Basel.
19. Knibestol, M., and Valibo, A. B. (1970): Single unit analysis of mechanoceptor activity from the human glabrous skin., *Acta Physiol. Scand.,* 80:178–195.
20. Kugelberg, E. (1962): Polysynaptic reflexes of clinical importance. *Electroencephalogr. Clin. Neurophysiol. (suppl.),* 27:103–111.
21. Kugelberg, E., Eklund, K., and Griby, L. (1960): The electromyographic study of the nociceptive reflexes of the lower limb. Mechanisms of the plantar responses. *Brain,* 23:349–410.
22. Lance, J. W., Nielson, P. D., and Tassinari, C. A. (1968): Suppression of the H-reflex by peripheral vibration. *Proc. Aust. Assoc. Neurol.,* 5:45–49.
23. Lloyd, D. P. C. (1943): Reflex action in relation to pattern and peripheral source of afferent stimulation. *J. Neurophysiol.,* 6:421.
24. Lundeberg, T. (1983): Long-term results of vibratory stimulation as a pain relieving mea-sure for chronic pain. *Pain,* 20:13–23.
25. Melzack, R., and Wall, P. D. (1965): Pain mechanism: A new theory. *Science,* 150:971–979.
26. Ottoson, D., Ekblom, A., and Hansson, P. (1981): Vibratory stimulation for the relief of pain of dental origin. *Pain,* 10:37–45.
27. Pinelli, P. and Valle, M. (1960): Studio fisiopatologico dei riflessi muscolari nelle paresi spastiche (sui tests per la misura della spasticitá). *Arch. Sci. Med. (Torino),* 109:106–120.
28. Shahani, B., and Young, R. P. (1971): Human flexor reflexes. *J. Neurol. Neurosurg. Psychiatr.,* 34:616–627.
29. Sherrington, C.S. (1910): Flexion reflex in the limb, crossed extension reflex and reflex stepping and standing. *J. Physiol. (Lond.),* 40:28–129.
30. Wall, P. D., and Cronly-Dillon, J. (1960): Pain, itch and vibration. *AMA Arch. Neurol.,* 2:365–375.
31. Wernicke, C. (1881): Lehrbuch der gehirnkrankheiten fur aerzte und studirende. *Kassel,* Vol. 1.
32. Willer, J. C. (1975): Influence de l'enticipation de la douleur sur les frequences cardiaques et respiratoires et sur le reflex nociceptif chez l'homme. *Physiol. Behav.,* 15:411–415.
33. Willer, J. C. (1977): Comparative study of perceived pain and nociceptive flexion reflex in man. *Pain,* 3:69–80.
34. Willer, J. C., Boureu, F., and Albe-Fessard, D. (1979): Supraspinal influences on nocicep-tive flexion reflex and pain sensation in man. *Brain Res.,* 179:61–69.

Advances in Pain Research and Therapy,
Vol. 10. Edited by M. Tiengo et al.
Raven Press, Ltd., New York © 1987.

Treatment of Pain in Spinal Cord Lesions

*M. Tiengo, *V. Moschini, and **G.C. Pastorino

*Cattedra di Fisiopatologia e Terapia del Dolore, Università degli Studi di Milano, 20122 Milan, Italy; and **Servizio di Neurofisiopatologia, Emanuela dalla Chiesa Setti Carraro, Istituti Clinici di Perfezionamento, 20122 Milan, Italy*

In order to obtain a more rational therapeutic approach to pain in patients with spinal cord lesions, we have studied the incidence, gravity, and the quantitative characteristics of the pain phenomenon in 170 patients.

Moreover, we have analyzed the effectiveness of the various therapeutic treatments for 22 patients who were directly observed. Through the recording of the evoked potentials to stimulate the common peroneal nerve, recording at scalp level in 20 of the patients, and by a close neurophysiopathological examination, we have studied the eventual relationships between the pain characteristics and the neurophysiological and clinical data.

From a first analysis of the data, we can denote a certain discrepancy between the pain characteristics and the clinical, neurological, and instrumental data of the patients.

The complex question of the treatment of pain in patients with spinal cord lesions and the high failure rate reported in this field by a number of workers (4,12,14,16,18,21) have, in recent years, led to a closer clinical and neurophysiopathological examination of the pain phenomenon in patients suffering from spinal cord lesions (5,13). In order to start a therapy which would be as rational as possible, we studied such patients by means of a questionnaire; a smaller group was then observed from a clinical and neurophysiological point of view through the recording of somatosensory evoked potentials.

MATERIALS AND METHODS

The epidemiological data pertaining to the pain phenomenon were obtained by sending a questionnaire to patients suffering from spinal cord lesions; of the questionnaires sent out, 170 complete ones were returned (17). The questions contained in the questionnaire were intended to explore in terms, as clear as possible, some characteristics of the phenomenon under study. It was divided into three parts: the first regarding mainly the whole of the clinico-anamnestic data, the second examining the pain symptom, the third the therapeutic aspects. Altogether the questionnaire contained 33 questions, some to be answered freely and others by multiple choice; in any case they always were easy for the patient to understand. In defining the qualitative aspects of the pain symptomatology, the patients could choose among some words proposed on the basis of various published works on the "language of pain."

Our study was then carried on by a direct observation of patients of the Paraplegic Division of the C.T.O. of Milan. We treated with drugs 22 patients aged between 22 and 59 years, inclusively, who had been suffering with complete spinal cord lesion for a period between 1 and 23 years, in all cases of a traumatic origin, and predominantly caused by road accidents.

The intensity of the pain was assessed by using a points scale: 1, no pain; 2, mild pain; 3, moderate pain; 4, strong pain; and 5, very strong pain. The quantitative assessment was repeated after one cycle of therapy using the same scale.

Essentially three therapeutic protocols were applied:

1. For pain of articular and myofascial origin: nonsteroid antiinflammatory analgesics (seven patients);
2. For contractures or fasciculations: dantrolene sodium or baclofen in association with benzodiazepines (eight patients);
3. For pain of central origin: psychotropic drugs and amino acids (chlordiazepoxide + amitriptyline chloridrate + tryptophan) (seven patients).

In order to obtain a better assessment of patients we finally used the recording of the somatosensory evoked potentials in 20. The common peroneal nerve was stimulated at the knee by surface electrodes with a frequency of 4 Hz and of an intensity such as to give a visible contraction of the muscle. The potential was recorded from the scalp by surface electrodes; the active electrode was positioned on the midline 2 cm posterior to Cz (International System 10–20) with reference to the ear lobe. For the recording the Amplaid MK10 System was used with time analysis of 100 msec and bandpass of 10 to 2,500 Hz. Two tests of 500 trials each were always carried out. In case a valid response was not visible, at least 2,000 trials were carried out. The peak latency of the components P 27 and N 35 was calculated.

We assessed the replies obtained on a statistical basis.

RESULTS

Among the 170 patients of the questionnaire 140 (82.4%) were men and 30 (17.6%) women; the average age was 41.2 ± 1 (SE) for the men and 36.7 ± 2 (SE) for the women; 128 (75.3%) presented pain and 42 (24.7%) were without pain; among them 106 (82.8%) were men and 22 (17.2%) women. The etiology of the spinal cord lesion was for most cases (94.6%) of a traumatic nature (Table 1).

TABLE 1. *Characteristics of patients with spinal cord lesions*

Patient description	Patients with pain	Patients without pain
Total number	128 (75.3%)	42 (24.7%)
Males	106 (82.8%)	34 (80.9%)
Females	22 (17.2%)	8 (19.1%)
Average age	41.2 ± 1[a]	36.7 ± 2[a]
Traumatic etiology	121 (94.6%)	36 (90.5%)
Nontraumatic	7 (5.4%)	6 (9.5%)
Presence of vertebral pathology	12 (9.4%)	2 (4.7%)
Resulting in paraplegia	101 (78.9%)	33 (78.5%)
Resulting in tetraplegia	27 (21.0%)	9 (21.4%)
Loss of consciousness accompanying the trauma	61 (47.6%)	19 (45.2%)

[a] Mean ± SE.

With regard to the location of the pain there is a substantial agreement between our data and that of Alabama University (16), with elective localization in the lower extremities, trunk, and pelvis. The general collocation of the pain seems to be acute and piercing and there is a notable difference that can be observed as regards the term "burning" (Table 2). The surveys report high percentages of definitions of "burning" while our data are much lower. Approximately 87% of the patients were able to indicate a precise location of their pain. In 57% of the cases the pain was localized in the lower extremities. Some patients indicated pain in a number of places. In 62.5% of them the pain was defined as piercing, in 20% dull.

With regard to the quantitative aspects of pain, in a high percentage of cases the pain is continuous, disturbs sleep, and prevents social relations and

TABLE 2. *Characteristics of pain*

Type of pain	Milan	Alabama	Victoria
Sharp, piercing	65%	48%	—
Dull	19%	25%	—
Burning	6%	50%	64%
Throbbing	6%	20%	20%
Paresthesias	85%	20%	—
Localized pain (decubitus ulcers)	35%	—	50%

work. It seemed to us that we could define the pain as serious when at least three of these four aspects were present. This was true in 46% of the cases.

As for the therapeutic protection used by the patients, 30% of them were undergoing physiotherapy; of these 50%, equal to 15% of the total, obtained relief from the pain; 56% were undergoing drug therapy. Among the drugs indicated as being effective, anti-inflammatory analgesics account for 35%; antispastics and myorelaxants 26% and 25%, respectively; analgesic drugs 7.5%; neurotropic drugs 5%; and anticholinergics 2.5%.

The quantitative analysis performed on the patients directly observed with pain of myofascial origin or with contractures or fasciculations showed a fairly good difference between the intensity of the pain before and after the treatment (Fig. 1)

The statistical elaboration of the data revealed a pretherapy situation characterized by an average score of 3.75 ± 1.965, corresponding to a mod-

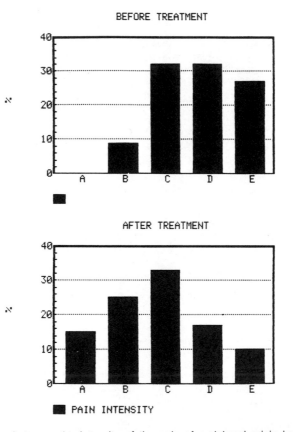

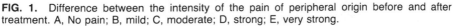

FIG. 1. Difference between the intensity of the pain of peripheral origin before and after treatment. A, No pain; B, mild; C, moderate; D, strong; E, very strong.

erate to strong pain. After therapy the average score recorded was of 2.75 ± 1.215, corresponding to a mild to moderate pain. The Student's *t*-test revealed a good effectiveness of the therapeutic treatment ($p < 0.05$). To the contrary, no significant statistical difference was observed in the patients with pain of central origin.

As for the neurophysiological study carried out in 19 patients out of 20 with plegia and total anesthetic below the level of the spinal lesion, it was not possible to note the evoked potentials. In one case with deafferentation pain the sensory evoked potential (SEPS) was present with normal latency and reduced amplitude, thereby suggesting the presence of a residual spinal function which was clinically unnoticeable.

DISCUSSION

Pain in the paraplegic is generally classified schematically into three categories:

1. Somatic root pain localized at the level of or near the spinal lesion.
2. Indistinct, vague visceral cramp pain accompanied by a dilation of the bladder and/or intestine.
3. Pain spread in various parts with a loss of sensitivity ill-defined as localization.

The first two categories are classified as pain of a peripheral origin, the third as pain of a central origin. The data to be found in various studies seem to agree on two basic aspects concerning deafferentation pain.

1. The pain must not be secondary to the stimulation of the nociceptors.
2. It is presumed that secondary processes involving the excitatory or inhibitory system are taking place (21,25)

It is thought that, in paraplegics, the pain depends on the activity of the structures above the spinal section. In these structures the lack of interaction between superspinal regions and the separate areas of the lesion produces a model of activity which, as a whole, generates the feeling of phantom pain and real pain (2). The incidence of the pain phenomenon in these patients is different for various investigators, whereas as regards the qualitative characteristic and the latency time between the lesions and the appearance of the symptomatology, there is a basic agreement. They report an incidence of the pain phenomenon which is extremely variable. Our data come between the two extremes registering an incidence of 75%. It must be observed, however, that this result might be overestimated, because it seems likely that the subjects with pain were more motivated to compile and send back the questionnaire, and that among more than 400 patients who did not answer it, a large number of them were without pain. On the other hand, one of the most important studies carried out in the same way as ours, the one already mentioned performed by Alabama University, also reports a high percentage of patients with pain (16).

The results of drug treatment (4,14,21) are at variance and, on the whole, disappointing, while we met with total failure as regards neurosurgical lesions except for the dorsal root entry zone (DREZ) lesion (21). In one survey, whereas we obtained good results in the treatment of pain of a myofascial or articular origin by means of mild analgesics, and in the control of contractures and fasciculations by association with dantrolene sodium or baclofen with benzodiazepines, we had poor results in the drug treatment of pain of a central origin. Moreover, apart from a tranquilizing, sedative, and hypnotic effect, the benzodiazepines seem to exert a greater spasmolytic effect on paraplegics than dantrolene sodium (8). They also have a direct analgesic effect due to an increase in the serotoninergic activity, correlated to that of chlordiazepoxide (20), and they seem to facilitate the inhibitory activity of γ-aminobutyric acid (GABA). The association of chlordiazepoxide, amitriptyline, and tryptophane find a rational base in the now-confirmed activity of the increase of superspinal inhibition induced by amitriptyline and other antidepressants and tranquilizers. Such an effect seems to contrast with the autonomous discharge and loss of descending inhibition as cause of the deafferentation pain. The use of tryptophane should stimulate the inhibition action of the descending system (23).

The focal destruction of the gelatinous structures (DREZ) seems promising; further confirmation is required (21). The surgery is intended to rebalance the relations between stimulation and inhibition of the spinal cord by depressing the spontaneous activity of the neurons of the surface lamina.

Transcutaneous electrostimulation (TENS) can be performed only on patients who present a certain number of unimpaired myelinic fibers, otherwise it is ineffective and painful (11,12,21).

Electrostimulation of the posterior horns of the spinal cord, effective in other types of deafferentation pain, does not seem to give particular results in patients with spinal cord lesion (19).

An indispensable presupposition for a more accurate therapeutic approach appears, therefore, to be a close examination of the neurophysiopathological information in patients with spinal cord lesions. In our case the presence of SEPSs constrasted with the clinical and neurological survey of total plegia and loss of sensitivity in the lower extremities, suggesting the presence of a residual spinal function (24). Many contributions have been made in published studies on the use of the SEPS in patients with spinal cord lesions (3,6, 9,10,15) with particular reference to their use in a prognostic sense in the phases immediately following the occurrence of the lesion (19), and in the assessment of the functional integrity of the spinal cord (4,7). There are not, however, as far as we know, published data regarding their use for an assessment of the anatomical damage of the spinal cord in relation to the presence of pain and its characteristics. Deafferentation pain must not, indeed, be secondary to the stimulation of the nociceptors, and it is generally localized in places where there is a loss of sensitivity. Such characteristics should therefore involve the SEP for the usual approach and for an intensity of stimulation such as to excite the fibers of smaller diameter delegated to the transmission of the painful stimuli. In conclusion, from the continuation and development of our research that points out some interesting and surprising discrepancies between the presence and characteristics of pain, neurological examination, and evoked potentials, we hope to derive some useful suggestions in the as yet ill-defined field of diagnostic background and therapy.

REFERENCES

1. Burke, D. C. (1973): Pain in paraplegia. *Paraplegia,* 10:297–313.
2. Carli, G. (1984): Fisiopatologia del dolore da deafferentazione. *Algos,* 4:42–48.
3. Chabod, R., York, D. H., Watts, C., and Waugh, W. A. (1985): Somatosensory evoked potentials evaluated in normal subjects and spinal cord injured patients. *J. Neurosurg.,* 63:554–561.
4. Cuocolo, R., Amantea, B., Belfiore, F., and Savoia, G. (1984): Concetti generali di terapia del dolore da deafferentazione. *Algos,* 4:49–59.
5. Dorfman, J., Perkash, I., Bosley, M., and Cummings, K. L. (1980): Use of cerebral evoked potentials to evaluate spinal somatosensory function in patients with traumatica and surgical myelopathies. *J. Neurosurg.,* 52:654–660.
6. Drechsler, F., and Schrappe, O. (1981): Somatosensory evoked potentials in above-knee amputees with phantom and stump pain. In: *Phantom and Stump Pain,* edited by J. Siegfried and M. Zimmermann, pp. 32–41. Springer-Verlag, New York.
7. El Negamy, E., and Sedgwick, E. M. (1978): Properties of a spinal somatosensory evoked potential recorded in man. *J. Neurol., Neurosurg. Psychiatry,* 41:762–768.
8. Glasse, A., and Hanna, A. (1974): A comparison of Dantrolene sodium and diazepam in treatment of spasticity. *Paraplegia,* 12:170–176.
9. Gruninger, W., and Ricker, K. (1981): Somatosensory cerebral evoked potentials in spinal cord diseases. *Paraplegia.* 19:206–215.
10. Kaplan, P.E., and Rosen, J.S.(1981): Somatosensory evoked potentials in spinal cord injured patients. *Paraplegia,* 19:118–122.
11. Karavel, Y., and Sindou, M. (1983): Anatomical conditions of efficiency of transcutaneous electrical neurostimulation in deafferentation pain. In: *Advances in Pain Research and Therapy, Vol. 5,* edited by J. J. Bonica, U. L. F. Lidblom, and A. Iggo, pp. 763–766. Raven Press, New York.
12. Klinger, D., and Kepplinger, B. (1981): Transcutaneous electrical nerve stimulation in the treatment of chronic pain after peripheral nerve lesion. In: *Phantom and Stump Pain,* edited by J. Siegfried and M. Zimmermann, pp. 103–106. Springer-Verlag, New York.
13. Loeser, J. D. (1983): Definition, etiology and neurological assessment of pain originating in the nervous system following deafferentation. In: *Advances in Pain Research and Therapy, Vol. 5,* edited by J. J. Bonica, U. L. F. Lidblom, and A. Iggo, pp. 701–711. Raven Press, New York.
14. Mazars, G. J., and Choppy, J. M. (1983): Revaluation of the deafferentation pain syndrome. In: *Advances in Pain Research and Therapy, Vol. 5,* edited by J. J. Bonica, U. L. F. Lidblom, and A. Iggo, pp.769–773. Raven Press, New York.
15. Nacimiento, A. C., Bartels, M., and Loew, F. (1986): Acute changes in somatosensory evoked potentials following graded experimental spinal cord compression. *Surg. Neurol.,* 25:62–66.
16. Nepomuceno, C., Fine, P. R., Richards, S. J., Gowerns, H., Stover, S. L., Rantaunabol, V., and Houson, R. (1979): Pain in patients with spinal cord injury. *Arch. Phys. Med. Rehab.,* 60:605–609.

17. Ranucci, M., Codeleoncini, S., Iorno, V., Marchetti, A., Moschini, V., Ravanelli, A., and Tiengo, M. (1985): Incidenza, gravità e caratteristiche qualitative del fenomeno dolore nel paziente con lesioni spinali. *Acta Anaesthesiol. Ital.*, 36:105–113.
18. Tasker, R. R., Tsuda, T., and Hawrylyskyn, P.(1983): Clinical neurophysiological investigation of deafferentation pain. In: *Advances in Pain Research and Therapy, Vol. 5*, edited by J. J. Bonica, U. L. F. Lidblom, and A. Iggo, pp.713–738. Raven Press, New York.
19. Tasker, R. R.(1984): Deafferentation. In: *Textbook of Pain*, edited by P. D. Wall and R. Melzack, pp.119–132. Churchill Livingstone, London.
20. Thiebot, M. H., Hamon, M., and Soubriè, P. (1982): Attenuation of induced anxiety in rats by chlordiazepoxide: role of raphe dorsalis benzodiazepine binding sites and serotoninergic neurons. *Neuroscience*, 7:2287–2294.
21. Tiengo, M., Calzà, L., and Rigoli, M. (1985): Il dolore da deafferentazione nella ricerca e nell'assistenza. *Algos*, 3:260–267.
22. Wall, P. D., and Melzack, R. (1982): *The Challenge of Pain*. Penguin, New York.
23. Weil Fugazza, J., Godefroy, F., Coudert, D., and Besson, J. M. (1980): Total and free serum tryptophan levels and brain 5-hydroxytriptamine metabolism in arthritic rats. *Pain*, 9:319–325.
24. Young, W. (1982): Correlation of somatosensory evoked potentials and neurological findings in spinal cord injury. In: *Early Management of Acute Spinal Cord Injury*, edited by C. H. Tator, pp.153–165. Raven Press, New York.
25. Zimmermann, M. (1983): Deafferentation Pain Chairman's introduction. In: *Advances in Pain Research and Therapy, Vol. 5*, edited by J. J. Bonica, U. L. F. Lidblom, and A. Iggo, pp.661–662. Raven Press. New York.

Advances in Pain Research and Therapy,
Vol. 10. Edited by M. Tiengo et al.
Raven Press, Ltd., New York © 1987.

Expression of Motility in Patients Treated with Pharmacological Neuromodulation

*G. Mocavero, *U. Cugini, *V. Paladini, *M. Scalia, and
**E. Campailla

*Department of Pain Therapy and ** Department of Traumatology, University of
Trieste, Trieste, Italy

Motion can be defined as the biomechanical translation, by the locomotor apparatus, of a central message arising either from the brain or the spinal cord. When decomposed, motion is equal to the vectorial summation of the singular angular movement of the articulations. Motion is made possible by a basal tone, in which muscles are contracted in an isometric fashion, and on which the phasic contractions take place: They are isotonic contractions, in which muscles are shortened. The integration of these functions is needed to reach a perfect balance of contractile activity, from which motility originates. Several structures are responsible for this integration: The primary motor cortex controls the ideation of the voluntary movement; from the primary cortex, the corticonuclear and the corticospinal long fibers originate. The cortical secondary areas, together with the striated body, the thalamus, the mesencephalic gray substance, the reticular formation, and the cerebellum, allow the elaboration of the movement on the basal tone, its adjustments and maintainance. At spinal level, tone is maintained by the stretch reflexes which are evoked by peripheral afferents, but are inhibited or facilitated by afferents from the already mentioned supraspinal motor centers. Peripheral afferents, mainly the subcortical ones, reach each neuronal station in charge of the movement; they can be autonomically elaborated to give an absolutely automatic and stereotyped motor response, just like a polysynaptic reflex. Thus, when lesions are limited to the peripheral compartment, motility wil be affected in an absolutely foreseeable fashion: A lesion of the brachial plexus will lead to flaccid paralysis with muscular atrophy of the upper limb. A central compartment lesion, on the contrary, modulated by redundance phenomena (i.e., many systems controlling one function) will present a more complex and unexpected behavior. Because of the suppression of a reciprocal inhibitory control among different structures, the symptoms will be those of a polyfunctional and hyperfunctioning lesion. A lesion of the internal capsule, for example, will cause spastic hemiplegia due to the interruption of most of the cortical fibers, thus releasing the subcortical centers. An interruption at the bulbar pyramid level causes flaccid paralysis, whereas a lesion limited to the primary motor cortex will affect the execution of fine and intentional movements; this pathology usually improves when auxiliary circuits become activated. Once the problem of motility is set against an anatomofunctional background, it is possible to emphasize the role of pharmacological neuromodulation in dealing with pain and motility. The pain therapist aims to improve the patient's quality of life through the control of pain and the improvement, or at least the preservation, of the motor function; the authors feel that this aim limits the use of neurolesive techniques. When looking at a pain syndrome associated with a motility impairment, the pain therapist must differentiate between two symptomatological aspects. The irreversible component of the motor disturbance is due to the permanent lesion of the motor fibers from the center to the muscle. In this case one could only employ some physiotherapy in order to create alternative schemes of movement, still bearing in mind the necessity to control pain. The reversible component of the motor impairment is referrable to reflex (subcortical) and behavioral (cortical) mechanisms triggered by peripheral or central pain. When pain interferes with movement, the analgesia improves the motor performance.

CLINICAL NOTES

To integrate the theoretical introduction, the authors present some clinical cases which have come to their attention. It is felt that it is advisable to consider surgery or similar techniques when possible. A vertebral collapse due to metastasis can be stabilized with Harrington bars. A pathological fracture of the humeral diaphysis secondary to breast cancer can be treated with metallic osteosynthesis. Orthopedic surgery for metastatic pathologies finds growing consensus thanks to the increased availability of prosthesis, cementing substances, and osteosynthesis techniques.

SEGMENTARY SPINAL NEUROMODULATION

Sometimes surgery is not sufficient, or presents technical difficulties, or does not find any indication in the light of the patient's conditions.

POLYARTHRITIS

A severe, overtreated polyarthritis will cause a hampered movement secondary to the altered articular dynamics, to a stenosed vertebral canal and to pain evoked by movement. Pain only can be improved through pharmacological neuromodulation, and motility is often improved just partially. In this case a continuous analgesic epidural blockade with buprenorphine is applied.

A malignancy is often complicated by the infiltration of the peripheral nervous structures, as, for example, in the Pancoast syndrome. In the first stage, the neoplastic growth does not involve peripheral receptors and is asymptomatic. In the second stage, pain is caused by the involvement of the healthy tissue surrounding the neoplastic mass. In the third stage, two different moments can be distinguished: (a) pain evoked by the inflammation of the perineoplastic tissue; and (b) pain due to the involvement of the nervous fiber. The latter can be defined as neuropathic pain.

In the fourth stage, pain is mainly of the neuropathic type, and is caused by the lesion of the nervous fiber by the neoplastic infiltration, or by the compression on a nerve root caused by vertebral collapse (incident pain).

NEURONAL MECHANISMS IN NEOPLASTIC PAIN

Phase 1: silent.

Phase 2: pain triggered by tissue distention.

Phase 3: 3a pain is due to the inflammation of the perineoplastic tissue; 3b pain is due to the inflammation of the nervous structure.

Phase 4: neuropathic pain due to neural infiltration or to incident pain.

PULMONARY APEX CANCER

In a patient affected by pulmonary apex cancer the site of application of pharmacological neuromodulation is the cervical spine, in order to reach both the posterior gray horns (segmental component) and the paleospinothalamic fibers (lower spinal component). The epidural route, moreover, has the advantage that it does not allow any communication with the liquoral spaces; by this route can be administered an opioid local anesthetic-steroid combination which acts in synergy in the incidental and the deafferentation pain. Hydrosoluble drugs, such as morphine, have shown a transdural passage with active concentrations producing analgesia through the interaction with thalamic and periaqueductal receptors of the descending inhibitory system for nociceptive afferents. Opioids that are administered by the spinal route do not show any effect on motor neurons in healthy patients at therapeutic dosage.

TETANUS

When dealing with tetanus, the epidural administration of buprenorphine did not act on the spontaneous excitability of the motor neuron, as shown by the identical electromyographical trace before and after the infusion. Yet the muscular rigidity is dramatically improved as well as the evoked pain, while the hyperkinetic sympathetic syndrome is avoided. The blockade of A δ- and C-fibers on sensitive afferents caused by the opioid could possibly affect the reflex activation of the somatic and autonomic motor neurons, which are already in an hyperexcitable state secondary to the tetanic neurotoxin. Spinal opioids improve spontaneous and reflex spasticity in paraplegias due to spinal lesions.

CEREBROVASCULAR LESION

Sometimes, as in painful spasticity due to an infarctual lesion of the internal capsule, the pharmacological neuromodulation abolishes pain but does not improve motility, probably because the patient's muscular tone is strictly dependent on peripheral afferents after the suppression of activating impulses from the brain.

CENTRAL NEUROMODULATION

Segmentary or high spinal analgesia might not be sufficient in severe pain syndromes following neoplastic polyfocal metastasis. An indication is found here for the administration of analgesic drugs directly into the subarachnoidal cerebral areas in order to act on those neurons which are responsible for the central control of pain. These neurons are found in the intralaminar nuclei of the thalamus, in the periductal gray substance, in the raphe magnum nucleus, and in the reticular substance of the brainstem. The catheter, inserted at low cervical level, can be threaded into the cisternal space or into the ventricular system through the foramen of Magendie.

In these cases it is advisable to employ a closed system of administration obtained by connecting to the subcutaneous reservoirs used and perfected in our institute.

PELVIC CANCER

A patient affected by a pelvic cancer involving the use of a stoma, previously confined in bed and dependent on other people, after pharmacological neuromodulation was able to walk and gain sufficient autonomy, improving his quality of life.

Further applications of the pharmacological neuromodulation to motility disturbances involving the presence of pain are part of our experience; among these are same musculoskeletal pathologies with which we are so often confronted.

The most frequently observed pain syndromes affecting the lumbar spine are those arising from radicular compression and associated with arthrosis with periodical "relapses." Pain and movement improve rapidly after a few epidural infusions of opioids, steroids, and local anesthetic mixtures.

Some degenerative pathologies of the articulations, such as the scapulohumeral or the coxofemoral, respond to the peri- or intra-articular injection of the above-mentioned mixture. Finally we emphasize how a laminectomy operation for herniated disc can be complicated by the inflammation of the epidural space. In this case, too, the local infiltration of an analgesic-steroid mixture proved its efficacy.

CONCLUSIONS

As many others in pain therapy we started with neurolesion and ended with neuromodulation. Although neurolesion is still indicated in various cases, we emphasize that when a motility impairment is associated with pain, the best results are obtained with a minimal damage to the motor structure and its fibers. On the sensorial side, in many recent papers, such as that of Sanes (1988), the importance of a complete afferent of the large sensorial fibers in the control of voluntary movement is emphasized.

REFERENCES

Cousins, M. J., and Mather, L. E. (1984): Intrathecal and epidural administration of opioids. *Anesthesiology*, 61:276–310.

Chauvin, M., Samii, K., and Viars, P. (1984): Les morphiniques administrés par voies péridurale et sous-arachnoidienne. *Encicl. Med. Chirurg.*, 36324 B. 10.

Gourlay, G. K., Cherry, D. A., and Cousins, M. J. (1985): Cephalad migration of morphine in CSF following lumbar epidural administration in patients with cancer pain. *Pain*, 23:317–26.

Kepes, E. R., and Duncalf, D. (1985): Treatment of backache with spinal injections of local anesthetics, spinal and sistemic steroids. A review. *Pain*, 22:33–47.

Mocavero, G. (1984): Dalla neurolesione alla neuromodulazione in terapia antalgica. *Federaz. Medica*, 37/6:547–556.

Moore, R. A., Bullingham, R. E. S., McQuay, H. J. et al. (1982): Dural permeability to narcotics: *in vitro* determination and application to extradural administration *Br. J. Anaesth.*, 54:1117–28.

Racagni, G., Nobili, M., and Tiengo, M. (1985): *Farmaci Nella Terapia del Dolore.* Edi Ermes, Milano.

Sanes, J. J., Mauritz, K. H., Evarts, E. V., et al. (1984): Motor deficits in patients with large-fibers sensory neuropathy. *Proc. Natl. Acad. Sci. USA*, 81:979–82.

Struppler, A., Burgmayer, B., Ochs, G. B. et al. (1983): The effect of epidural application of opioids on spasticity of spinal origin. *Life Sci.*, 33:607–10.

Yakhs, T. L., and Hammond, D. L. (1982): Peripheral and central substances involved in the rostrad transmission of nociceptive information. *Pain*, 13:1–86.

Yakhs, T. L., and Noueihed, R. (1985): The physiology and pharmacology of spinal opiates. *Annu. Rev. Pharmacol. Toxicol.*, 25:433–62.

Wall, P. D. (1984). Cancer pain: neurogenic mechanisms. *Pain,* suppl. 2:S197.

*Advances in Pain Research and Therapy,
Vol. 10.* Edited by M. Tiengo et al.
Raven Press, Ltd., New York © 1987.

Motility in Patients Treated with Chronic Peridural Catheter

*M. Trompeo, **G. Cerutti, **R. Cavallo, **E. Manno, **L.
Azzarà, **M. Carbone, **M. Sciuto, **M. Riva, and **L.
Ceretto

*Reanimation and Intensive Care Unit, and **Department of Anesthesiology and
Reanimation, University of Turin, Turin, Italy*

The use of the peridural area for administering drugs for the control of chronic pain is relatively new, even though this anatomic area had been successfully used in the past to control pain incurred under surgery.

The peridural area (Fig. 1) is a virtual cavity which surrounds the dural sac containing the medulla immersed and protected by the cerebrospinal fluid. In this area, the anterior and posterior spinal roots extend laterally from the medulla, and, joining level with the vertebral foramen, extend from the spine as metameric roots.

In their extramedullar, however, still intraspinal, tract, the spinal roots are, at first, protected by the medullar dura mater and then, on passing through the vertebral foramen toward the outside, are free. It must be noted, therefore, how substances injected into the peridural area can interfere with the neuronal transmission activity of the spinal root.

The practical application of this particular anatomic-functional conformation was realized as far back as 1885 by the American neurologist, James Corning, but was first clinically used by Sicard in 1901, who utilized the epidural area, reached through the sacral hiatus as a way through which it was possible to introduce an anesthetic substance—cocaine—to control pain incurred under surgery.

The lack of drugs suited to this purpose inhibited the use of this technique which was, however, limited to the sacral epidural area. Only in 1921 did the Spaniard, Fidel Pages, attempt to inject substances to control pain incurred under surgery into the lumbar peridural area. The lack of suitable instruments, perfectly sterile drugs, together with a certain amount of improvisation in the application technique, did not allow for a correct clinical evaluation of what this way of administering might represent in surgery.

Only in 1931 did Achille M. Dogliotti give a precise and scientifically accurate description of the peridural area as a place to introduce local anesthetics, at the same time illustrating the advantages and disadvantages, and

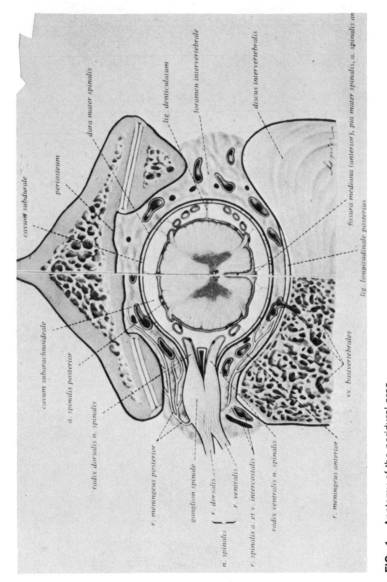

FIG. 1. Anatomy of the peridural area.

hypothesizing an action mechanism to explain the clinical result of administering the drug.

In 1933, the new technique, already accepted in its essentials, was published in the American Journal of Surgery. American surgeons and anesthetists immediately realized the highly revolutionary importance of this technique and adopted it widely, contrary to what was happening in Europe.

In 1941, Rees and Abajian proposed and adopted the continual sacral epidural anesthesia.

In 1949, Curbello started the continual peridural anesthesia era by introducing a little ureteral catheter through a Tuoy needle into the peridural area. Thus, the usual time limits of the single peridural injection of a local anesthetic were bypassed.

In 1954, Philip Bromage, re-examining the physiopathology of the peridural area, explained, systematically and organically, the action of drugs administered to this part, confirming and, of course, expanding on what Dogliotti had, 20 years earlier, understood and expressed when he presented this new analgesic technique.

Having reached its heyday, and when it seemed set on a path of unstoppable ever-expanding use, peridural anesthesia was ousted by modern polypharmacologically balanced narcosis which was utterly changed by the introduction of curare, tracheal intubation, mechanical artificial ventilation, and made more secure and comfortable by means of new halogen anesthetics.

In analgesic therapy, too, masterly set out by Bonica in his treatise in 1954, the peridural technique was considered most effective; it was, however, limited as regards chronic pain by the necessity of repeated injections which rendered the method rather unpleasant for the patient.

On the other hand, continual peridural, which allowed for lengthy surgical operations, could not be utilized in the treatment of chronic pain as the materials with which the small catheters were made presented certain drawbacks, and caused irritation and damage to the delicate balance of the peridural area when kept in for more than a period of 48 to 72 hr.

It was only in the 1970s, with the introduction of biocompatible peridural catheters into clinical practice, that the analgesic continual peridural asserted itself as an extremely efficacious technique in many forms of chronic pain, especially those of neoplastic origin.

The biocompatibility of the catheter, which allowed for the latter to be kept in the peridural area for lengthy periods, however, gave rise to new problems for those who were caring for the patients. They had to find a solution to the problem of algia, at the same time allowing the patient to have an almost normal quality of life and human relationships and hence sufficient motility, so that the patients were not regarded as being handicapped.

Such a premise imposed a series of preliminary considerations which at first conditioned and restricted the extended adoption of the technique. It immediately seemed obvious that the use of local anesthetics (even if nonirritating and nondamaging both to the anatomic structure and to connective tissue structures of the peridural area) had to be restricted to those patients whose primary illness prevented them from leading a normal life and who were consequently bedridden.

It is, moreover, well known how the administering of local anesthetics into the peridural area compromises motility regarding both strength and motor coordination in that the action of the drug not only involves the posterior root, but also, to a greater or lesser degree, the anterior motor root.

Moreover, the interruption of the nervous conduction affects the sympathetic activity, and upsets the pressure balance of the systemic cycle; even very serious postural hypotension can occur. It was therefore necessary to use other drugs in the peridural area, suitable for reducing the negative effects of local anesthetics, at the same time, however, obtaining the same analgesic results.

From examination of this problem it seems obvious that the peridural area is a particularly selective and specific pharmacologic introduction site for those products with a more marked action on the central nervous system.

In particular, it was inferred that a drug introduced into the peridural area can act in two ways (see Fig. 2):

1. Direct action on the emerging fibers with a consequent modification of nerve conductivity. This action is shown when the drug penetrates the fiber and a more or less reversible link is formed, as happens with local anesthetics; or a superficial membrane alteration, as happens with substances with either very alkaline or acidic pH values regardless of their structure.
2. Receptor-action on medullar structures subjected to high relative concentration dialyzes drugs through the dura mater and runs into the cerebrospinal fluid. This action mechanism imposes pharmacokinetic analysis of the peridural area according to the various drugs used.

The destination of a drug injected into the peridural area, regardless of the mechanism with which its pharmacological action develops, is illustrated by Fig. 3 which indicates all the hypotheses proposed up to the present day, each of which explains the activity previously illustrated. In particular, the diffusion of the drug in the subdural area, and hence its dispersion in the cerebrospinal fluid, irrefutably explains the pharmacological activity of a receptor-drug.

The laws followed by a receptor-drug are numerous and involve both physicochemical and biological features. Among the physicochemical features are the following:

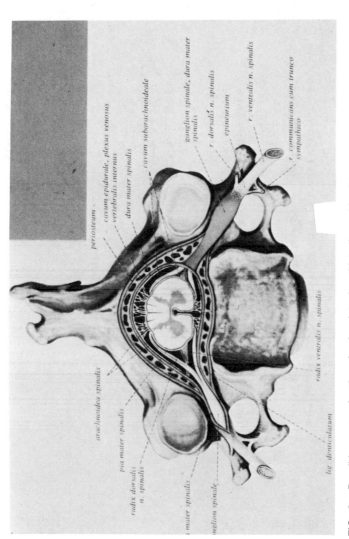

FIG. 2. Possible course of action of a drug introduced into the peridural area.

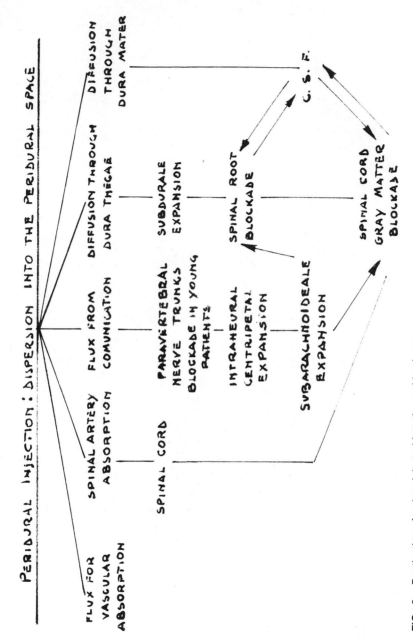

FIG. 3.   Destination of a drug injected into the peridural area.

1. The concentration of the drug injected.
2. Lipo- and hydrosolubility: The velocity of dialysis through the membrane increases as the coefficient of hydrosolubility becomes higher, whereas this velocity will decrease when liposolubility prevails. The reverse occurs regarding the medulla: The therapeutic effectiveness and the reaction time of lipo-soluble drugs is higher and longer-lasting, whereas the opposite occurs with higher hydrosolubility drugs which are not only less effective and long-lasting, but also develop a greater central toxicity due to migration of the fluid in the cerebral regions.
3. Molecular weight: The transit velocity is inversely proportional to the molecular weight (increased weight corresponds to less velocity).
4. Regional vascularization: It is well known how the vascular quota of the medullar dura mater decreases with age. It can, however, also vary (at times greatly) in the presence of regional inflammation or in the presence of neoplastic local or perifocal localizations.

The main biological features are:

1. The number of specific receptor-sites or the regional concentration of these on the medulla.
2. The elasticity of the dural structure which can accelerate or reduce the velocity of the diffusion of a drug. The elevated elasticity, typical of youth, allowing for a rhythmical variation of pressure according to arterial pressure and according to the respiratory rhythm and amplitude, facilitates the diffusion of the drug through the dural meninx. The opposite occurs when the dura mater becomes hardened with age or with previous ionizing treatment.
3. Cerebrospinal fluid pressure: This parameter is influenced by many factors such as the choroid plexuses' ability to produce cerebrospinal fluid, or its reabsorption in the caudal region, as well as the speed with which this circulation occurs in both a backward and forward direction. Forward circulation, considered by some as only a form of mixing, is responsible for the central toxicity of drugs injected into the peridural area. (For labeled morphine there is a mixing time in normotensive subjects and thus central toxicity of approximately 6 hr. This time does, however, vary greatly from subject to subject).

The systemic absorption of a drug injected into the peridural area is similar to that of an average vascularization tissue, such as muscular tissue.

Cerebrospinal fluid absorption is, on the other hand, approximately ten times more selective. It is, therefore, possible to obtain the same medullar response, to reduce the doses of drug injected into the peridural area to one-tenth and obtain the same therapeutic result as with a full-dosage systemic administering.

The following considerations are the main reasons why receptor-action drugs are used in the peridural area. Drugs used today belong to the following three groups: (a) opiates; (b) benzodiazepines (Midazolam); and (c) α–β lytics (Labetolol).

The analgesic effects are naturally greater with opiates, with variables as regards the intensity and duration of the analgesic action differing from product to product. The general reactions are, however, similar regarding normal quality of life and motility. Thus, we can make a general discussion with the exception of slight variants which could be referred to other groups of substances.

Analgesic treatment does, in fact, propose to not only eliminate pain, but also to restore the patient's normal life and human relationships with as little jeopardy as possible to his functional motility.

It is for these reasons that it is not possible, as we mentioned earlier, to use a local anesthetic as a specific drug, in that it seriously jeopardizes motility when the effective dosage is reached because of interference with the motor fibers of the anterior roots.

The jeopardy is dose-dependent, with the variable that it is greater, the dose being the same, the lower the level of concentration of solution; that is to say, when the volume is greater than the capacity of the peridural area and the anesthetic leaks from the vertebral foramen.

When opiates are used, some considerations regarding the lesion of the primary illness are required to evaluate the possible jeopardy to motility. It is, in fact, evident how motility may be jeopardized regardless of the drug used when the primary lesion involves motor zones, that is plexuses or articular regions which are fundamental to normal human relationships. When, on the other hand, the motor regions are undamaged, it is possible to show the effect of the analgesic drug injected.

Recorded data on the subject are rather modest, and we too, not being able to carry out experiments on humans, have come up with results which, although few in number, are sufficient to confirm what had previously been set down in the literature.

Motility was assessed using a dynamometrical method for working strength and a neurological test for motor coordination. To complete the study, research was then carried out on reaction time in order to evaluate possible cortical jeopardy. To evaluate motor jeopardy, a 2-kg dumbbell was used. Patients having high thoracic pain of the Pancoast type were asked to raise the dumb-bell rhythmically with the flexor muscles of the arm. Measurements were taken alternatively on the injured and healthy sides. The data gathered showed how, prior to administering the drug, the injured side only managed three slow movements before stopping the exercise, due to the advent of pain, while on the healthy side as many as twelve movements were possible before having to stop the exercise because of fatigue (see Fig. 4).

After these measurements were taken, 1 mg morphine chlorohydrate di-

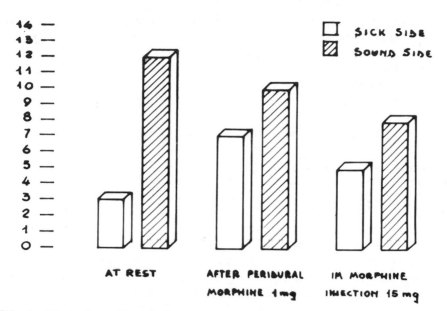

FIG. 4. Effects of morphine injection.

luted in 3 ml 5% glucose solution was administered in the peridural region $C_7–D_1$. One hour after administering the analgesic, when the pain had completely disappeared, motor performances were assessed, and the values recorded were, respectively, seven for the injured side and ten for the healthy side.

In order to underline the merits of the analgesic peridural block with opiates, according to the general administering of the same drug, a dose of morphine chlorohydrate able to remove the pain in the patient was administered intramuscularly. The dose necessary to obtain the analgesic result was 15 mg morphine.

The patients stated that they had always stopped doing the exercise because of muscle fatigue and not because of pain. Substituting morphine chlorohydrate with a 0.1-mg dose of Buprenorfine, jeopardy to motility of upper limbs was practically identical.

The neurological test carried out 60 min after administering, showed a lower motor coordination, which was more evident in the area where the drug was administered. This phenomenon is not of tantamount importance, but nevertheless cannot be neglected because it jeopardizes spontaneous motility, due to the sense of insecurity it causes. The coordination alterations remained for approximately 2 hr and then gradually decreased until they disappeared completely after 4 to 6 hr, even though a certain level of analgesia still remained.

On these grounds, administering of smaller and more frequent doses of the drug could be considered, although the risk of toxicity would be higher. This problem could be overcome by using an infusion micro-pump, keeping the receptor saturation level constant, and keeping motor jeopardy and coordination alterations to a minimum.

The study of psychomotor responsiveness, through the analysis of reaction times, was added to the two above-mentioned criteria for the evaluation of motility.

The technique we have illustrated in previous pharmacological papers, consists of measuring the reaction time necessary to switch off a lamp, switched on by the operator at random. The muscular movement being negligible, the time measured to a thousandth of a second by an electronic timer was supposed to correspond to pure reaction time. The value read is the average value of ten tests carried out in 2 min. Administering an opiate in the peridural area, the reaction time of the healthy side, before and after the injection, is approximately 20 to 25% slower.

The psychic behavior shows a slight euphoria, independent of the dose, without drowsiness occurring at the same time. Drowsiness, however, always occurred when morphine was administered intramuscularly.

No measurements were taken with higher doses, as we did not wish to cause the negative side effects of administering opiates in peridural area. However, we were interested in the cyclo-instrumental evaluation of motor jeopardy with minimum doses of analgesics.

The critics' estimates of the experimental results show a series of important considerations, at the end of a very precise and important antalgic therapy using the peridural method. In fact, one can come to the conclusion that contrary to earlier opinion, use of an opioid was able to interrupt the painful perception that usually compromises the motor activity and neuropsychic state of the patient, above all the motor coordination, the patient's behavior, and the reduction of the reaction time. The motor compromise is less, however, when the drug is injected into the peridural area than when given parenterally. The main motor compromise of the parenteral administration is tied up partly with the compromise of the motoneuron and partly by the state of surveillance. This particular behavior leads us to define the antalgic peridural treatment as a risk, not only regarding the possible injections, but also the neuropsychic state of the patient.

Therefore, we can deduce the necessity for a constant control of the patients during their relationship with the hospital and even more so at home. A constant watch would have to be organized by the relatives or helpers, inasmuch as some motor activity is potentially dangerous; for instance, stair-climbing and car-driving are to be avoided when a patient is under antalgic peridural treatment and above all during the first few hours after the injection.

Note that the psychomotor compromises may seem to discourage the use of the peridural method of anesthetic administration, but simply needs a series of precautions and controls particularly with accurate assistance.

The usefulness of the method must always be carefully evaluated, above all now that this relatively simple method helps to cure patients in their own homes and to become part of an almost normal life, although not so normal as to be able to take part in new job surroundings, especially under the same conditions as other individuals. Also, psychologically these patients cannot be considered completely healthy, in fact, if we should expose ourselves to this type of superficiality, we could find ourselves yet again face to face with very critical results.

REFERENCES

1. Bapat, Kshirsager, and Bapat, R. D. (1979): Aspects of epidural morphine. *Lancet,* 2:584.
2. Beher, M., Olshang, D., and Davidson, J. T. (1979): Epidural morphine in treatment of pain. *Lancet,* 1:527.
3. Bromage, P. R. (1975): Mechanism of action of epidural analgesia. *Br. J. Anaesth.,* 47:209.
4. Causins, M. J., and Glynn (1980): New horizon. In: *Neural Blockade in Clinical Anesthesia and Management of Pain,* edited by Causins and Bridenbaugh, pp. 699–719. Lippincott, Philadelphia.
5. Causins, M. J., and Mather, L. E. (1984): Intrathecal and epidural administration of opioids. *Anesthesiology,* 60:276–310.
6. Chauvin, M., Samii, K., Schermann, J. M., Sandauk, P., Bourdan, R., and Viars, P. (1981): Plasma concentrations of morphine after intramuscular, epidural and intrathecal administration. *Br. J. Anaesth.,* 53:911.
7. Cherry, D. A., Gourlay, G. K., McLachlan, M., and Cousins, M. J. (1985): Diagnostic epidural opioid blockade and chronic pain: Preliminary report. *Pain,* 21:143–152.
8. Cheyen, M., S., Rudik, V., and Borvine, A. (1980): Pain control with epidural injection of morphine. *Anesthesiology,* 53:338.
9. Davies, G. K., Tolhurst-Cleaver, C. L., and James, T. L. (1980): CNS depression after intrathecal narcotics. *Anaesthesia,* 35:1080–1083.
10. Gustefsson, L., Schildt, and Jacobsen (1982): Adverse effects of epidural and intrathecal opiates. *Br. J. Anaesth.,* 54:479–486.
11. Jorgensen, B. C., Andersen, M. B., and Engquist, A. (1981): CSF and plasma morphine after epidural and intrathecal application. *Anesthesiology,* 55:714.
12. Kanto, J., and Erkkola, R. (1984): Epidural and intrathecal opiates in obstetrics. *Nat. J. Clin. Pharmacol. Ther. Toxicol.,* 22:316–323.
13. McCaughey, W., and Graham, J. L. (1982): The respiratory depression of epidural morphine; Time course and effects of posture. *Anaesthesia,* 37:990–995.
14. Onofrio, B. M., Yaksh, T. L., and Arnold, P. G. (1981): Continuous low dose intrathecal morphine administration in the treatment of chronic pain of malignant origin. *Mayo Clin. Proc.,* 56:516–520.
15. Nordberg, G., Hedner, T., Mellstrand, T., and Delstrom, B. (1984): Pharmacokinetic aspects of intrathecal morphine analgesia. *Anesthesiology,* 60:448–454.
16. Roy, R., and Tunks, E. (editors) (1982): *Chronic Pain: Psychosocial Factors in Rehabilitation.* William & Wilkins, Baltimore.
17. Rucci, F. S., Cardamone, M., and Migliori, P. (1985): Fentanyl and bupivacaine mixtures for extradural blockade. *Br. J. Anaesth.,* 57:275–284.
18. Samii, Keret, Herari, and Viars (1979): Selective spinal analgesia. *Lancet,* 1:1142.
19. Yaksh, T. L. (1981): Spinal opiate analgesia: Characteristics and principles of action. *Pain,* 11:293–346.

Advances in Pain Research and Therapy,
Vol. 10. Edited by M. Tiengo et al.
Raven Press, Ltd., New York © 1987.

Which Opiates Are Indicated for Spinal Administration?

*Renato Cuocolo, *Bruno Amantea, *Gennaro Savoia, *Ciro
Esposito, *Francesco Belfiore, **Gianfranco Formicola,
†Antonio Savanelli, and ††Goffredo Acampora

*Istituto di Anestesia e Rianimazione e Terapia Intensiva, **Clinica Urologica, and
†Clinica Chirurgica Pediatrica, II Facoltà di Medicina e Chirurgia, Università degli
Studi di Napoli, 80131 Naples, Italy; and ††Ospedale Fondazione Senatore Pascale,
Istituto per la Diagnosi e Cura dei Tumori, 80131 Naples, Italy*

When opiates are administered in the subarachnoid space, their distribution in the cerebrospinal fluid (CSF) can really influence both therapeutic and secondary effects.

Many factors influence the opioid CSF distribution (Table 1). Among these, the most important are: the mechanisms of CSF movement in the subarachnoid space, the physical features of CSF, and the characteristics of the administered drugs.

The actual knowledge about CSF dynamics shows that CSF is principally produced by the choroidal ventricular plexi, while its absorption is carried out principally via the arachnoid granulations in the cerebral sinuses and, second, in the spinal subarachnoid space. Secretion rate is on an average of 500 ml/day (0.35 ml/min); CSF total volume in man is approximately 150 ml, and an average of 50% of CSF is situated in the spinal subarachnoid space (2).

CSF moves in craniocaudal direction, however, a slow CSF circulation in caudocranial direction has been also suggested.

Therapeutic and secondary effects of opioids, when they are administered in the subarachnoid space, are greatly affected by their distribution in the CSF. This is supported by the demonstration that a number of substances, such as radionuclides and metrizamide, when injected in the lumbar subarachnoid space gradually reach the fourth vetricle and lateral ventriculi within a period lasting 3 to 6 hr (2). This slow upward flow is possibly influenced by (7): (a) transabdominal and transthoracic pressure variations, (b) turbulence produced in the CSF by injection volumes superior to 10% of the CSF spinal volume (>7 ml); (c) CSF physical characteristics; and (d) physical characteristics of the solution injected in the lumbar subarachnoid space.

TABLE 1. *Factors affecting intrathecal distribution of opiates*

Factors related to the patient
    Age, sex, height
    Thoracoabdominal pressure
    Anatomical features
    Position
Factors related to the technique
    Injection rate
    Barbotage
    Injection site
    Density and pressure of the solution
    Liposolubility
    Injected dose and volume
    Use of vasoactive drugs epidurally

As the specific weight of CSF is equal to 1, CSF distribution for hypobaric (<0.9990), or hyperbaric (>1.0015), but not for isobaric, solutions is correlated to patient position.

Epinephrine can influence spinal opiate distribution, mainly after epidural administration, because the vasoconstriction produced by the drug reduces drug vascular clearance from the epidural space and indirectly enhances opiate CSF concentrations.

A 7.4 pH level is necessary to obtain the linkage between the opioid and the receptor. Shulmann et al. (10) showed that an alkaline pH enhances cerebral uptake of radiolabeled morphine in the cat hippocampus.

Another important opiate characteristic is the constant of dissociation. pK_a values close to pH 7.30 are important to obtain the opioid movement through the biological membranes (Table 2).

The clinically useful opiates (morphine, fentanyl, and meperidine) have a tertiary amine group that is ionized at physiological pH. Ionization ratio results from the dissociation constant and from the environmental pH.

Morphine, because of the presence of two ($OH-$) groups, is a hydrophilic molecule compared to the more lipophilic compounds, such as meperidine, fentanyl, and buprenorphine.

The most important factors that influence transmembrane diffusion rate are the octanol/water distribution coefficient and the dissociation constant (pK_a).

A high liposolubility at physiological pH increases the passage of a non-ionized drug through the cellular membrane.

OPIATE PHARMACOKINETICS AFTER SPINAL ADMINISTRATION

In man, when morphine and other opioids are injected directly into the CSF, they reach higher concentrations compared to those obtained by sys-

TABLE 2. *Physical-chemical characteristics of clinical opiates*

Opiate	pK$_a$ at 37° C	% Ionization[a]	Distribution coefficient octanol/water[a]	% Initial spinal cord linkage
Morphine	7.9–9.6	76	1.4	3.8
Meperidine	8.5	95	39	70
Fentanyl	8.4	92	77	95.8

[a] At pH 7.4.

temic or epidural administration (7). When the drug is directly administered into the CSF, there is a 100% bioavailability, and because there is not a systemic absorption, the concentration peak is rapidly reached after the injection.

Opioid clearance in the CSF depends on a liposolubility bioexponential pattern; there is a general agreement about this opinion.

Compared to the intrathecal route, opioid pharmacokinetics, after administration in the peridural space, are influenced by three conditions:

1. Difficult penetration through the dura depending on opioid molecular weight and conformation; Cousins (2) suggests that opioids can reach the medulla not only through the dural barrier, but also through the posterior radicular arteria;
2. Deposit in the epidural fat, principally for the lipophilic substances; and
3. Systemic vascular absorption that is faster and of remarkable entity for the lipophilic substances (meperidine, fentanyl, and heroin).

The vascular absorption occurs via the epidural venous plexus that discharges directly into the azygos vein or the Batson basivertebral venous plexus, and a discharge into cerebral venous sinus (2).

Plasma concentrations that are reached in the first 2 hr after opiate epidural administration are comparable to those obtained after intravenous or intramuscular administration.

After epidural administration, the analgesia is obtained by the activation of spinal sites complemented by the involvement of supraspinal sites, because there is a systemic absorption. However, vascular absorption can improve analgesia only for a short period of time (2–3 hr); after this period, analgesia is related only to the spinal component (3). The pharmacokinetic model of Cousins et al. (2) is actually the most reasonable theory.

When opioids are in the CSF, they can spread rostrally. In a study with sheep models (8), in which the lumbar subarachnoid space and the magna cisterna were connected by a catheter system, it was demonstrated that the opioid caudorostral movement in CSF depends on the substance liposolubility and on the CSF bulk flow. After intrathecal lumbar administration of the drug cocktail (morphine, 1 mg; methadone, 1 mg; and radiolabeled sucrose), morphine and sucrose simultaneously reached a peak level in the cisterna after 90 min. Methadone was completely removed prior to reaching the higher levels, so that it was not detected in cisternal CSF. In this study, morphine sulphate and methadone hydrochloride have been used, respectively, as hydrophilic and lipophilic drugs, while sucrose, an hydrophilic molecule, has been used as a CSF inert marker.

Also, in man, a CSF rostral distribution of hydrophilic opioids has been shown. In a study on 14 neoplastic patients, Gourlay et al. (5) detected significant drug concentrations at the cervical level after 10 mg of morphine administration at the lumbar level (L_2-L_3). After 60 min, CSF concentrations reached 300 ng/ml, and 3 hr later they reached 600 ng/ml.

In a clinical study on 20 neoplastic patients with chronic pain, we have administered intrathecal morphine (0.5 mg) to ten patients; in the rest (ten patients), we administered epidural morphine (4 mg in 5 ml saline solution); then we tested CSF concentrations at lumbar (L_3-L_4) and cervical (C_7-D_1) levels.

By the intrathecal route, after 60 min high concentrations can be detected at the cervical level, whereas by the epidural route significant cervical levels were reached 2 hr after the administration (Fig. 1). At the steady state, there was a CSF concentration gradient lumbar/cervical (2/1) with both methods, and a level of 300 ng is raised, enough to obtain analgesia.

After lumbar-spinal administration, high opioid concentration in cervical or cisternal CSF represents CSF bulk flow, however, they are not correlated to other mechanisms for drug movement in CSF.

This phenomenon is not explained by diffusion, because substance diffusion from the subarachnoid lumbar level to magna cisterna needs days rather than minutes. Likewise, this phenomenon cannot be explained by vascular redistribution in the magna cisterna by systemic absorption, because blood concentrations measured after intrathecal administration are very small.

The early onset of itching and vomiting after spinal administration of opioids suggests that the high cervical and cisternal concentrations of opioids depend on the rapid absorption through the Batson basivertebral venous plexus, but this hypothesis can be repeated because the opioids movement (1–6 hr) in liquid is not similar to the rapid movement through the basivertebral plexus (2).

In summary, the CSF bulk flow is the only mechanism that can explain the duration time necessary for opioids to spread rostrally and to reach the high levels detected after lumbar spinal administration. This mechanism also explains the side-effects onset (nausea, vomiting, itching, sedation, and respiratory depression), in particular after spinal administration of hydrophilic opioids. Particular attention must be paid to the respiratory depression after intrathecal opioid administration, because it can be affected by many factors such as:

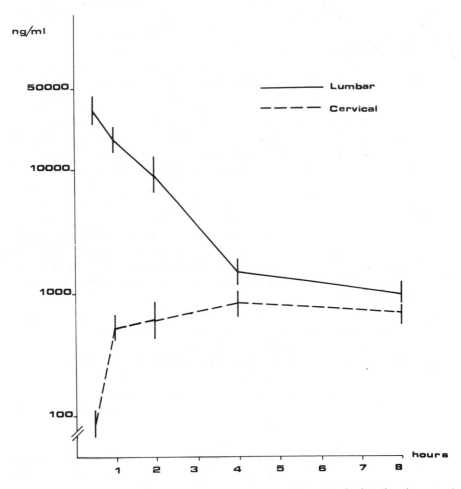

FIG. 1. CSF concentrations of morphine (0.5 mg) administered in the intrathecal space at lumbar level.

1. Use of hydrophilic opioids;
2. Use of high doses;
3. Marked changes in thoracoabdominal pressure;
4. Advanced age;
5. Concomitant administration, by other routes, of opioids or other CNS depressant drugs.

Respiratory depression occurs most frequently in the postoperative period, in particular in *naif* subjects. To prevent respiratory depression, the following protocol is now accepted:

1. Use of low opioid doses;
2. Dilution volume must not exceed 10% of spinal CSF volume;
3. Sitting position reduces the incidence of respiratory depression;
4. Avoidance of parenteral administration of opioids after spinal injection;
5. If necessary, use naloxone infusion for postoperative pain treatment.

Particular consideration must be given to urinary retention (9), the most frequent side effect (15–90% incidence) due to spinal morphine administration. A higher frequency is found in young volunteers, rather than in other patients. Among these, the incidence is higher in naive subjects undergoing postoperative pain relief because morphine administration causes a rapid detrusor relaxation in 15 to 30 min, so that bladder capacity and urinary retention increase; however, spontaneous recovery of bladder function occurs after 14 to 16 hr, and in chronically treated patients when they have not shown opioid tolerance. However, postoperative urinary retention is influenced by the type and the anatomic site of surgery, the supine position, the nursing care, the peri- and postoperative hypovolemia, deep sedation, etc. The influence of these factors seems to be shown by the failure of reversal of retention following naloxone.

These side effects are not dose-related and their reversal is rapid after naloxone administration; they are different from those caused by intravenous or intramuscular morphine administration.

In a recent trial, urodynamic alterations in ten patients (5 naive and 5 nonnaive) affected by neoplastic or vascular pain were studied (Cuocolo et al., *unpublished data*). Monitoring was performed as follows: under normal conditions; 90 min after epidural morphine (4.0 mg); and after naloxone (i.v., 0.4 mg) (these were administered just when urodynamic changes occurred).

Figure 2 shows the behavior of a naive patient, afflicted with prostatic hypertrophy; in such a case, the use of morphine results in a partial detrusor relaxation, while the bladder capacity is unmodified. Naloxone administration increased detrusor contraction, sufficient to induce urinary output. In nonnaive patients, receiving oral or parenteral morphine chronically, the administration of epidural morphine (4 mg) did not result in a significant effect with respect to the basal values; Fig. 3 shows urodynamic monitoring obtained in one of these patients.

To explain the mechanism of urinary retention after spinal morphine administration, three hypotheses have been suggested:

1. Supraspinal inhibitory effect at the pons, where the primary center for micturition and the receptors for opioids exist. Such a hypothesis is in accord with the rostral drug distribution in the CSF, until the supraspinal structures. However, the time necessary for drug diffusion in the CSF is higher than the 15 to 30 min necessary for morphine to cause relaxation of the bladder detrusor;

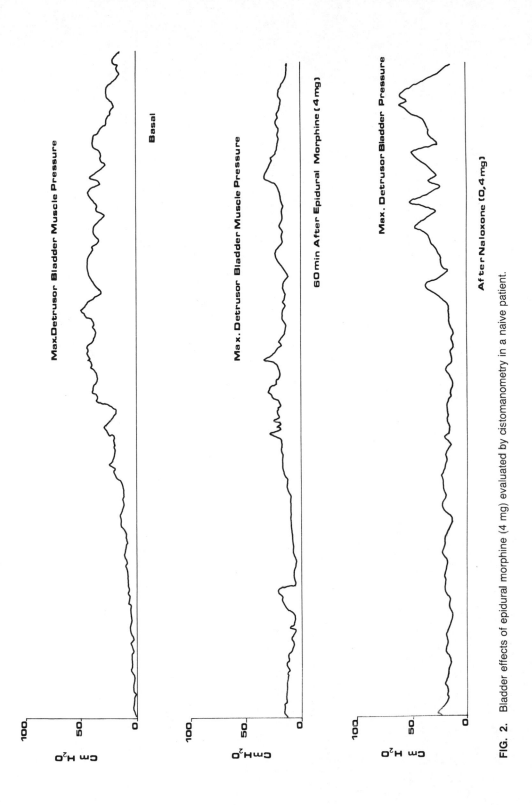

FIG. 2. Bladder effects of epidural morphine (4 mg) evaluated by cistomanometry in a naive patient.

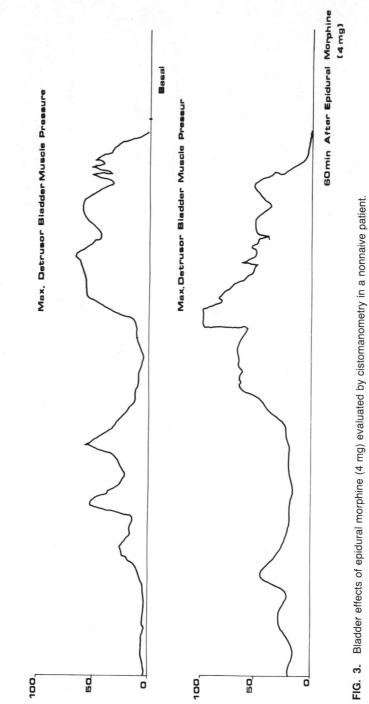

FIG. 3. Bladder effects of epidural morphine (4 mg) evaluated by cistomanometry in a nonnaive patient.

2. Presence of opioid receptors in the urinary bladder, as well as in deferens vessels and in the ileum of animals. Such a hypothesis is in opposition to the lack of changes of bladder function found after parenteral morphine administration;
3. Presence of a spinal action site, demonstrated by a rapid onset of detrusor relaxation. Autonomic inhibition should be caused by morphine effects on the parasympathetic sacral mechanism.

Detrusor relaxation and analgesia onset both occur within 30 min after spinal morphine injection, and they suggest the hypothesis of a common action site at spinal level, whereas the other side effects appear later and seem to be related to morphine supraspinal diffusion.

CORRELATIONS BETWEEN PHARMACOKINESIA AND ANALGESIA

Hydrophilic opioids such as morphine, hydromorphone, D-ala-D-leu-enkephaline (DADLE), and β-endorphine, have a significative rostral distribution after spinal administration. They slowly penetrate the dura, and are adsorbed in epidural veins, reaching systemic blood levels that can be redistributed at the supraspinal and spinal analgesic sites. Liposoluble opioids such as methadone, meperidine, fentanyl, and buprenorphine have a limited rostral CSF distribution. Liposoluble opioids reach high plasma levels when spinally administered but they produce fast analgesia within the first 2 hr so that the supraspinal opioids redistribution can only potentiate the analgesia.

Theoretically, the ideal opioid for spinal administration should have the following characteristics:

1. High lipid solubility: This allows a rapid uptake from the CSF to the spinal cord and produces a rapid onset of analgesia; in this way, a small amount of opioid spreads over rostral regions;
2. A lower pK_a in the CSF at the physiological pH: Opioids, which are largely nonionized at this pH would penetrate the lipophilic spinal cord more efficiently than ionized opioids. However, the commonly administered opioids get a high pK_a and are largely ionized at the normal CSF pH;
3. Linkage affinity and tenacity for spinal cord receptors: To produce analgesic effect practically, we could give a smaller amount of selective agonist, such as the DADLE, rather than a nonselective agonist, as morphine.

Payne (8) suggests that the intrathecal administration of a smaller but more effective dose of DADLE could decrease CSF and plasma drug concentrations and minimize the effects at supraspinal analgesic sites, activated as a result of vascular or CSF redistribution of the opioid.

However, in this case, the greatest selectivity alone is not sufficient to reduce selective spinal effects; in fact, DADLE is a hydrophilic agonist that is associated with supraspinal redistribution and with toxic effects similar to morphine.

Relatively, buprenorphine seems to be an ideal drug because it connects liposolubility with tenacity for spinal cord receptors, but it is not specific for them. It has a lower incidence of respiratory depression compared to hydrophilic opioids. However, when buprenorphine is given epidurally, the analgesia is less lasting in comparison with morphine. Actually, opioids with low liposolubilty (e.g., morphine) are best for subarachnoid or epidural administration to obtain pain relief in chronic and acute pain. They are able to reach high concentrations in the CSF with a slow and constant penetration of the drug from the CSF to the spinal cord.

Nevertheless, these characteristics can cause undesirable side effects. Alternatively, continuous infusion or frequent boluses of lipophilic opioids can be helpful to obtain relief from acute pain.

SPINAL OPIATES AND MOTILITY

The advantages of spinal administration of opioids in the management of acute and chronic pain are a result of the selectivity of the spinal analgesia which does not involve, generally, other functions, such as sensorial and motor.

The preservation of the efferent sympathetic activity was studied by specific tests as sudomotor activity and vasoconstrictor sympathetic activity, measured by venous occlusion plethysmography after ice application to the skin of the involved dermotomic area. This means that sudomotor activity and vasoconstrictor sympathetic activity are unaffected by epidural meperidine.

Bromage et al. (1) found that the psychogalvanic response and the arterial pressure response to Valsalva's maneuver were not abolished after hydromorphine epidural administration. On the contrary, after epidural morphine the changes of blood pressure in response to immersion of lower limbs in ice water are calmed, and this means a reduction "firing" along the afferent side of pressure reflex.

As far as nervous conduction rate is concerned, after application of opioids directly to nervous roots, it was shown that only high concentrations of meperidine (1–2%) are able to cause a peripheral nerve block.

With regard to motor function in the animals, the specific-acting μ- and Δ-opioids, spinally administered, exert an inhibitory effect on the firing of α-motor neurons, evoked by muscle stretch (6). These effects are not evident in humans.

In our recent trial, we have studied the changes of the H reflex in five naive patients, with chronic pain after epidural administration of morphine (4 mg) at the lumbar level (L_3–L_4).

The technique involved stimulating the sciatic nerve on the apex of the poples, and recording electric muscular activity by surface electrodes on the soleus muscle. By increasing stimulus intensity, a first wave (M) was recorded, that is, the direct response of the motor unit; after a time space (termed H-M), we recorded a second wave (H) that proves a reflex response

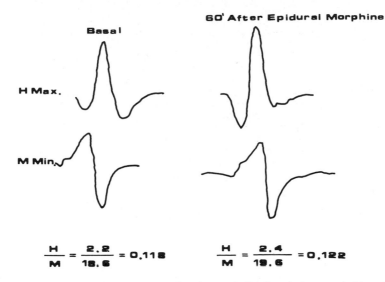

FIG. 4. H reflex responses. Epidural morphine does not alter the electromyographic pattern (see the text).

of muscle. We have also considered: (a) the threshold to evoke the H wave; (b) the H- and M-wave's maximal amplitude; and (c) the ratio between the maximal level of H and M waves. We have not found any significant changes of these parameters in our subjects 1 hr after epidural morphine (Fig. 4). This means that opiates at clinical doses do not alter motor function.

CONCLUSIONS

The results of a great deal of research in these past years concerning applications of the technique described show the importance of a better comprehension of spinal cord functions. For many years we have not been able to manipulate spinal cord functions by a foreseeable model. Only a good comprehension of spinal cord pharmacology will allow a specific action on pain pathways.

REFERENCES

1. Bromage, P. R., Camporesi, E., and Leslie, J. (1980): Epidural narcotics in volunteers sensitivity to pain and to carbon dioxide. *Pain,* 9:145–160.
2. Cousins, M. J., Lawrence, E., and Mather, L. E. (1984): Intrathecal and epidural administration of opioids. *Anesthesiology,* 61:276–310.
3. Cuocolo, R., Amantea, B., Savoia, G., Belfiore, F., and Esposito, C. (1985): Farmacocinesia degli oppiacei per via spinale. *Atti VIII Congresso Nazionale A.I.S.D.* Grafica Zeta Verona, 1986 (*in press*).

4. Glynn, C. J., Mather, L. E., Cousins, L. J., Graham, J. R., and Wilson, P. R. (1981): Peridural meperidine in humans: analgetic response, pharmacokinetics and transmission into CSF. *Anesthesiology,* 55:520–526.
5. Gourlay, J. K., Cherry, D. A., and Cousins, M. J. (1985): Cephalad migration of morphine in CSF following lumbar epidural administration in patients with cancer pain. *Pain,* 23:317–326.
6. Krivoy, W., Kroeger, D., and Zimmermann, E. (1973): Actions of morphine in the segmental reflex of the decerebrate spinal cat. *Br. J. Pharmacol.,* 47:457–464.
7. Nordberg, G. (1984): Pharmacokinetic aspects of spinal morphine analgesia. *Acta Anaesthesiol. Scand.,* (Suppl. 79) 28:1–37.
8. Payne, R., and Inturrisi, C. E. (1985): Distribution of morphine, methadone and sucrose after intrathecal injection. *Life Sci.,* 37:1137–1144.
9. Rawal, N., Mollefors, K., Axelsson, K., Lingardh, G., and Widman, B. (1983): An experimental study of urodynamic effects of epidural morphine and of naloxone reversal. *Anesth. Analg.,* 62:641–647.
10. Shulman, D. S., Kaufmann, J. J., Eisenstein, M. M., and Rapaport, S. I. (1984): Blood pH and brain uptake of 14-C-Morphine. *Anesthesiology,* 61:540–543.

Advances in Pain Research and Therapy,
Vol. 10. Edited by M. Tiengo et al.
Raven Press, Ltd., New York © 1987.

Pain as the Cause of Limitation of Joint Movement in Degenerative Lesions of Arthrosis

Giovanni Peretti

Clinica Ortopedica Dell'Università degli Studi di Milano—III Cattedra, Milan, Italy

In the title of this chapter are present three key words: arthrosis, pain, and movement; they represent many tightly connected and interdependent phenomena.

As it is true that arthrosis is the cause of pain and of limitation of the articular function, it is also true that pain determines a functional limitation and, as direct consequence, an increase of the degenerative lesions. Thus, it is evident that articular movements and their functional limitation determine an improvement or a worsening of the degenerative processes and consequently a mitigation or an increase of the articular pain.

Arthrosis, as we know, is a chronic degenerative process that always reveals itself with many local reactions that determine cellular and tissue regeneration and local inflammation. It is therefore not only a passive event, but also an active phenomenon, where regeneration and phlogosis exist together and alternate with the degenerative articular processes.

All the articular components are involved with these events, from the articular cartilage to the subchondral bone, to the synovial membrane, the articular capsule, the tendons, and the muscles of the involved joint.

The articular cartilage is initially damaged into the overcharged seats and proliferates in the free regions; the subchondral bone presents aspects of necrosis with the formation of geodes and takes an active part in the formation of sclerotic bone. The synovial membrane shows processes of degeneration or of hypertrophy, with phlogosis and an increase of its secretive and reabsorption activity. The capsule is also involved with articular inflammation, while muscles and tendons play a role only later and determine the limitations of the articular movements by diminishing its dynamic function and increasing its static one. The pain in the joint caused by arthrosis comes from the subchondral bone which can be deformed from the pressure, the irritated periosteum, the articular capsule, the irritated tendons, and from muscles submitted to excessive work. Pain is also derived from the peripheral nerves (as in the arthrosis of the interapophyseal joints of the spine) compressed by the osteophytes and the periarticular inflammatory tumor.

The articular receptors consist of four types:

Type 1: static and dynamic meccanoceptors.
Type 2: dynamic meccanoceptors (low threshold).
Type 3: meccanoceptors (very high threshold).
Type 4: nociceptors (with amyelinated fibers).

The function of these receptors is multiple and it is especially addressed to the control of the static and dynamic of the joint by means of the activation of simple or polysynaptic reflexes: The arthrostatic reflexes are driven from the type 1 receptors; the arthrodynamic reflexes are driven from type 1, 2, and 3 receptors; the algogenic reflexes are driven from type 4 receptors (more or less combined with the impulses coming from type 1, 2, and 3 receptors).

The nociceptive stimuli arrive at the spinal cord through a first-order neuron with partially myelinated δ-fibers (high-speed conduction) and through amyelinated C fibers (slow conduction); from the spinal cord, with second- and third-order neurons they join with the spino-thalamic and thalamocortical pathways; the cortex realizes, hence, the consciousness of the pain; the intermediate neurons allow the realization of simple reflex arches (to the spinal cord) or polysynaptic reflex arches (to the thalamus).

The articular pain can be exactly localized at the seat of the lesion or at a distance from this (referred or radiated pain) because the nerve fibers follow the afferent pathways originating from other areas.

Whereas the pain originating from superficial joints is exactly localized, the pain originating from deep joints is not; the muscle pain is generally diffused to all the involved muscle and often is referred to a distance from the muscle itself.

The pain induced from arthrosis can be of two different types: mechanical and chemical. The mechanical pain is generally due to the tension of the capsule of the joint or of its ligaments, to the pressure on the periosteum, to the muscular and tendon tension, and to the compression of the peripheral nerves.

The chemical pain can originate from these structures as a consequence of accumulation of chemical algogenic substances. In arthrosis, as in other events, whatever the cause and the seat of pain might be, to the somatic component is always added a psychological component, more or less clear with reference to the age of the patient, the sex, the personal and family culture, the behavior of the doctor, and other circumstances. This psychological component becomes more and more important, even becoming preeminent when the pain becomes chronic. According to Bonica, this is due to the persistence of the lesive stimulus on the nociceptors or to their sensibilization, or to both, in the periphery, in the spinal cord, or in the psychological make-up of the patient.

The movement in the arthritic joint is generally decreased, and this limitation is first because of a mechanical effect due to the alteration of the joint surfaces, or the production of marginal osteophytes, or the modification of the form of the articular bone ends. But even if it is the initial cause, other components play their role in inhibiting or limiting the articular movement. Among them are the lesions of all the other articular components: the nerve compression, the concomitant muscular lesion, and especially the presence of algogenic, phlogistical reflexes that determine a reflex inhibition of the muscle activity that drives the movements of the joint. The muscular activity can be excited or inhibited in reflex reply to the articular pain, or as a consequence of compression or irritation of the receptors or by pain within the same muscle or groups of muscles.

The algogenic reflexes rarely follow the stimulation of nociceptors alone, but are generally the results of stimulus afferent from different articular receptors; as a consequence, the articular replies are disordered and cause pathological alterations whether of the articular status or of the dynamic status. Irregular movements and incorrect postural attitudes follow. In turn, a symptomatology of pain results due to accumulation of catabolites in the involved muscles and the persistent tension in corresponding tendineal insertions to the skeleton, where many sensitive and nociceptive endings are localized.

Other alterations are added to the above, due to facilitation or inhibition of peripheral motoneurons as response to nociceptive afferents; these prevail over the normal reflex responses to stimuli originating from nociceptors.

This phenomenon grows more severe when the phlogistic stimulus becomes chronic and the capsule is particularly sensitive to the nociceptive stimulation.

When the pain is chronic, very often there are simple reflex responses causing alterations of peripheral tissues that may create a reflex contracture of skeletal muscles; these excite the afferent pathways and contribute to create a vicious circle consisting of pain–muscular excitation–pain.

The continuous algic afferents determine also a reflex sympathetic hyperactivity, with consequent vasospasm, ischemia, and cellular necrosis; hence there is liberation of algogenic factors, sensibilization of nociceptors, and a further increase of secretion of norepinephrine at the level of nerve endings. The circle closes with an increased discharge in small sensory fibers and an increase of muscle excitability.

The alteration of the articular movements can be the consequence of an alteration of the muscular response to afferent stimulations, with muscular uncoordination, or functional muscular limitation as a consequence of muscular pain.

The muscle can be the seat of referred pain, but it is often the seat of pain in arthrosis, as a consequence of postural change, of tendinous irritation, of phlogosis of the muscle itself, or of scant blood supply related to the vasospasm due to symptomatic stimulation.

Particularly important is the postural pain because the condition of persistent muscular hypertonicity creates a compression on capillary vessels with consequent diminution of oxygen supply and accumulation of lactic acid. As a consequence, muscle and tendon receptors are excited and the consequent further stimulation increases the muscle tone, with the completion of a further vicious circle. The excitation of nociceptors determines, in fact, the reflex activity of agonist and antagonist muscles, with stimulation of muscle spindle fibers and consequent reflex hypertonicity.

Thus, we have had the opportunity to observe that arthrosis is the cause of limitation of movement and pain. The limitation of movement produced by algogenic stimuli is a cause of pain and of further limitation of movement, with muscular hypertonicity and consequent articular overcharge. As the absence or the limitation of movement is one of the factors that increases articular degeneration, together with the articular overcharge, our brief considerations take us to the conclusion that the arthrosis is the cause of pain and pain is the cause of worsening of the arthrosis.

Thus closes a vicious circle that brings us to the three key words of the title of this chapter: arthrosis, pain, and movement: These terms are strictly joined and interdependent and suggest that the therapy of the arthrosis must seek to break the vicious cycle that only can worsen. Decrease of pain, decrease of phlogosis and of muscular hypertonicity, and increase of movement are the main objectives to prevent the progressive worsening of the degenerative processes of the arthrosis.

Advances in Pain Research and Therapy,
Vol. 10. Edited by M. Tiengo et al.
Raven Press, Ltd., New York © 1987.

Clinical Aspects of Heart Pain

Paolo Procacci and Marco Maresca

Institute of Medical Clinic, Pain Center, University of Florence, 50134 Florence, Italy

The concept of cardiac pain has been differently considered in different times. According to the medicine of the ancient Mediterranean civilizations, the heart was the center of sensibility. This concept was accepted by most Greek philosophers and especially stressed by Aristotle. For some centuries the Aristotelian Schools considered the heart as the center of all types of sensibility, i.e., the sensorium commune (15,27). The concept of pain originating from the heart was present in the *Corpus Hippocraticum* (12). Caelius Aurelianus (3), Roman physician of the fifth century A.D., used the term of passio cardiaca propria to indicate specific heart pain.

During the sixteenth, seventeenth, and eighteenth century different authors (2,4,8,17,22) described cases characterized by chest pain, which was interpreted as having an origin from the heart. In 1768 Heberden presented his precise description of angina pectoris. It must be noted that the term pectoris (i.e., of the breast) is a purely descriptive term, which does not imply a definite pathogenetic interpretation. In fact, Heberden could not identify a pathologic alteration that could be considered the cause of pain. With the term angina (formerly used to indicate all the diseases characterized by a sense of strangling), Heberden intended to stress the quality of pain, indicating that a strong, constrictive pain was experienced by the patients, with a sense of choking and strangling, accompanied by a terrible anxiety and anguish (angor animi) (9,10).

In the nineteenth century different pathophysiological interpretations of angina pectoris were opposed. According to one theory, this syndrome was due to coronary sclerosis; according to other theories, other mechanisms (such as cardiac distention or cardiac neuralgia) played a fundamental role in the genesis of pain (28). A revival of these polemics occurred in recent years. The importance of mechanical factors and of nervous alterations in the genesis of pain of ischemic heart disease has been stressed by some authors (20,30). As regards nervous alterations, the development of an ischemic neuropathy of heart nerves has been especially considered: The damage of myelinated fibers, less resistant to ischemia, provokes an imbalance of afferent input, with a prevalence of C-fiber discharge; such an unbalanced input opens the central gate mechanisms which control the transmission of afferent impulses (30).

Pain is a very important symptom in cardiac diseases, especially in ischemic heart disease. However, a differential diagnosis between cardiac pain and pain due to diseases of other thoracic organs is often difficult. Heberden (10) distinguished angina pectoris, characterized by a sense of strangling, anguish, and anxiety, and dolor pectoris, which comprised all the other kinds of chest pain. The difficulties in differential diagnosis especially concern aortic diseases (aneurysms, aortic dissection, and syphilitic aortitis), sometimes mediastinal and lung diseases, pleurisy, and oesophageal diseases. An intrigue of problems is often present, as we consider later.

Apart from pain of angina pectoris and myocardial infarction, other causes of cardiac pain must be considered:

1. Inflammatory diseases of the heart: Pain can be present in endocarditis, myocarditis, and pericarditis, but it is more frequent in pericarditis, as the pericardium has a high algogenic sensibility. It must be noted that these diseases are often associated. Pericarditis is often characterized by a deep substernal pain, sometimes by a precordial pain. Pain can be continuous, exacerbated by deep inspiration, cough, and lateral movements of the chest. It may radiate to the left shoulder, scapula, and arm, to the neck, and to the epigastrium. Sometimes it may appear during exertion, resembling angina. Chronic pericarditis is often painless; in some cases a deep, dull, slight pain or a sensation of heaviness or fullness in the chest may be reported.

2. Mitral stenosis: The occurrence of pain in mitral stenosis was considered rather frequent by Hope (13). Vaquez (32) identified a myalgic area on the left interscapulovertebral region, particularly evident in the early phases of mitral stenosis. This pain differs from that of angina: It is located in the left interscapulovertebral area, it is deep and crushing; it is accompanied by deep and/or superficial tenderness in the same area (30). The evolution is typical, because pain begins with the increase of atrial pressure, when the compliance of atrial wall is still unchanged, i.e., in the initial phases of the disease. We may note that today, with the development of cardiac surgery, this type of pain is rarely observed.

3. Aortic stenosis: Pain is described as a typical effort angina and is related to many mechanisms, such as insufficient perfusion of the hypertrophic cardiac muscle, excitation of mechanoreceptors, and possible coronary narrowing. However, we have never observed patients with this type of pain. The occurrence of pain is also described, as a very rare event, in aortic insufficiency; for this type of pain also, which we never observed, we must refer to the literature (6).

4. Cor pulmonale: In chronic cor pulmonale, the occurrence of pain similar to anginal pain is described. Spontaneous or exertional pain in this disorder is characterized by an increase of cyanosis (angor coeruleus). This type of pain is rare.

Pain of angina pectoris and myocardial infarction is commonly called "ischemic pain." However, many pathogenetic aspects are still the object of discussion. As considered above, the importance of mechanical factors and of an ischemic neuropathy has been recently stressed. As regards myocardial infarction, the relationship between coronary thrombosis and myocardial necrosis has been especially discussed. Criticisms have been leveled against the concept that myocardial infarction is always a consequence of coronary thrombosis (1). The biochemical component of pain in ischemic heart disease has also been studied. Different biochemical mechanisms have been considered: increase of lactic acid, release of potassium ions, production of kinins and other pain-producing substances which probably act in concert (30). According to Keele and Armstrong (16), similar biochemical phenomena are active in myocardial infarction and in the diseases due to myonecrosis of skeletal muscles, such as idiopathic myoglobinuria, Haff disease, and sea-snake poisoning. In all these conditions, characterized by a severe long-lasting pain, the fundamental pain-producing mechanism could be the release of pain-producing substances from the necrotic tissue. According to Lunedei (19), the main pain-producing mechanism in angina pectoris is a metabolic disturbance which shows similarities with the mechanism of pain from fibrositis of skeletal muscle: Both in fibrositis and in angina pectoris algogenic conditions may be easily induced by the release of pain-producing substances. On the basis of this concept, an analgesic therapy with aspirin may be especially useful in ischemic heart disease to block the activation of pain-producing substances.

A coronary obstruction with sudden death in patients with angina pectoris was described by Obrastzow and Straschesko (24) in 1910 and by Herrick (11) in 1912. So the nosographic entity of myocardial infarction appeared. It could seem strange that it had never been considered before. However, it is interesting to note that at postmortem examination of patients who were suffering from angina pectoris some authors (5,14,25) had previously observed "scars" in the heart or a particular alteration, called polysarcia adiposa cordis (i.e., a thickening of cardiac wall with fatty infiltration): It may be suggested that these authors had really observed myocardial infarction.

The clinical features of pain in angina pectoris and in myocardial infarction are presented in classical schematic descriptions reported by most textbooks of cardiology. Schematics are useful, but they have not an absolute value. Our school has especially studied this argument (26,29–31). First, it must be considered that a continuum of sensations is observed from the absence of any sensation (as in painless myocardial infarction) to the excruciating pain, with all the possible degrees of pain intensity between these two extremes. Moreover, in myocardial infarction, but sometimes in angina pectoris too, some "common" visceral sensations may be present, such as a sense of malaise or fullness of the stomach, so that the patients may describe their illness as an "indigestion."

Visceral algogenic conditions may give rise to two main types of pain with different characteristics: true visceral pain and referred pain. True visceral pain is often the first type of pain felt by the patients: It is deep, vague, poorly localized, and not well defined; it is frequently accompanied by neurovegetative phenomena, such as nausea, vomiting, and profuse sweating, and by a strong psychic alarm reaction. When a painful process affecting a viscus recurs frequently or becomes more intense and prolonged, the location becomes more exact and the painful sensation is progressively felt in more superficial structures: This phenomenon is usually called "referred pain." Referred pain may be accompanied by hyperalgesia in the skin and in deep somatic structures. In the genesis of referred pain two different mechanisms may be active which, at least in part, overlap: a central convergence of somatic and visceral afferent impulses and the activation of viscerocutaneous and visceromuscular reflexes which induce algogenic conditions in the periphery.

PAIN IN MYOCARDIAL INFARCTION

Pain can arise with different modalities, sometimes suddenly, sometimes preceded by a vague feeling of chest discomfort. This early pain is deep, central, anterior, and sometimes also posterior; it shows the characters of true visceral pain. This kind of pain is present in approximately 80% of patients. It is central, often behind the lower sternum, less frequently in the epigastrium. In approximately 15% of the patients, anterior pain is concomitant with a central back pain; in 1% of the cases, the pain is only posterior. Pain is often accompanied by vegetative symptoms, i.e., nausea, vomiting, and diffuse sweating. A strong alarm reaction is present.

In a following phase, after a period that varies from 10 min to a few hours, pain is referred to the parietal structures, assuming the characteristics of deep somatic pain. In approximately 20% of the patients this is the first perceived pain. In many others, only with a careful anamnesis we can recognize the first episode of true visceral pain. This somatic pain is more exactly localized than visceral pain. It is often accompanied by sweating, but rarely by nausea and vomiting. Pain is often felt in the precordial area, spreading frequently to both upper limbs, more frequently to the left one, rarely only to the right. This radiation can be accompanied by paresthesias, such as tingling, numbness, and sense of constriction of the elbow and wrist. A less common radiation is to the jaw, to the neck, or temporomandibular joints on both sides simultaneously. Pain is sometimes referred also to the back, to the interscapulovertebral region, and may radiate to the ulnar side of the left arm.

Only in 20% of the patients the superficial (dermatomeric) referred pain, described as classical in many textbooks, is present. It is localized in the dermatomes C_8–T_1, that is, in the ulnar side of the left arm and forearm.

In the areas of referred pain a cutaneous primary hyperalgesia, i.e., a lowered pain threshold to nonnoxious stimuli, and a typical muscular tenderness with myalgic spots are often found. It is important to note that there are no correlations between the localization of the infarction and the pattern of pain.

PAIN IN ANGINA PECTORIS

We must note that in effort angina (or stable angina) pain is generally somatic, sometimes superficial, with the same qualities and radiations as those described in myocardial infarction. The intensity and duration are less and the alarm reaction is less intense. In unstable angina, also known as preinfarction angina, pain shows characteristics intermediate between those of infarction and those of stable angina. We can observe a deep visceral pain, but generally less intense than in myocardial infarction. We have, however, observed many cases in which attacks of angina pectoris could not be distinguished, on the basis of the pain felt by the patients, from a myocardial infarction, which occurred later in the same patients, sometimes after months or years. This may explain why astute physicians, as Heberden, Fothergill, Parry, Laënnec, and Trousseau did not distinguish, on the basis of the symptoms, angina pectoris from myocardial infarction (28). Moreover, it is well known that in clinical practice a differential diagnosis of angina pectoris and myocardial infarction based on the characters of pain is sometimes extremely difficult. Only typical ECG changes and the increase of plasma levels of some enzymes, when present, can allow the distinction between a clear angina pectoris and a clear myocardial infarction.

In our investigations we have also considered two problems: (a) mnemonic traces in cardiac pain; (b) intricate syndromes.

As regards mnemonic traces, it has been demonstrated that the mnemonic process is easier if the experience to be retained is repeated many times or is accompanied by pleasant or unpleasant emotions. It has also been demonstrated that pain, as other sensory modalities, is, at least in part, a learned experience (21). This is not a memory in the sense that it can be called to the conscious mind by action of the will. Therefore, the processes of retained painful experience were appropriately termed by Melzack (21) memory-like processes. Nathan (23) observed that in some subjects different kinds of stimuli could call to mind forgotten painful experiences.

We observed that in patients who had suffered from a previous myocardial infarction and in patients with angina pectoris, who were absolutely normal to a complete examination of sensibility, ischemia induced in the arms at rest could provoke an attack of angina pectoris or a pain similar to that perceived during the infarction. Our observations demonstrate that even a nonpainful stimulus, such as ischemia induced by a pneumatic cuff in the limbs at rest, may activate mnemonic traces. Obviously, such mnemonic traces induce a facilitation not only of memory, but also of reflexes; therefore, they may facilitate the onset of further attacks (26,29,31).

The concept of "intricate syndromes" (angors coronariens intriqués) was introduced by Froment and Gonin (7). It has been observed that angina pectoris and even myocardial infarction are more frequent in subjects with another disease in the same or other metameres. The clinical interpretation of these patients is sometimes difficult for a physician. In some cases there is a typical anginal pain, but in many cases there are different patterns of pain, varying from subject to subject, extremely difficult to interpret. As regards the pathogenesis, a summation of painful stimuli arising in the heart and in different structures may occur at a spinal level, as in cervicothoracic painful osteoarthritis and in fibrositis of the muscles of the chest. In other cases, as in osteoarthritis without pain, in hiatal hernia and nonpainful cholecystitis, long-lasting somatovisceral and viscerosomatic reflexes are surely important. These reflexes can induce, more often than is generally thought, a vicious circle: periphery—central nervous system—periphery, as observed in the classical reflex dystrophies. A well-known case is that of scapulohumeral periarthritis following infarction, treated with good results 50 years ago by Leriche and his group with a sympathetic block (18). We have observed that these subjects present many myalgic areas (trigger points) in the muscles of the chest, shoulder, and arm. They also have a low threshold to pain measured with mechanical, thermal, or electrical algometers. This can facilitate, of course, the onset of a vicious circle. On the other hand, when we observe myalgic spots, we must suppose that the peripheral conditions leading to pain, i.e., the release of algogenic substances such as prostaglandins, kinins, histamine, and others, are easier to induce. This is proved by the good results of a therapy with aspirin. The problem that our school and other researchers posed is whether this easier induction of pain-producing substances is limited to the voluntary muscles or is present also in the heart. This point seems important not only from a pathogenetic point of view, but above all from a therapeutic one. In other words, we must consider whether a therapy with aspirin-like drugs is acting on different structures, visceral and somatic. Further investigation is necessary on this point. This demonstrates that heart pain must be considered from a holistic point of view, pathogenetic, clinical, and therapeutic.

REFERENCES

1. Baroldi, G. (1976): Coronary thrombosis: facts and beliefs. *Am. Heart J.,* 91:683–688.
2. Bonet, T. (1700): *Sepulchretum sive Anatomia Practica ex Cadaveribus Morbo Denatis.* Cramer et Perachon, Geneva.
3. Caelius Aurelianus (1722): *De Morbis Acutis et Chronicis.* Wetsteniana, Amsterdam.
4. Castelli, B. (1598): *Lexicon Medicum Graeco-latinum ex Hippocrate et Galeno Desumptum.* Breae, Messanae.
5. Fothergill, J. (1783): *Complete Collection of the Medical and Philosophical Works.* Dilly, London.

6. Friedberg, C. K. (1956): *Diseases of the Heart,* 2nd ed. Saunders, Philadelphia.
7. Froment, R., and Gonin, A. (1956): *Les Angors Coronariens Intriqués.* Expansion Scientifique Française, Paris.
8. Harvey, W. (1766): *Opera Omnia a Collegio Medicorum Londinensi Edita.* Bowyer, London.
9. Heberden, W. (1772): Some account of a disorder of the breast. *Med. Trans. R. Coll. Phys. Lond.,* 2:59–67.
10. Heberden, W. (1802): *Commentaries on the History and Cure of Diseases.* Payne, London.
11. Herrick, J. B. (1912): Clinical features of sudden obstruction of the coronary arteries. *JAMA,* 59:2015–2020.
12. Hippocratis medicorum omnium facile principis opera omnia quae extant. Chouët, Geneva, 1657.
13. Hope, J. (1832): *A Treatise on the Diseases of the Heart.* William Kidd, London.
14. Hunter, J. (1794): *A Treatise on the Blood, Inflammation and Gun-shot Wounds.* Nicol, London.
15. Keele, K. D. (1957): *Anatomies of Pain.* Blackwell, Oxford.
16. Keele, C. A., and Armstrong, D. (1964): *Substances Producing Pain and Itch.* Arnold, London.
17. Lancisi, J. M. (1707): *De Subitaneis Mortibus.* Buagni, Roma.
18. Leriche, R. (1949): *La Chirurgie de la Douleur.* Masson, Paris.
19. Lunedei, A. (1967): Problemi attuali sulla patogenesi della cardiopatia ischemica. *Sett. Med.,* 55:737–739.
20. Malliani, A., and Lombardi, F. (1982): Consideration of the fundamental mechanisms eliciting cardiac pain. *Am. Heart J.,* 103:575–578.
21. Melzack, R. (1973): *The Puzzle of Pain.* Penguin, Harmondsworth.
22. Mercurialis, H. (1627): *Praelectiones Patavinae de Cognoscendis et Curandis Humani Corporis Affectibus.* Junta, Venetiis.
23. Nathan, P. W. (1962): Pain traces left in the central nervous system. In: *The Assessment of Pain in Man and Animals,* edited by C. A. Keele and R. Smith, pp. 129–134. Livingstone, Edinburgh.
24. Obrastzow, W. P., and Straschesko, N. D. (1910): Zur Kenntnis der Thrombose der Koronararterien des Herzens. *Z. Klin. Med.,* 71:116–132.
25. Parry, C. H. (1799): *An Inquiry into the Symptoms and Causes of the Syncope Anginosa, Commonly Called Angina Pectoris.* Cadell and Davis, London.
26. Procacci, P., Buzzelli, G., Voegelin, M. R., and Bozza, G. (1968): Esplorazione della funzione sensitiva degli arti superiori in soggetti con pregresso infarto miocardico. *Rass. Neurol. Veg.,* 22:403–418.
27. Procacci, P., and Maresca, M. (1984): Pain concept in Western civilization: a historical review. In: *Advances in Pain Research and Therapy, Vol. 7,* edited by C. Benedetti, C. R. Chapman, and G. Moricca, pp. 1–11. Raven Press, New York.
28. Procacci, P., and Maresca, M. (1985): Historical considerations of cardiac pain. *Pain,* 22:325–335.
29. Procacci, P., Passeri, I., Zoppi, M., Burzagli, L., Voegelin, M. R., and Maresca, M. (1972): Esplorazione della funzione sensitiva degli arti superiori in soggetti con angina pectoris. *Giorn. Ital. Cardiol.,* 2:978–984.
30. Procacci, P., and Zoppi, M. (1984): Heart pain. In: *Textbook of Pain,* edited by P.D. Wall and R. Melzack, pp. 309–318. Churchill Livingstone, Edinburgh.
31. Procacci, P., Zoppi, M., Padeletti, L., and Maresca, M. (1976): Myocardial infarction without pain. A study of the sensory function of the upper limbs. *Pain,* 2:309–313.
32. Vaquez, H. (1922): *Malattie del cuore.* UTET, Turin.

Advances in Pain Research and Therapy,
Vol. 10. Edited by M. Tiengo et al.
Raven Press, Ltd., New York © 1987.

Cancer Pain and Motility

Vittorio Ventafridda, Augusto Caraceni, Luigi Saita, Alberto
Sbanotto, Elio Spoldi, and Franco De Conno

*Istituto Nazionale per lo Studio e la Cura dei Tumori, Servizio di Terapia del Dolore
20133 Milan, Italy*

Pain is a significantly important symptom of neoplastic disease, the incidence of which increases as the disease progresses. The prevalence of pain in advanced stages of cancer can be estimated at 60% to 80% with solid tumors (3,8). Physical disability caused by or associated with pain produces a worsening in the quality of life of a patient. In fact, the quality of life is less affected by physical pain when performance is normal, than when the suffering interferes with the individual's mobility.

Table 1 shows a list of the principal conditions that cause pain associated with motor deficiency in cancer patients, with the exclusion of causes unrelated to the tumor or to its therapy. It is evident that sensory and motor disturbances can be associated with many of these painful conditions, since the nervous and skeletal structures which respond to these diverse functions are often involved.

Moreover, it is obvious that both the factors inherent in tumor diseases and the iatrogenic factors cause an involvement of the same structures, in particular the nervous system, which are at the origins of the pain symptom and motor deficiency.

On the basis of these considerations we discuss some different syndromes (bone infiltration, peripheral neuropathies, brachial plexus syndromes, lumbosacral syndrome, epidural compression) with particular emphasis on the forms with typical characteristics on the clinical and etiological plane.

BONE METASTASES

The most common cause of pain in the advanced cancer patient is undoubtedly bone involvement (1,8).

Quite different from the primary bone tumor which is relatively rare in man, the secondary bone localization is a frequent and common event in most neoplasms. They are particularly frequent in cancer of the breast, prostate, lung, kidney, and thyroid, which are the causes of 80% of bone metastases; whereas the remaining 10% to 20% are due to cancer of the colon, pancreas, stomach, bladder, uterus, and esophagus.

TABLE 1. *Pain syndromes in patients with cancer*[a]

Pain associated with direct tumor involvement
  Tumor infiltration of bone
    Base-of-skull metastases
      Jugular foramen
      Clivus
      Sphenoid sinus
    Vertebral-body metastases
      Subluxation of the atlas
      C_7–T_1 metastases
      L_1 metastases
      Sacral metastases
  Tumor infiltration of nerve
    Peripheral neuropathy
    Brachial, lumbar, sacral plexopathy
    Meningeal carcinomatosis
    Epidural spinal cord compression
  Tumor infiltration of hollow viscus

Pain associated with cancer therapy
  Pain occurring postsurgery
    Postthoracotomy pain
    Postmastectomy pain
    Postradical neck pain
    Phantom limb pain
  Pain occurring postchemotherapy
    Peripheral neuropathy
    Postherpetic neuralgia
    Steroid pseudo-rheumatism
    Aseptic necrosis of bone
  Pain occurring postradiation therapy
    Radiation fibrosis of the brachial plexus and lumbar plexus
    Radiation myelopathy
    Radiation-induced peripheral nerve tumors

---

[a] From ref. 8.

The bone localizations that can most frequently affect motility are the most significant. In fact, the spina, pelvis, and proximal extremities of the long bones are the most affected sites in relation to not only the nociceptive stimulus, but also the functional impotence which derives from the bone segments involved.

More or less serious concomitant neurological lesions are frequent and often manifest themselves as specific syndromes which cause alterations in the postural capacity of the patient. Metastases at the base of the skull are characterized by pain, and often give rise to neurological clinical manifestations:

1. Jugular foramen syndrome: Cranial nerves IX, X, XI, and XII are involved and produce pain at the top of the head, in the shoulder, and in the homolateral arm, with dysartria, dysphagia, palpebral ptosis, weakness of the neck and shoulder according to the nerves involved;

2. Metastases of the clivus: The pain produced may be at the top of the head exacerbated by movement of the neck and involvement of the cranial nerves V to XII;

3. Metastases of sphenoidal sinus: The pain produced may be an intense bifrontal headache radiating to both temples, with retro-orbital intermittent pain which is, in general, the characteristic symptom of this condition. Unilateral or bilateral paralysis of the cranial nerve VI indicates the diagnosis (8).

Vertebral metastases which are frequent also produce pain, which becomes more acute with movement, functional impotence, and both sensorial and motor neurological dysfunction. In particular, vertebral collapse can cause neurological deficiency which can be irreversible as far as para- and tetraplagia according to the involved level. Clinical signs vary considerably when either the roots or the spinal cord are involved. Involvement of the roots can be recognized by the localization of pain at the metameric level and by dysesthesia which are generally unilateral, as well as by the weakness of some groups of muscles. Involvement of the spinal cord is much more serious due to the often irreversible consequences, both as regards motility and the control of the sphinteric muscles, as discussed below.

NEUROPATHY DUE TO THE TUMOR

Involvement of the peripheral nerves in cancer disease can be caused in several ways: through the direct action of the tumors as in cases of compression, diffuse infiltration, and paraneoplastic syndromes, or as a side effect of therapy. Invasion of the large nerve trunks by a tumor is a fairly rare event with regard to solid tumors (28). In the majority of cases, infiltration is confined to the epinerve, and the bundles can be encapsulated by the tumor without being invaded. The nervous fibers can be completely undamaged or undergo degenerative transformation both by demyelinization and axonic degeneration. Infiltration of the peripheral nerves is more frequent in lymphoma and leukemia conditions. Invasion of the nerve trunks is diffused but not uniform in these diseases, it is concentrated in the subperineural space and along the endoneural septa, and as a principal consequence a Wallerian degeneration is seen which obviously causes atrophy of the skeletal muscles (13).

In the case of nasopharyngeal tumors and those of the paranasal sinuses, the trigeminal nerve can be affected. A case has been described of invasion of the trigeminal branches by a basaloma of the face (18). In these cases motor symptoms can serve to differentiate initial tumor invasion from a simple neuralgia.

Moreover, metastases that involve the base of the skull can cause various syndromes with painful symptoms and associated sensory deficiency. Unsold

(23) reports a case in which all the nerves of a cavernous sinus were affected by a tumor of unknown origin.

It is also obvious that primary bone tumors or metastases situated in strategic positions can occasionally involve an adjacent nerve. Peroneal paralysis with metastases in the fibula is an example (13).

Sensorimotor neuropathy can be experienced as the distant effect of carcinoma, myelomas, and, more seldom, lymphomas (paraneoplastic syndromes). The most frequent sensorimotor form is weakness, increasing often until autonomous movement is impossible, with ataxia and loss of sensation: In 59% of the cases pain is present (7). These polyneuropathies are clinically manifest in approximately 2% to 5% of all patients with cancer; lung tumor is responsible for 50% of sensorimotor neuropathies and of 75% of the purely sensitive forms (6).

NEUROPATHIES OF IATROGENIC ORIGIN

Neuropathies Due to Chemotherapy Drugs

In relation to this assortment of special situations, peripheral neuropathies caused by chemotherapy are much more regular. The drugs which most frequently cause neuropathy are the vinca alkaloids, cisplatin, procarbazine, and, more rarely, misonidazole, and hexamethylamine. Clinical manifestations most frequently to be seen are painful paresthesias, dysesthesias, and burning. The polyneuropathy is most often of a sensorial nature, whereas the motor dysfunction is rare, though areflexia or hyporeflexia are almost constantly present.

Vinca alkaloids in the peripheral nerves cause the destruction of the microtubuli, an accumulation of neurofilaments, and alteration of the axoplasmatic transport. They can cause paresthesias and dysesthesias in up to 100% of the patients treated (24,27). They cause a dose-dependent axonopathy, which is, generally, though not always, reversible when the patients stop taking the drugs. With very low doses of up to 4.5 mg as the total dose of vincristine (5), one can encounter paresthesia and loss of the profound reflexes; muscular pain is another early symptom which is followed by loss of sensibility, this stage is often followed by weakness and muscular atrophy. Electrodiagnostic tests can show a slight reduction in both sensorial and motor conduction velocity and can prove normal where there are clear subjective symptoms (5,19).

Neuropathy as a result of vincristine administration is more common in the elderly patient and in those who suffer from other lesions of the peripheral nervous system. The principal lesion is that of axonal Wallerian degeneration. This condition affects both the large fibers and the thin fibers, and it is more pronounced distally so as to suggest a dying-back phenomenon (12). Muscular biopsies show atrophy due to varying degrees of denervation.

Both cisplatin and procarbazine also produce peripheral neuropathy. High doses of intravenous procarbazine produce some neuropathy in 10% to 15% of cases. Conditions of paresthesia, hyporeflexia, proximal myalgia, and weakness gradually manifest themselves.

A sensorimotor neuropathy can be caused by cisplatin at normal doses with the same manifestations as those caused by vincristine and procarbazine (27).

Neuropathies Due to Surgery and Radiotherapy

Some particular specific and demanding surgery can cause intensely painful syndromes; an example of this is the pain that results from radical dissection of the neck due to the resection of the cervical nerves, with the added complication of motor deficiency from exeresis of the neck muscles. Postmastectomy pain is due mainly to a lesion of the intercostal brachial nerve, whereas lasting or recurrent postthoracotomy pain is often a sign of the return of the neoplastic disease. Irradiation has proved toxic for peripheral nerves in animal models. Radiation-induced insurgence of tumors of the peripheral nerves has been reported in the literature (10).

BRACHIAL PLEXOPATHY

A lesion of the brachial plexus of cancer patients can have various causes:

1. Trauma during anesthesia and surgery;
2. Direct metastatic involvement of the plexus;
3. Irradiation damage;
4. Cancer of the plexus induced by radiotherapy.

Involvement of the brachial plexus in a patient who has been treated by radiotherapy also on the plexus always presents the problems of differentiation of the diagnosis between recurrence of the disease and irradiation-induced plexopathy. The problem has been discussed by many authors from the point of view of the clinical aspects as well as the data provided by several diagnostic tools (16,17). No clinical or instrumental criteria exist by which diagnosis of plexopathy can be established absolutely as neoplastic or as caused by irradiation; even a surgical exploration is sometimes not able to answer this question (16). It seems to us that some factors may be usefully presented for a diagnosis of probability.

Neoplastic infiltration of the brachial plexus derives most commonly from breast cancer as well as from a broncogenic tumor (20). As far as the relationship between plexopathy and irradiation is concerned, it has been observed that patients with irradiation-induced tumors had generally undergone radiation in excess of 6,000 rad, and that an interval of more than a year between therapy and first symptoms related positively to irradiation-

TABLE 2. *Clinical signs in lumbosacral plexopathy secondary to cancer[ab]*

Leg weakness	86%
Sensory loss	73%
Reflex asymmetry	64%
Focal tenderness	55%[c]
+ Direct SLRT[d]	53%
Leg edema	47%
+ Reverse SLRT	45%
Rectal mass	39%
Dysesthesias	15%
Decreased sphinteric tone	12%
Fasciculations	12%

[a] $n = 85$.
[b] From ref. 14.
[c] Bilateral in 18%.
[d] SLRT = staight leg-raising tests.

induced plexopathy (2,16). The initial symptoms seem to bear particular significance for these two situations. Pain is the dominating symptom in neoplastic invasion and it tends to worsen and persist, whereas it is present less frequently and is nonlasting with irradiation-induced tumors. Paresthesia seems to be predominant in irradiation-induced lesions; motor deficiency as an early symptom is not frequent, but it is more or less constant in the progression of both forms. Emphasis has been laid on the prevalence in patients with radiation-induced plexopathy of involvement, mainly, of the C_5-C_6 innervated muscles, and for patients with neoplastic forms involvement of the muscles innervated from C_8-T_1 (16). The Claude-Bernard Horner syndrome is much more frequent in the neoplastic forms, whereas lymphoedema appears to be slightly more frequent in the irradiation-induced forms. Another frequent symptom is reduced sweating.

Of the instrumental methods of diagnosis, the computerized tomography (CT) scan can provide sufficiently clear images of the tumor masses which invade the plexus areas, but it cannot provide incontrovertible facts in the case of irradiation-induced lesions. Electromyography identifies atrophied muscles; and in irradiation-induced plexopathy patients, greater frequency in spontaneous activity manifested as fasciculations and myokimia has been reported (17).

We would point out that tumoral involvement of the plexus can also develop an epidural invasion which can be revealed by CT scan or by myelograph.

LUMBOSACRAL PLEXOPATHY

One of the most disabling complications in pelvic tumors is the lesion of the lumbosacral plexus, as it causes motor deficiency even as far as a plegic

TABLE 3. Clinical symptoms in lumbosacral plexopathy secondary to cancer[a,b]

Symptom	At presentation (%)	During disease course (%)
Pain	91	98
Numbness	18	42
Weakness	15	60
Paresthesias	13	33
Incontinence	5	9
Impotence	11[c]	11[c]

[a] n = 85.
[b] From ref. 14.
[c] Men only.

state, and it is accompanied by intense pain. Primary tumors causing lumbosacral plexopathy are colorectal cancer followed by sarcoma, cancer of the breast, and cancers affecting the genitourinary tract (14).

For a differential diagnosis of sacral plexus lesions with regard to epidural, caudal, or nerve root compression, the clinical and instrumental tools should be assessed (CT scan, bone scintigraphy with examination of the spine, myelography, electromyography).

The symptoms and the clinical features present with different frequencies (Tables 2 and 3). Pain is the initial manifestation in the typical evolution of symptoms; in some patients it is the only symptom. Pain presents according to three modalities: local, referred, or radicular, followed by loss of sensibility, parasthesia, asymmetry of the reflexes, or muscular weakness, which in many cases may develop into focal muscular paralysis which can arise weeks or months from the onset of symptoms. The progressive worsening of symptoms and other features discussed develop along with the progression of the disease. It should be noted that in a smaller number of cases extrapelvic tumor metastases can also provoke the compression of the plexus.

Epidural involvement was seen on myelographs in 45% of the cases at T_{10} level or lower, lesions above the conus medullaris are rather rare (16% of cases) (14). Invasion of the lumbosacral plexus presents a bad short-term prognosis. When epidural infiltration is suspected, the most useful diagnostic method is myelography for this type of disease.

EPIDURAL COMPRESSION

Involvement of the spinal cord is a fairly frequent complication of systemic neoplasias (5%–10%) (13), damage to the spinal cord can be caused by tumor growth in the epidural space, or by direct invasion of the parenchyma. Epidural metastatic compression is significantly more frequent than the latter case.

TABLE 4. *Karnofsky performance status scale*

Patient status	Performance status	Description
Able to carry on normal activity and to work; no special care is needed.	100	Normal; no complaints; no evidence of disease.
	90	Able to carry on normal activity; minor signs or symptoms of disease.
	80	Normal activity with effort; some signs or symptoms of disease.
Unable to work; able to live at home and care for most personal needs; a varying degree of assistance is needed.	70	Cares for self; unable to carry on normal activity or to do active work.
	60	Requires occasional assistance, but is able to care for most of own needs.
	50	Requires considerable assistance and frequent medical care.
Unable to care for self; Requires equivalent of institutional or hospital care; disease may be progressing rapidly.	40	Disabled; requires special care and assistance.
	30	Severely disabled; hospitalization is indicated although death not imminent
	20	Hospitalization necessary, very sick, active supportive treatment necessary
	10	Moribund; fatal processes progressing rapidly.
	0	Dead.

The tumors that most frequently cause epidural compression, generally following vertebral involvement, are breast, lung, and prostate cancer; lymphomas and sarcomas: The growth of paravertebral tumors through the intervertebral foramina is a rare event, but is characteristic of lymphoma and neuroblastoma progression.

In the clinical picture, regularly 90% of patients present back pain localized at the affected area and, in the majority of cases, associated with radicular pain (4,11). The disease develops after days or weeks towards motor deficiency which progresses to paraplegia. If the state of paraplegia is reached rapidly, a weak paralysis may set in, with reduced or abolished reflexes. When progression to paraplegia is less acute, a spastic state develops and reflexes are increased (13). Sensorial symptoms such as paresthesia and sensory deficiency are less common at the beginning.

The examination of choice in the case of epidural compression is myelography. Differential diagnosis is performed with intraspinal cord metastases, dislocated discs, radiation-induced myelopathy, epidural hematomas, and abcesses.

TABLE 5. *Eastern Cooperative Oncology Group (ECOG)
performance status score*

Score	Description
0	Normal activity.
1	Symptoms but nearly fully ambulatory.
2	Some bed time, but needs to be in bed less than 50% of the normal daytime.
3	Needs to be in bed greater than 50% of normal daytime.
4	Unable to get out of bed.

PRINCIPLES OF THERAPY

The control of pain in advanced cancer patients is one of the most difficult tasks in modern medicine. When pain is accompanied by motor deficiency, an extra special effort is required.

The essential step in starting on therapy is the assessment of pain. As well as the symptom of pain itself, emotional, socioenvironmental, and performance factors must be considered. The most simple instrument for the assessment of the performance of the patient is the Karnofsky scale (15) (Table 4) and the Eastern Cooperative Oncology Group (ECOG) test (Table 5). The numerical codification that should be allocated at the first visit and at subsequent checks of the performance status is of great importance because these values should be kept elevated in the therapeutic strategy.

Undoubtedly, pain interferes considerably with a person's mobility, as has been shown in our study which has examined the assessment parameters of pain and the overall conditions of the patients (21). The correlation between

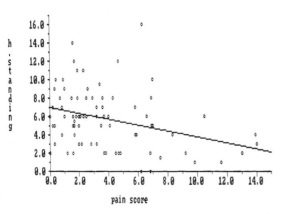

FIG. 1. Relationship between the pain score and the hours of standing of 81 patients. Regression equation: $y = 7.03 - 0.03 x$. The slope of this line is significantly different from 0 ($p < 0.01$).

the number of hours spent standing and the score which integrates the values of intensity and duration of pain (25) on 81 patients show how a lower capacity of mobility corresponds to the greater intensity of pain ($r = -0.32$, $p < 0.01$, Pearson's correlation) (Fig. 1).

Following a careful assessment of the suffering and its interference with motor activity, therapeutic strategy foresees as a first step the analgesic treatment planned as follows:

1. The gradually sequential application of the drugs, from the anti-inflammatory drugs through the weak opioids to the strong opioids, paying particular attention to the various ways of administrating opioids and the indications for their use. Moreover, adjuvant steroid and psychotropic drugs are also associated (9,22,26). In the meantime, any specific or palliative anticancer treatment like hormonal chemotherapy or radiotherapy should be carried out if necessary;
2. The interruption of the pain pathways with neurolesive techniques selective for the sensitive routes whenever the clinical situation demands.

The objectives of this type of intervention, in order of importance are: (a) an increase in the hours of sleep; (b) an increase in the static pain-free hours, for example, with mobilization in a wheel chair; and (c) an increase in incidental pain-free hours, both for spontaneous deambulation and with the use of orthopedic prostheses.

Moreover, in order to guarantee surgery aimed specifically at pain and the preservation of motility, even though reduced, it is necessary to:

1. Carry out a depistage of possible pathological fractures;
2. Guarantee a lower load position, both in the active and in the passive state;
3. Immobilize, where necessary, with orthopedic aids, in a wheel chair, or in bed, paying particular attention to bed sores;
4. Educate towards a palliative rehabilitation which will give the patient the possibility of leading a possibly autonomous life with mechanical means;
5. Provide for physiotherapy, when indicated, based on suitable motor rehabilitation exercises, massage therapy, and thermal applications (hot and cold packs).

When undertaking neurolesive treatment the sensorial and motor dysfunctions that can result must be borne in mind. Among the techniques performed most frequently are percutaneous cervical cordotomy, chemical sacral rhizotomy, glossopharyngeal and trigeminal rhizotomies, and the alcoholization of the celiac ganglion. Each technique is selected according to the site of the nociception, the general condition of the patient, and the response to the drugs.

A review of world literature from 1979 to 1983 has been done and on the basis of a study of 76 works the following data were extrapolated:

1. Percutaneous cervical cordotomy (714 patients and 835 operations): paralysis, 1%; paresis, 11%; ataxia, 4%.
2. Sacral rhizotomy (961 patients and 1,118 operations): motor deficiency, 5.5%; sphinteric deficiency, 3%; paresthesia, 0.5%.
3. Glossopharyngeal or trigeminal rhizotomy (494 patients and 160 operations): sensorial deficiency, 37.5%; swallowing problems, 37.5%.
4. Alcoholic gangliolysis of the celiac ganglion (494 patients and 551 operations): orthostatic hypotension, 53%.

Considering the low percentages, the question of motor side effects due to antipain intervention seems not very important, but, at the same time, it should not be underestimated if one is treating pain and wishing to guarantee the patient a good quality of life, and consequently his spontaneous mobility.

CONCLUSIONS

Chronic pain in the cancer patient is a sign of a reduced span of survival, there is a decrease in the physical capacity of these patients due to the irreversible biological process. Immobilization and the need to live with this state can last for weeks or even months. In these cases, therefore, the therapeutic approach cannot of itself be the answer to these situations if it is not accompanied by adequate assistants capable of maintaining communication with the patient, and overall continuous care.

REFERENCES

1. Baines, M., and Kirkbam, S. (1984): V. Carcinoma involving bone and soft tissue. In: *Textbook of Pain,* edited by P. D. Wall and R. Melzack, pp. 453–459. Churchill Livingston, Edinburgh.
2. Basso-Ricci, S., Della Costa, C., Viganotti, G., Ventafridda, V., and Zanolla, R. (1980): Report on 42 cases of postirradiation lesions of the brachial plexus and their treatment. *Tumori,* 66:117–122.
3. Bonica, J. J. (1985): Treatment of cancer pain: Current status and future needs. In: *Advances in Pain Research and Therapy, Vol. 9,* edited by H. L. Fields, F. Dubner, and F. Cervero, pp. 589–616. Raven Press, New York.
4. Brice, J., and McKissock, W. S. (1965): Surgical treatment of malignant extradural spinal tumours. *Br. Med. J.,* 1:1339–1342.
5. Casey, E. B., Jellife, A. M., LeQuesne, P. M., and Millet, Y. L. (1973): Vincristine neuropathy. clinical and electrophysiological observations. *Brain,* 96:69–86.
6. Croft, P. B., and Wilkinson, M. I. P. (1965): The incidence of carcinomatous neuromyopathy in patients with various types of carcinoma. *Brain,* 88:427–434.
7. Davis, L. E., and Drachman, D. B. (1972): Myeloma neuropathy: successful treatment of two patients and a review case. *Arch. Neurol.,* 27:507–511.
8. Foley, K. M. (1979): Pain syndromes in patients with cancer. In: *Advances in Pain Research and Therapy, Vol. 2,* edited by J. J. Bonica and V. Ventafridda, pp. 59–74. Raven Press, New York.
9. Foley, K. M. (1985): The treatment of cancer pain. *N. Engl. J. Med.,* 313:84–95.

10. Foley, K. M., Woodruff, J. M., Ellis, F. T., and Posner, J. B. (1980): Radiation-induced malignant and atypical peripheral nerve sheath tumors. *Ann. Neurol.*, 7:311–318.
11. Gilbert, K. W., Kim, J. H., and Posner, J. B. (1978): Epidural spinal cord compression from metastatic tumours diagnosis and treatment. *Ann. Neurol.*, 3:40–50.
12. Guiheneuc, P., Ginet, J., and Groelau, J. Y. (1980): Early phase in vincristine neuropathy in man. Electrophysiological evidence of dying-back phenomenon, with transitory enhancement of spinal transmission of monosynaptic reflex. *J. Neurol. Sci.*, 45:355–366.
13. Henson, R. A., and Urich, H. (1982): *Cancer and the Nervous System. The Neurological Manifestations of Systemic Malignant Disease*. Blackwell, Oxford.
14. Jeackle, K. A., Young, D. F., and Foley, K. M. (1985): The natural history of lumbosacral plexopathy in cancer. *Neurology*, 35:8–15.
15. Karnofsky, D. A., and Burchenal, J. H. (1949): The clinical evaluation of chemotherapeutic agents in cancer. In: *Evaluation of Chemotherapeutic Agents*, edited by C. M. McLeod, pp. 191–205. Columbia University Press, New York.
16. Kori, S. H., Foley, K. M., and Posner, J. B. (1981): Brachial plexus lesions in patients with cancer: 100 cases. *Neurology (NY)*, 31:45–50.
17. Lederman, R. J. and Wilbourn, J. (1984): Brachial plexopathy: Recurrent cancer or radiation? *Neurology*, 34:1331–1335.
18. Mark, G. J. (1977): Basal cell carcinoma with intraneural invasion. *Cancer*, 40:2181–2187.
19. McLeod, J. G., and Penny, R. (1969): Vincristine neuropathy: an electrophysiological and histological study. *J. Neurol. Neurosurg. Psychiatry*, 32:297–304.
20. Pancoast, H. K. (1932): Superior pulmonary sulcus tumour. *JAMA*, 99:1391–1396.
21. Tamburini, M., Selmi, S., De Conno, F., and Ventafridda, V. (1987): Semantic descriptors of pain. *Pain*, 25:187–193.
22. Twycross, R. G., and Lack, S. A. (editor) (1978): *Symptom Control Care of Terminal Cancer Patients*. Pergamon Press, London.
23. Unsold, R., Safran, A. B., Safran, E., et al. (1980): Metastatic infiltration of nerves in the cavernous sinus. *Arch. Neurol.*, 37:59–61.
24. Ventafridda, V. De Conno, F., Gallucci, M., and Ripamonti, C. (1985): Sequele e complicanze algiche in terapia oncologica. *Argomenti di Oncologia*, 6:249–258.
25. Ventafridda, V., De Conno, F., Di Trapani, P., Gallico, S., Guarise, G., Rigamonti, G., and Tamburini M. (1983): A new method of pain quantification based on a weekly self-descriptive record of the intensity and duration of pain. In: *Advances in Pain Research and Therapy, Vol. 5*, edited by J. J. Bonica et al., pp. 891–895. Raven Press, New York.
26. Ventafridda, V., Tamburini, M., and De Conno, F. (1985). Comprehensive Treatment in Cancer Pain. In: *Advances in Pain Research and Therapy, Vol. 9*, edited by H. L. Fields et al., pp. 617–628. Raven Press, New York.
27. Young, D. F., and Posner J. B. (1980): Nervous system toxicity of chemotherapeutic agents. In: *Handbook of Clinical Neurology*, edited by P. J. Vinken and G. W. Bruyen, pp. 91–129. North-Holland, Amsterdam.
28. Willis, R. A. (1973): *The Spread of Tumours in the Human Body*. Butterworth, London.

Advances in Pain Research and Therapy,
Vol. 10. Edited by M. Tiengo et al.
Raven Press, Ltd., New York © 1987.

Persistent Pain and Motor Behavior in Different Experimental Conditions

Giancarlo Carli

Institute of Human Physiology, 53100 Siena, Italy

Experimental pain in animals may be classified as transient or persistent pain according to the duration of the motor reactions and the presence and amount of tissue injury. Formalin is one the irritants which induce a class of edema characterized by insensitivity to both antiallergic and antirheumatic drugs, and there is some evidence that these edemas result from direct tissue damage (2). The formalin test is a convenient method for producing persistent nociceptive responses in freely moving animals. Pain intensity may be inferred from objective motor responses which are not only specifically related to the site of the stimulus, but may also indicate changes occurring in the general state of the animal. Recent experiments in anesthetized rats (19) have shown that cutaneous polymodal nociceptors are readily excited by formalin injection. This irritative response, which lasts a few minutes, is followed by a subsequent sensitization which is characterized by a transient but prominent increase in heat-evoked discharge and by a long-lasting decrease in the thermal threshold (19). In humans, formalin elicits a sensation similar to a bee sting, which is definitely pain and which lasts for a reasonable duration.

A series of recent experiments has shown that formalin, tail-flick, and hot-plate tests each reveal different components of the mechanisms of pain and analgesia. For instance, when the periaqueductal gray is stimulated, much less electrical current is necessary to produce analgesia in the formalin test than in the other tests (7). In general, the formalin test is more sensitive to the effects of some analgesic drugs or transmitters, while tail-flick and hot-plate are more resistant to others (8). Moreover, investigations in morphine-tolerant rats have shown a rapid tolerance in the tail-flick test, but little or no tolerance in the formalin test (1). It has been suggested that the results with the formalin test are clearly like those observed in people suffering chronic severe pain (1).

Our studies have focused on the effects of formalin pain on several models of integrative functions such as sleep-wakefulness patterns, tonic immobility, and exploratory activity. We have combined behavioral and electrophysiological methods, since, in freely moving animals they may provide crucial

TABLE 1. *Modifications of sleep stages latencies following persistent pain*[a]

Sleep stage[b]	Group A		Group B	
	Control	Day 1	Control	Day 1
LS	15.1 ± 21.5	213.7 ± 98.6	9.7 ± 10.6	121.5 ± 19.1
DS	23.3 ± 20.7	290.7 ± 165.2	24.7 ± 13.7	198.2 ± 85.8
REM	145.0 ± 91.8	1027.8 ± 364.3	89.5 ± 6.7	408.7 ± 149.5

[a] Sleep stage latencies (minutes).
[b] LS: light, slow-wave sleep; DS: deep, slow-wave sleep; REM: rapid-eye-movement sleep.

information about the changes in the excitability of the central nervous system. In several models we have also compared the effects of two different levels of pain intensity to test the hypothesis that the intensity of the stimulus may play a critical role in the quality of the response.

SLEEP

Acute and chronic pain is known to impede initiation and maintenance of sleeping state in humans. The purpose of this work is to investigate the sequence of modifications of sleep and pain parameters in a condition of persistent nociceptive stimulation.

In freely moving cats carrying implanted electrodes, continuous polygraphic and behavioral recordings were collected 24 hr/day for several consecutive days before and after treatment. Sleep stages were classified according to Ursin (21) as LS (light, slow-wave sleep), DS (deep, slow-wave sleep), and REM (rapid-eye-movement sleep). The amount of each sleep stage was expressed for each animal as a percentage of 24-hr recording time. Animals were grouped according to treatment: Group A was injected with 2 ml of 37% formalin, and group B received 0.5 ml of 8% formalin.

Formalin injection was followed by a period of continuous wakefulness which lasted a few hours (Table 1, latency of LS). In all animals of both groups the appearance of LS, DS, and REM was significantly delayed with respect to the controls (Table 1, paired t-test, $p < 0.005$). Although the latencies in group B on the day of injection (day 1) appeared shorter than in group A in all stages, they resulted significantly different only for REM (student t-test, $p < 0.025$).

In group A on day 1 of pain, the mean percentage of LS did not differ from controls, whereas DS and REM were greatly decreased (Table 2). Moreover, LS amount, as soon as present in absence of the other sleep stages, reached control levels. As for pain signs, at the site of injection there was a gradual development of edema which lasted 2 to 5 days. All animals displayed leg flexion, favoring of the injected foot, and limping during loco-

TABLE 2. *Effects of high pain on daily percentage of sleep stages[a]*

| Group | Sleep stage[b] | | | Total |
	LS	DS	REM	
Control	11.5 ± 3.0	34.7 ± 9.3	8.7 ± 2.9	54.9 ± 1.0
Day 1	10.3 ± 4.9	21.3 ± 5.6	2.3 ± 2.2	32.1 ± 1.5
Paired				
t-test	ns	$p < 0.025$	$p < 0.001$	$p < 0.001$

[a] High pain = Group A.
[b] LS: light, slow-wave sleep; DS: deep, slow-wave sleep; REM: rapid-eye-movement sleep.

motion. Episodes of licking and biting the injected foot, scored only when lasting more than 30 sec (1 unit = 30 sec), occurred during wakefulness initially and later in between sleep stages on day 1 and 2 of pain. Figure 1 shows that licking episodes gradually decrease while the total amount of sleep (LS + DS + REM) increases. The electromyogram (EMG) activity of the tibialis anterior muscle, the flexor muscle of the injected foot, showed a sharp increase in the early 4 to 6 hr after injection, thus indicating a condition of continuous nociceptive input. A moderate increase in the EMG could persist for 3 to 4 days during wakefulness, LS and DS, but was replaced by an atonia during REM.

In group B, sleep recovery occurred sooner and, on day 1, the amount of LS, DS, and REM did not differ from control levels. Moreover, LS resulted initially increased in absence of the other sleep stages. The behavioral and the local manifestations of pain were present only during day 1 of pain.

In conclusion, results suggest that (a) the absolute insomnia elicited by formalin pain is not long-lasting; (b) once present, LS amount is not reduced, and, initially, in absence of the other sleep stages may be actually increased when the level of pain is not too high as in group B; (c) signs of pain, such as increase in the EMG activity in the flexor muscle, may be present during some sleep stages; and (d) sleep stages' latency and amount are differentially affected by the treatment with painful stimuli, the REM sleep being the most vulnerable period.

TONIC IMMOBILITY

In several animal species (e.g., rabbits), transient physical restraint is a very effective stimulus to elicit tonic immobility. The immobility response, which may last several minutes and is often indicated as animal hypnosis, has been regarded as the last defensive resort that an animal displays against a predator (18). The emotional aspects of the immobility reaction have been recognized, and the response itself is favored by fear stimuli (12). The main

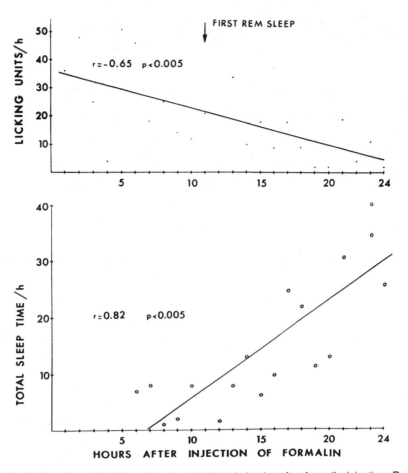

FIG. 1. Temporal modifications of pain and sleep behavior after formalin injection. Results from a single experiment (cat no. 6), Group A (2 ml of formalin at 37%). **Top:** licking units/hr. **Bottom:** total sleep time (LS + DS + REM). Note that the absolute insomnia lasted approximately 6 hr and that the first episode of REM occurred only 11 hr after the formalin injection.

physiological characteristics of animal hypnosis in the rabbit are: (a) tendency to develop high-voltage slow waves in the electrocorticogram (ECoG) (4,15); (b) reduction in frequency and amount in the hippocampal rhythmic activity (θ-rhythm) (10); (c) depression of cerebral glucose utilization (17); (d) decreased levels of serotonin (5-HT) in the brain (9); and (e) depression of spinal mono- and polysynaptic reflexes (4).

It was the purpose of the present work to study the effects of different levels of pain on the duration of the immobility response.

Experiments were performed on freely moving rabbits carrying implanted electrodes for recording the ECoG and EMG of the tibialis anterior muscle.

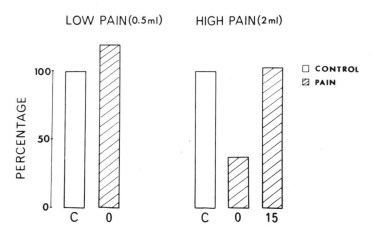

FIG. 2. Effects of pain on the duration of tonic immobility. Changes in duration are expressed as percentage of the mean duration of tonic immobility in control condition (C). Two different groups of animals. Induction of immobility occurred immediately after formalin injection (O) and after 15 min (15). **Right** (high pain): the duration of trial O is significantly reduced (paired *t*-test, *p* < 0.05).

Persistent pain was elicited by formalin by using the two doses previously described in sleep studies.

As in cats, the injection of formalin-saline (0.5 ml at 8%) in rabbits produced long-lasting ECoG low-voltage fast waves typical of wakefulness, accompanied by licking and shifting movements, tonic increase in the EMG activity of the tibialis anterior muscle of the injected limb, as well as thumping behavior. If the procedure of immobility induction was applied immediately after the induction, the response could be easily induced and all the pain reactions were suddenly suppressed. The duration of the immobility and the amount of high-voltage slow waves in the ECoG during the immobility reached similar values as that in control conditions in absence of the pain stimulus (Fig. 2, left). Moreover the tonic increase in the EMG activity of the tibialis anterior muscle was temporarily abolished and hypotonia was recorded. After the end of the immobility response all the pain reactions immediately resumed (6).

In a second group of animals the larger dose of formalin (2 ml, 37%) was followed by the induction of two immobility responses, the first immediately after the injection, the second 15 min later. The first postinjection episode of immobility was characterized by a shorter duration and a decreased amount in the EEG high-voltage slow waves than in the control condition (Fig. 2, right). In the second postinjection episode the duration of the immobility response and the amount of EEG high-voltage slow waves were again at basal levels (Fig. 2, right). In both episodes of immobility the reduction in the EMG activity of the tibialis anterior muscle was recorded (6).

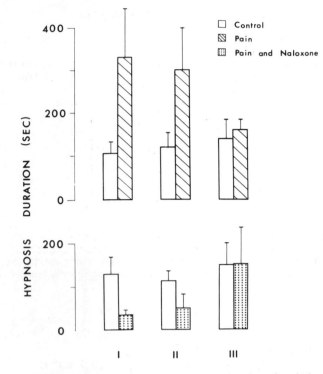

FIG. 3. Effects of pain and pain plus naloxone on the duration of tonic immobility (animal hypnosis). I, II, III: mean duration of postinjection trials compared to the corresponding trials of the control day. **Top:** prolonged nociceptive stimulation (2 ml, 37%) potentiated immobility duration of trials I and II (paired *t*-test, *p* < 0.05). Trial I was induced 5 min after formalin injection. **Bottom:** different group of animals. Naloxone (5 mg/kg, i.m.), injected 3 min after formalin and 2 min before trial I, strongly reduced the duration of trial I (*p* < 0.001) and II (*p* < 0.05). Note that both pain and pain + naloxone did not affect the duration of trial III. (From ref. 5.)

In another group of animals, injected with the larger dose of formalin, three uninterrupted episodes of immobility were elicited starting 5 min after injection (5). In this instance, a clear-cut short-lasting (approximately 10 min) potentiation in the duration occurred in the two postinjection trials, while the last trial was again at basal levels (Fig. 3, top). This potentiation in duration was abolished when animals were pretreated with naloxone (5 mg/kg, i.m.) and replaced by a short reduction (Fig. 3, bottom). In absence of pain, the same doses of naloxone did not affect the duration of the immobility and only higher doses (15 mg/kg) could reduce the response (5).

Results provide the following indications about the mechanisms of pain and tonic immobility: (a) the immobility response may be elicited in a condition of persistent pain; (b) during tonic immobility all behavioral and polygraphic parameters related to the pain response are temporarily abolished; (c) high pain is able to elicit a biphasic effect, an initial decrease followed by a potentiation, thus suggesting that two opposite mechanisms may be triggered with a different latency and/or may depend on pain intensity; (d) the potentiation in immobility duration might be due to an opiate mechanism which is silent or very weak in normal conditions, and is triggered by some levels of persistent pain during tonic immobility.

EXPLORATORY ACTIVITY

Exploratory behavior in animals has been associated with attention and emotionality and a relationship between fear and emotionality has also been proposed (13). Novel stimuli seem to be effective not only in generating orienting responses, exploration, and anxiety, but also inhibition of ongoing behavior as well as increment in arousal and attention. The hippocampus seems to be essential for exploratory behavior (16) and the hippocampal rhythmic slow activity (RSA) has been related to arousal, selective attention, orienting response, learning, and voluntary movements (13). In some animal species RSA occurs only during voluntary movements, but in rabbits a low-frequency RSA may be recorded also during immobility.

In a previous research we have used rabbits in a simultaneous study of their behavioral and neural activity in three different experimental situations containing components of novelty and fear (11). In particular the activity of the dorsal hippocampus was recorded in the following experimental situations: (a) novel environment (NE) consisting of the experimental cage; (b) the same environment with an object (O); (c) the same environment with a stuffed sparrow hawk (SP). At the same time behavioral elements were collected and then analyzed in two main categories: exploratory elements directed towards the environment and exploratory activity elicited by the stimulus (11). RSA was also analyzed during movements and during spontaneous immobility. The same experimental model has been adopted to study the effects of persistent pain.

During control conditions, in absence of pain, rabbits displayed in NE a certain amount of exploratory activity which was expressed by the total number of elements and their duration. The exploratory activity was reduced when an object (O), a cup full of cabbage, was introduced in the experimental cage and remained at lower levels when the object was removed and replaced by an SP. Animals were divided in two groups according to treatment, i.e., low and high doses of formalin as in the experiments on sleep and tonic immobility. Low pain increased the duration of exploratory elements during NE. Such an increase, however was suppressed during O and SP. As for the hippocampus, RSA did not change in frequency and amount both during movement and during spontaneous immobility. On the contrary, in the high-pain group, exploratory activity was sharply reduced in all three experimental conditions.

Summing up, exploratory activity is affected by emotional influences and by persistent pain. Low and high pain elicit opposite modifications on exploratory activity. The mechanisms involved have not yet been investigated and only working hypotheses may be proposed. The increase in exploratory activity by low pain could be due to the activation of some arousing stimuli, as suggested by the increase in the frequency of hippocampal RSA. The reduction in exploratory activity, on the other hand, could be related to a release of some endogenous opiates, which is known to occur following stress and/or pain (20) and to reduce general motor activity (3,14).

CONCLUSIONS

Results show that persistent pain greatly affects sleep patterns, tonic immobility, and exploratory activity. These modifications are not univocal and depend on several mechanisms differentially activated by the level of pain intensity.

REFERENCES

1. Abbott, F. V., Melzack, R., and Leber, B. F. (1982): Morphine analgesia and tolerance in the tail-flick and formalin tests: Dose-response relationships. *Pharmacol. Biochem. Behav.,* 17:1213–1219.
2. Bonta, I. L. (1969): Microvascular lesions as a target of anti-inflammatory and certain other drugs. *Acta Physiol. Pharmacol. Neerl.,* 15:188–222.
3. Bloom, F., Segal, D., Ling, N., and Guillemin, R. (1976): Endorphins: Profound behavioral effects in rats suggest new etiological factors in mental illness. *Science,* 194:630–632.
4. Carli, G. (1969): Dissociation of electrocortical activity and somatic reflexes during rabbit hypnosis. *Arch. Ital. Biol.,* 107:219–234.
5. Carli, G., Farabollini, F., and Fontani, G. (1981): Effects of pain, morphine and naloxone on the duration of animal hypnosis. *Behav. Brain Res.,* 2:373–385.
6. Carli, G., Lefebvre, L., Silvano, G., and Vierucci, S. (1976): Suppression of accompanying reactions to prolonged noxious stimulation during animal hypnosis in the rabbit. *Exp. Neurol.,* 53:1–11.
7. Dennis, S. G., Choinière, M., and Melzack, R. (1980): Stimulation-produced analgesia in rats: assessment by two pain tests and correlation with self-stimulation. *Exp.Neurol.,* 68:295–309.
8. Dennis, S. G., Melzack, R., Gutman, S., and Boucher, F. (1980): Pain modulation by adrenergic agents and morphine as measured by three pain tests. *Life Sci.,* 26:1247–1259.
9. Farabollini, F., Carli, G., and Lupo, C. (1984): Changes in brain serotonin and 5-hydroxyindolacetic acid levels in the rabbit following tonic immobility. *Physiol. Behav.,* 32:205–209.
10. Fontani, G., Grazzi, F., Lombardi, G., and Carli, G. (1982): Hippocampal rhythmic slow activity (RSA) during animal hypnosis in the rabbit. *Behav. Brain Res.,* 6:15–24.
11. Fontani, G., Farabollini, F., and Carli, G. (1984): Hippocampal electrical activity and behavior in the presence of novel environmental stimuli in rabbits. *Behav. Brain Res.,* 13:231–240.
12. Gallup, G. C. (1977): Tonic immobility: the role of fear in predation. *Psychol.Rec.,* 27 (Suppl. 1):41–61.
13. Gray, J. A. (1982): *The Neuropsychology of Anxiety: An Enquiry into the Functions of the Septo-hippocampal system.* Oxford University Press, Oxford.
14. Jacquet, Y. F., and Marks, N. (1976): The C-fragment of β-lipotropin: an endogenous neuroleptic or antipsychotogen? *Science,* 194:632–635.

15. Klemm, W. R. (1966): Electroencephalographic-behavioral dissociations during animal hypnosis. *Electroencephalogr. Clin. Nuerophysiol.,* 21:365–372.
16. O'Keefe, J., and Nadel, L. (1978): *The Hippocampus as a Cognitive Map,* pp. 163–190. Oxford University Press, Oxford.
17. Passero, S., Carli, G., and Battistini, N. (1981): Depression of cerebral glucose utilization during animal hypnosis in the rabbit. *Neurosci.Lett.,* 21:345–349.
18. Ratner, S. C. (1967): Comparative aspects of hypnosis. In: *Handbook of Clinical and Experimental Hypnosis,* edited by J. E. Gordon, pp. 550–587. MacMillan, New York.
19. Reeh, P. W., Handwerker, H. O., and Carli, G. (1987): Effects of formalin on cutaneous nociceptors (*in press*).
20. Rossier, J., French, E. D., Rivier, C., Ling, N., Guillemin, R., and Bloom, F. (1977): Foot-shock induced stress increases β-endorphin levels in blood but not brain. *Nature,* 270:618–620.
21. Ursin, R. (1968): The two stages of slow wave sleep in the cat and their relation to REM sleep. *Brain Res.,* 11:347–356.

Advances in Pain Research and Therapy,
Vol. 10. Edited by M. Tiengo et al.
Raven Press, Ltd., New York © 1987.

Peripheral Nerve Deafferentation Affects Brain and Spinal Cord Neuropeptides: Lateralization and Pharmacological Treatments

Alberto E. Panerai, Paola Sacerdote, Anna Brini, Mauro
Bianchi, Lucio Rovati, and Ennio Cocco

Deparment of Pharmacology, University of Milan, 20129 Milan, Italy

One of the most challenging pain syndromes is, from both a pathophysiological and therapeutic point of view, the one present in subjects who underwent an accidental or iatrogenic lesion of peripheral nerves, such as the phantom limb, or postherpetical syndromes.

It is well known that peripheral nerve lesions induce in the experimental animal neurophysiological and behavioral changes, such as an extension of the sensitive fields and self-mutilation (autotomy) of the body region affected by the lesion (3,7,8).

In the search for a better knowledge of the biochemical changes underlying these modifications, the behavioral correlates, and a possible pharmacological approach to its therapy, we evaluated, after the section of mixed somatic and motor nerves (i.e., the sciatic or the brachial plexus) or purely somatic nerves (i.e., the sural or saphenous nerves) (5), the changes in the concentrations of brain and spinal cord neuropeptides. These neuropeptides included the opioid peptides β-endorphin (βE), met-enkephalin (ME), and dynorphin (DYN), and the nonopiate peptide substance P (SP), one of the alleged "pain messengers" of primary sensory neurons, and somatostatin (SRIF), a peptide of which the involvement in pain modulation was suggested by studies in the experimental animal and the human (6).

In order to evaluate a possible lateralization of biochemical changes in the brain due to the section of the peripheral nerves, the concentrations of the neuropeptides were evaluated in brain areas ipsilateral or contralateral to the peripheral lesion. Moreover, with the aim of better evaluating the therapies most commonly used in deafferentation pain, rats bearing the section of the right sciatic nerve were treated with either the tricyclic antidepressants chlorimipramine and nortriptyline, the serotonin precursor 5-hydroxytryptophan, diphenylhydantoin, or baclofen.

MATERIALS AND METHODS

Rats and Surgery

Over 100 CD Sprague-Dawley (SD) male rats weighing 150 to 200 g (Charles River, Calco, Italy) were used in this study. Rats were housed at 22 ± 2°C, with a 10:14-hr light:dark cycle and had water and dry pellets ad libitum. Animals were anesthetized with pentobarbital (40 mg/kg) and underwent the section of the right, left, or both sciatic nerves, or the right branch of the other nerves described above, while one experimental group had the lumbar spinal cord transected. The lesions were performed cutting away 1 cm of nerve starting, when possible (i.e., the sciatic nerve and the brachial plexus), from the point of entrance in the spinal column.

Rats were killed at 6, 12, 24 hours; 2, 7, 14, 28, 35 days, and 4 months after the lesions. At least eight rats were used in each experimental group and anesthetized, and sham-operated rats served as controls in all experiments.

Measurement of Peptides

We measured βE, met-enkephalin, substance P, somatostatin, and dynorphin concentrations at different times after sham operation or deafferentation.

Rats were killed by microwave irradiation with a method previously described and validated (18). The use of microwave is suggested by the necessity of denaturing all the enzymes that could induce a postmortem degradation of the peptides. The hypothalamus, hindbrain, midbrain, striatum, and cortex were dissected according to Glowinski (4) and then divided into the right and left side. The spinal cord was dissected into the cervical (C_1–C_7), thoracic (T_1–T_2), and lumbosacral (L_1–S_5) tracts. In a group of rats, the spinal cord was transected at the level of S_1 and rats were killed 1 week thereafter. The tissues were homogenized in 2 ml 1N acetic acid (1) and centrifuged; the pellet was used for protein determination (9), while the supernatant was frozen until radioimmunoassay was performed. All samples from a single experiment were evaluated in the same assay.

For the measurement of βE concentrations, we used an antiserum obtained in our laboratory in the rabbit against a glutarhaldehyde conjugate of camel-βE (that is identical to the rat peptide) and bovine serum albumin. All the other antisera used in our work were obtained by us by the same method used for βE. The ME antiserum shows 1% cross-reactivity with leu-enkephalin and 100% cross-reactivity with the proenkephalin-A precursor, but not with the other peptides, hormones, or drugs listed above.

The antisera against SRIF and SP did not show any cross reactivity with the same substances tested for βE. The radioimmunoassay methods for βE, ME, SRIF, and SP were previously described in detail (11,17).

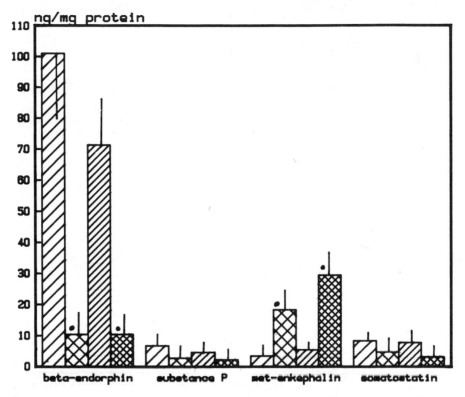

FIG. 1. Hypothalamic concentrations of β-endorphin, somatostatin, met-enkephalin, and substance P in the left hypothalamus of sham-operated (large diagonal) and deafferentated (large crosshatch) rats, and in the right hypothalamus of sham-operated (small diagonal) or deafferentated (small crosshatch) rats.

Drug Treatment

Starting the day of surgery, 50 rats were treated for 35 days with either the tricyclic antidepressants chlorimipramine (CIM; Ciba-Geigy, Origgio, Italy) or nortriptyline (NOR; Recordati, Milan, Italy) 20 mg/kg twice daily; the serotonin precursor 5-hydroxytryptophan (5-HTP; Sigma-Tau, Pomezia, Italy) 30 mg/kg twice daily; diphenylhydantoin (DPH; Dilantin, Recordati, Milan, Italy) 30 mg/kg twice daily; or baclofen (BCL; Ciba-Geigy, Origgio, Italy) 10 mg/kg twice daily. None of the drugs used can be defined as absolutely specific in its mechanism of action, however, CIM is considered to be a fairly selective blocker of serotonin reuptake, with minor effects on the noradrenergic and cholinergic systems (10); NOR is considered to be a fairly specific blocker of norepinephrine reuptake, with minor effects on the serotoninergic system (10); 5-HTP is a precursor of serotonin syntheses;

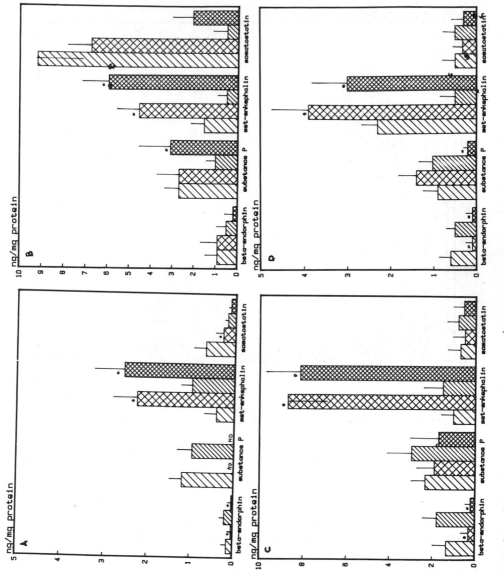

FIG. 2. Concentrations of β-endorphin, somatostatin, met-enkephalin, and substance P in the left or right cortex (**A**), striatum (**B**), midbrain (**C**), or hindbrain (**D**) of sham-operated (diagonal) or deafferentated (crosshatch) rats.

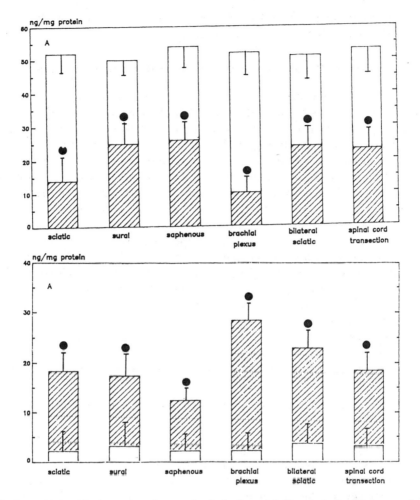

FIG. 3. β-Endorphin (**upper**) and met-enkephalin (**lower**) in the whole hypothalamus of rats that underwent sham operation (open box) or different deafferentations (diagonal).

DPH is an antiepileptic drug possibly acting through the GABAergic system (18), and BCL is a direct agonist of the β-GABA receptor (1). At the end of treatment, we measured βE, ME, DYN, SP, and SRIF concentrations in all the brain areas and spinal cord tracts listed above.

Statistical Analysis of Results

Statistical analysis of results was performed by ANOVA followed by Dunnet multiple range test for multiple comparisons when comparing values versus normal intact rats, while the Student's *t*-test was used for comparisons between sham-operated and deafferentated rats or values for the left or right side, at each given time after surgery.

Effect of Peripheral Nerves Section on Brain Neuropeptides

The effects of the section of the right sciatic nerve on βE, ME, SP, and SRIF concentrations in the left or right hypothalamus is reported in Fig. 1, while the concentrations in the left or right midbrain, hindbrain, striatum, and cortex are reported in Fig. 2. The data refer to 28 days after the lesion. It appears that in all brain areas, with the only exception of striatum, βE concentrations decrease significantly after the section of the peripheral nerve, while ME concentrations constantly increase, and while the concentrations of DYN or other peptides involved in pain modulation, such as SP or SRIF, changed significantly. From the data reported in the tables it also appears that lateralization of the neuropeptides does not seem to be present in SD rats: either in normal rats (sham-operated) or in those that underwent the monolateral section of the sciatic nerve. The lesion of either the left, right, or both sciatic nerves, the right brachial plexus, the right sural, the right saphenous or the transection of the spinal cord yielded the same results reported for the monolateral section of the sciatic nerve. Figure 3 shows, in the upper panel, βE, and in the lower panel ME hypothalamic concentrations 28 days after the lesions of different nerves or 1 week after the transection of the spinal cord in SD rats or their sham-operated controls.

Effect of Peripheral Nerve Section on Spinal Cord Neuropeptides

The different lesions performed yielded consistent results as far as the peptide affected is concerned, while they differ for the localization of the changes observed. As it is shown in Fig. 4, all lesions induced an increase of ME concentrations, while the other neuropeptides were apparently not affected. However, the regional distribution of the changes we observed seems to reflect the site of entrance of the interested sensory afferents. In fact, ME concentrations increased only in the lumbosacral tract after section of one or both sciatic nerves, the sural or saphenous nerve, while they increased only in the cervical tract when the brachial plexus was lesioned.

Time Pattern of the Changes in the Concentrations of the Neuropeptides

The time of the changes in the hypothalamic concentrations of βE and ME are reported in the upper and lower panel of Fig. 5, respectively. The data reported for the hypothalamus are representative of the data observed in all other brain areas and the spinal cord. As it is shown, ME concentrations were decreased 6 and 12 hr after the lesion; however, at these times they were not different from those of sham-operated anesthetized rats,

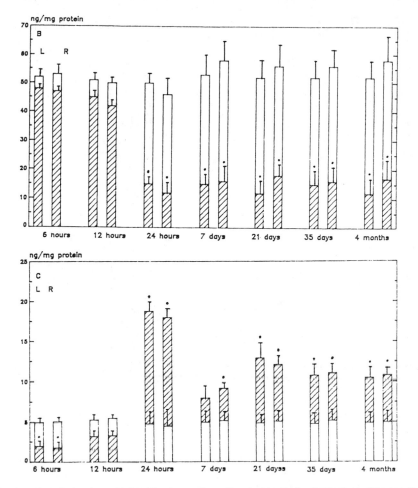

FIG. 4. Hypothalamic β-endorphin (**upper**) and met-enkephalin (**lower**) at different times after sham operation (open box) or section of the right sciatic nerve (diagonal).

which were also changed when compared to untreated rats. A significant increase was present starting on the first day after surgery and lasted up to 6 months thereafter. βE concentrations decreased starting 24 hr after surgery and remained significantly lower than the sham-operated controls up to 4 months after surgery. None of the other peptides we measured was modified at any of the times after surgery we considered (data not presented).

Lateralization

From the examination of the whole of the data we obtained, it appears that the brain concentrations of the neuropeptides underwent the same

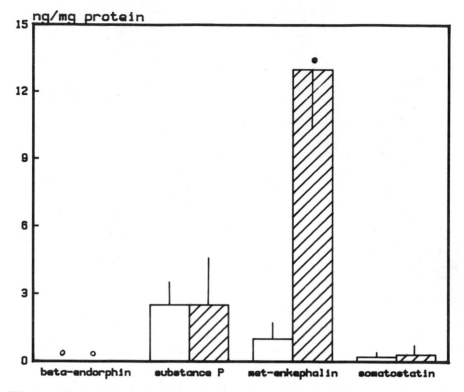

FIG. 5. β-Endorphin, substance P, met-enkephalin, and somatostatin concentrations in the lumbosacral spinal cord of rats that underwent section of the right sciatic nerve (crosshatch) or sham operation (open box).

modifications after the lesion of the right, left, or both sciatic nerves, or the right sural, saphenous brachial plexus. Besides, no differences were detected between right or left brain areas in any of the experimental conditions.

Effect of Drug Treatments

The treatment of SD rats with the serotoninergic drugs CIM and 5-HTP reversed in all brain areas the decrease of the concentrations of the peptide that follows the section of peripheral nerves, while the increase in ME concentrations was not reconducted to normality either in the brain or the spinal cord. None of the other drug treatments tested reversed the changes in ME and βE concentrations induced by deafferentation. In WL rats, to which only CIM was administered, ME concentrations that were increased after deafferentation, were not affected by the pharmacological treatment, while βE, that was not affected by deafferentation, was not modified also by treatment with CIM. The effects on βE hypothalamic concentrations of each

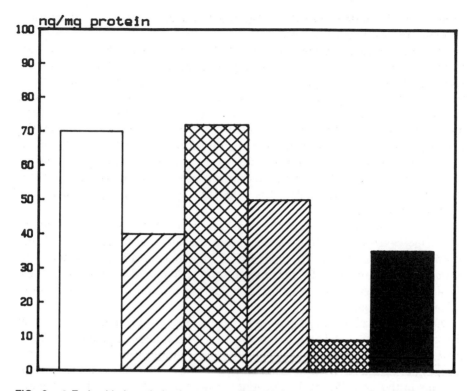

FIG. 6. β-Endorphin hypothalamic concentrations 28 days after section of the sciatic nerve in rats treated with saline (large diagonal), chlorimipramine (large crosshatch), baclofen (small diagonal), diphenylhydantoine (small crosshatch), or nortriptyline (solid box).

of the drugs we tested in SD rats that underwent the section of the right sciatic nerve is shown in Fig. 6, compared to treatment with saline.

It is important to point out that after treatment with CIM or 5-HTP, none of the SD rats developed autotomy, whereas this was still present in the animals receiving the other treatments.

DISCUSSION

The data presented are the first evidence of an effect of peripheral nerve lesions on the concentrations of some opioid neuropeptides in brain areas.

Before any further discussion of the results, it is important to point out that our rats looked well groomed, gained weight normally, and were not irritable, thus indicating the lack of a general discomfort, and therefore excluding a nonspecific stress as cause of the changes we observed.

The decrease of the brain concentrations of βE we observe reminds one of the decrease of the cerebrospinal fluid concentrations of this peptide observed in conditions of chronic pain such as recurrent low back pain or arthritis in the human (15,19) or in the brain areas of rats with chronic adjuvant induced arthritis (16).

The decrease in βE concentrations might be due to the lack of tonic inputs from the periphery to the hypothalamic regions of βE synthesis, through a spinal pathway. This hypothesis is consistent with the observation that a similar pattern is also present in rats treated neonatally or as adults with capsaicin (14), a neurotoxic agent for primary sensory neurons (21). In fact, also under these condition there is a lack of "pain messages" carried by the primary sensory neurons. Furthermore, the decrease of βE might be mediated by a serotoninergic pathway, since we have shown that drugs increasing the serotoninergic, but not other neurotransmitter systems, can bring hypothalamic concentrations of βE back to normal in rats bearing the section of the right sciatic nerve.

As far as ME is concerned, the concentrations of this peptide are significantly increased both in brain areas and in the spinal cord tracts specifically interested by the lesion. The increase in ME concentrations appears 24 hr after the lesion, while a decrease is present at 6 and 12 hr; however, anesthesia can reasonably account for this decrease, since it is present also in sham-operated rats.

Our data are also against the presence in rats of a clear lateralization in the brain areas of localization and function of the neuropeptides we evaluated, as opposed to what suggested by some authors for other neurotransmitters (12). In fact, we did not observe any difference between the concentrations in the areas of the left or right hemisphere in basal condition (sham-operated rats) or after lesions of right nerves (sciatic, brachial plexus, saphenous, or sural), or the left nerves or both sciatic nerves. However, since we did not dissect the spinal cord in a right and left region, lateralization at this level cannot be excluded.

A note of caution has to be put forward in the interpretation of the results we presented, but also of all the other studies based on the measurement of concentrations of neuropeptides. We do not know the real meaning of our numbers since a method for evaluating the turnover of the neuropeptides is not available. Molecular biology will be probably helpful in providing this parameter, but at the moment there is space for misinterpretations. As data are presented now, a decrease in concentrations can in fact be interpreted as a very accelerated turnover, as well as that the system is exausted: two opposite interpretations. The same holds for increased concentrations.

The only thing that can be said without fear of misinterpreting the data is that central nervous system neuropeptides are affected by peripheral nerve lesions.

This unexpected observation, which, however, appears to be very consistent in our experiments, opens the way to a better understanding of the multiple phenomena and/or symptoms that accompany peripheral nerve lesions, and can explain the effectiveness of some therapeutical approaches (e.g., the use of tricyclic antidepressants), or indicate new approaches in the attempt to re-establish the homeostasis of neuropeptides.

The data we obtained after pharmacological treatments confirm the important role of the serotoninergic system in the modulation of cerebral βE concentrations in human subjects and SD rats (2,20). It is particularly interesting to observe that, of the two antidepressants used, only CIM, which acts through the serotoninergic system, is effective, while NOR, which acts through the noradrenergic system, is ineffective. This observation is against the hypothesis that antidepressants are useful in deafferentation pain for their antidepressant effect, that is common to both drugs, while suggests that their effect can be reconducted to their pharmacological effects, i.e., the increased availability of amines (serotonin and/or norepineparine) at the synaptic cleft. Another observation that arises from our studies is that the normalization of the peptides we observe is limited to βE, while the increase in ME caused by deafferentation is not affected. The only partial reversal of the changes in brain and spinal cord neuropeptides induced by peripheral nerve deafferentation might be one of the reasons why none of the drugs we used is completely satisfactory in the clinical management of deafferentation pain.

In conclusion, we have shown that the concentrations of brain and spinal cord ME, and brain βE, are greatly modified after the deafferentation of peripheral somatic and sensitive nerves, and these modifications can be partially reversed by treatment with serotoninergic drugs.

REFERENCES

1. Bowery, N. G. (1982): Baclofen ten years on, *T.I.F.S.*, 3:400–403.
2. De Benedittis, G., Di Giulio, A. M., Massei, R., Villani, R., and Penerai, A. E. (1983): Effect of 5-hydroxytryptophan on central and deafferentation chronic pain. In: *Advances in Pain Research and Therapy*, edited by J. J. Bonica, U. Lindblom, and A. Iggo, pp. 285–304. Raven Press, New York.
3. Devor, M., and Wall, P. D. (1981): Plasticity in the spinal cord sensory map following peripheral nerve injury in rats. *J. Neurosci.*, 1:679–684.
4. Glowinski, J., and Iversen, L. L. (1966): Regional studies of catecholamines in rat brain. *J. Neurochem.*, 13:655–669.
5. Greene, E. C. (1983): *Anatomy of the Rat*, pp. 131. Hafner, New York.
6. Kurahishi, Y., Hirota, N., Sato, Y., Hino, Y., Satoh, M., and Takagi, H. (1985): Evidence that substance P and somatostatin transmit separate information related to pain in the spinal dorsal horn. *Brain Res.*, 325:294–298.
7. Lombard, M. C., Jarlet, M. A., and Daheb, S. (1984): Correlation between deafferentation, self-mutilation, neuronal rhythmical activity and sleep disturbances in the rat. *Pain (Suppl.)*, 2:S465
8. Lombard, M. C., Nasholds, B. S., and Albe-Fessard, D. (1979): Deafferentation hypersensitivity in the rat after dorsal rhizotomy: a possible animal model of chronic pain. *Pain*, 6:305–328.
9. Lowry, O. H., Rosebrough, N. J., Farr, A. L., and Randall, R. J. (1951): Protein measurement with the folin phenol reagent. *J. Biol. Chem.*, 193:265–275.
10. Maj, J., Przegalinski, E., and Mogilnicka, E. (1984): Hypotheses concerning the mechanism of action of antidepressant drugs. *Rev. Physiol. Pharmacol.*, 100:1–74.

11. Ogawa, N., Panerai, A. E., Lee, S., Forsbach, G., Havlicek, V., and Friesen, H. G. (1979): β-endorphin concentrations in the brain of intact and hypophysectomized rats. *Life Sci.*, 25:317–326.
12. Oke, A., Lewis, R., and Adams, R. M. (1980): Hemisperic asymmetry of NE distribution in rat thalamus. *Brain Res.*, 188:269–272.
13. Panerai, A. E., Martini, A., Abbate, D., Villani, R., and DeBenedittis, G. (1983): β-Endorphin, met-enkephalin and β-lipotropin in chronic pain and electroacupuncture. In: *Advances in Pain Research and Therapy, Vol. 5*, edited by J. J. Bonica, V. Lindblom, and A. Iggo, pp. 543–547. Raven Press, New York.
14. Panerai, A. E., Martini, A., Locatelli, V., and Mantegazza, P. (1983): Capsaicin decreases β-endorphin hypothalamic concentrations in the rat. *Pharmacol. Res. Commun.*, 15:825–832.
15. Panerai, A. E., Martini, A., Sacerdote, P., and Mantegazza, P. (1984): K receptor antagonists reverse "non opioid" stress induced analgesia. *Brain Res.*, 304:153–156.
16. Panerai, A. E., Sacerdote, P., and Mantegazza, P. (1987): Brain and spinal cord neuropeptides in chronic arthritis in rats. *Life Sci.* (in press).
17. Panerai, A. E., Salerno, F., Baldissera, F., Martini, A., Di Giulio, A. M., and Mantegazza, P. (1982): Brain β-endorphin concentrations in experimental chronic liver disease. *Brain Res.*, 247:188–190.
18. Patsalos, P. N. and Lascelles, P. T. (1981): Changes in regional brain levels of aminoacid putative neurotransmitters after prolonged treatment with the anticonvulsant drugs diphenylhydantoin, phenobarbitone, sodium valproate, etosuximide, and sulthame in the rat. *J. Neurochem.*, 36:688–695.
19. Puig, M. M., Laorden, M. L., Miralles, F. S., and Olaso, M. K. (1982): Endorphin levels in cerebrospinal fluid of patients with postoperative and chronic pain. *Anesthesiology*, 57:1–4.
20. Sacerdote, P., Mantegazza, P., and Panerai, A. E. (1987): A role for serotonin and β-endorphin in tricyclic antidepressants analgesia. *Biochem. Behav. Pharmacol.*, 26:153–158.
21. Virus, R. M., and Gebhart, G. F. (1979): Pharmacologic actions of capsaicin: apparent involvement of substance P and serotonin. *Life Sci.*, 25:1273–1284.

Advances in Pain Research and Therapy,
Vol. 10. Edited by M. Tiengo et al.
Raven Press, Ltd., New York © 1987.

Behavioral Effects of Intrathecally Administered Neuropeptides in the Rat

S. Spampinato, S. Candeletti, E. Cavicchini, P. Romualdi,
E. Speroni, and S. Ferri

Institute of Pharmacology, University of Bologna, 40126 Bologna, Italy

Anatomical studies have demonstrated that most of the recently characterized neuropeptides are present in neural components of the spinal dorsal horn: (a) the terminals of primary afferent neurons; (b) the terminals of neurons originating from descending brainstem pathways; and (c) intrinsic neurons (1,9). Multidisciplinary experimental approaches have demonstrated that spinal peptidergic systems may participate in the integration of nociceptive information (for review see ref. 7). Recent investigations suggest that neuropeptides, in addition to pain modulation, may play a role in the mediation of a variety of somatomotor and autonomic functions (6,22). Interestingly, several reports have shown that intrathecal administration of opioid and nonopioid peptides such as dynorphin A-(1–17) (11,15) and substance P analogs (14), respectively, causes motor dysfunction after doses above those producing antinociceptive effects. As regards dynorphin A-(1–17), we recently found, by using different analgesimetric procedures, that both effects are clearly distinguishable in time and mediated, at least in part, by a k-type opioid receptor (18).

Dynorphin A-(1–17) is generated, by cleavage of the precursor prodynorphin, together with a series of opioid peptides: dynorphin A-(1–32), dynorphin A-(1-8), dynorphin B-29, and dynorphin B. Immunoreactive dynorphin-like material has been detected in the spinal cord (20); and, recently, Civelli et al.(5) have isolated and sequenced in this tissue the prodynorphin gene. Moreover, at present, little has been explored about the effects of dynorphin-related peptides after intrathecal administration.

Our studies have focused on behavioral effects elicited in the rat by intrathecal administration of these peptides, as well as of the nonopioid peptides: somatostatin-(1-14), neurotensin, and calcitonin-gene-related peptide (CGRP), which may be of importance for the modulation of nociceptive information (9,12,23). In particular, studies on CGRP have been carried out with the aim of comparing with salmon calcitonin (s-calcitonin), a peptide that elevates the nociceptive threshold after intracerebroventricular (10) or intrathecal (19) administration and binds to specific sites throughout the neuraxis, including the spinal cord (13).

METHODS

Adult male Sprague-Dawley rats (300–350 g; Nossan, Italy; singly housed with 12-hr light cycle; food and water *ad libitum*) were used in all the experiments. The rats were implanted with chronic intrathecal catheters while under sodium pentobarbital anesthesia, as reported previously (18). All animals were allowed to recover for at least 1 week before the experiment, and any rats that showed neurological or motor deficits were discarded. At the end of the experiment the position of the catheter was verified by injection of Evans blue. Animals were habituated for 1 week to plexiglas restraining cylinders which would be used during test sessions. To ascertain alterations of the nociceptive threshold we used the hot plate (19), the tail-flick (18), and the vocalization test (where the reaction of the animal to an electrical stimulus is assessed from vocalization, keeping the rat restrained) (18).

Hind-limb function was graded as follows: 0, normal motor function; 1, mild paraparesis with ability to walk; 2, severe paraparesis; and 3, complete paraplegia. Peptides used in this study were purchased by Peninsula (San Carlos, California), except for s-calcitonin (a gift of Sandoz, Basel). Purity of the peptides was assessed by high performance liquid chromatography (18). MR 1452, $(-)$-N-(3-furylmethyl)-α-normetazocine methanesulfonate, was a gift of Dr. H. Merz (Boehringer, Ingelheim Am-Rhein).

Results were expressed as mean ± standard error of the mean. For each set of experiments six to ten animals per group were used. Statistical analysis of the data was performed by analysis of variance followed by single comparisons of means (two-tailed tests).

RESULTS

Behavioral Effects of Intrathecal Prodynorphin-Derived Peptides

Dynorphin A-(1-32)

Intrathecal injection of dynorphin A-(1-32) elevated the nociceptive threshold to a different extent in the tail-flick and vocalization tests. As shown in Fig. 1, the higher dose (25 nmol) produced maximal elevation of tail-flick latency lasting at least 4 hr, while the lower dose (12.5 nmol) caused a smaller change. The time-course curve obtained by the vocalization test gave a different result: The antinociceptive effect had worn off within 120 min with the higher dose injected (Fig.1). Animals treated with 25 nmol of the peptide showed a severe hind-limb paralysis and tail flaccidity within the first minutes after administration, and remaining unmodified for 4 to 6

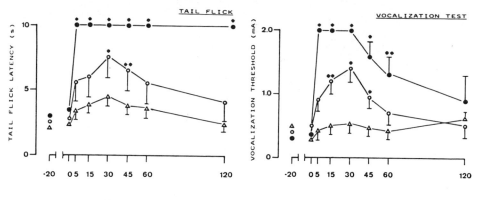

FIG. 1. Time course of the antinociceptive effect of dynorphin A-(1–32) injected intrathecally alone, or concomitantly with MR 1452. (○)Dynorphin A-(1–32), 12.5 nmol; (●)Dynorphin A-(1–32), 25 nmol; (△)Dynorphin A-(1–32), 12.5 nmol + MR 1452, 30 nmol. Each curve represents the mean and SEM from six animals; (*) $p < 0.01$; (**) $p < 0.05$ versus pretreatment values.

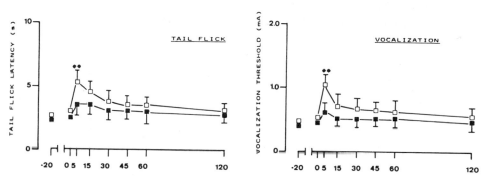

FIG. 2. Time course of the antinociceptive effect of dynorphin A-(1–8) injected intrathecally. (■)Dynorphin A-(1–8), 50 nmol; (□)Dynorphin A-(1–8), 100 nmol. Each curve represents the mean and SEM from six animals; (**) $p < 0.05$ versus pretreatment values.

hr. On the contrary, only a moderate reduction of motor function was elicited by the lower dose of the peptide in some animals (Fig.4), recovering within 1 hr. MR 1452 (30 nmol) prevented both the antinociceptive (Fig. 1) and motor effects (Fig. 4).

Dynorphin A-(1-8)

Dynorphin A-(1-8) caused a moderate and brief elevation of the nociceptive threshold only at the dose of 100 nmol [this effect was prevented by 60

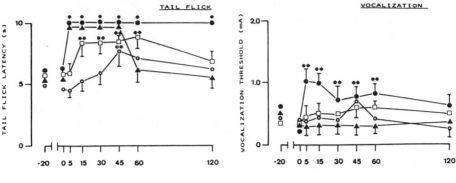

FIG. 3. Time course of the antinociceptive effect of dynorphin B-29 injected intrathecally at four different doses: (○) 12.5 nmol; (□) 25 nmol; (▲) 50 nmol; and (●) 100 nmol. Each curve represents the mean and SEM from six to eight animals; (*) $p < 0.01$; (**) $p < 0.05$ versus pretreatment values.

nmol of MR 1452 concomitantly administered (data not shown)], while the dose of 50 nmol was ineffective on both analgesimetric tests (Fig. 2). No signs of motor impairment were observed (Fig. 4).

Dynorphin B-29

Dynorphin B-29 (12.5, 25, 50, and 100 nmol) produced a dose-related elevation of the tail-flick latency. A statistically significant increase of the vocalization threshold occurred only with the dose of 100 nmol (Fig.3). Motor dysfunction was absent at 12.5 and 25 nmol, and mild with 50 nmol, and moderately severe with the dose of 100 nmol (Fig. 4).

Dynorphin B

Dynorphin B produced a small, short-lasting change in the nociceptive threshold, evaluated by tail-flick and vocalization tests, at the dose of 100 nmol only (data not shown), accompanied by a moderate impairment of motor function (Fig. 4).

Behavioral Effects of Intrathecal Nonopioid Peptides

Somatostatin-(1-14)

The intrathecal administration of somatostatin-(1-14) (12.5 and 25 nmol) elicited a dose-related elevation of the nociceptive threshold as assessed by tail-flick and vocalization tests (Fig. 5). In addition to nociception, somatostatin at the dose of 25 nmol produced hind-limb paralysis and tail flaccidity lasting up to 24 to 48 hr. When injected with half-maximal dose (12.5 nmol)

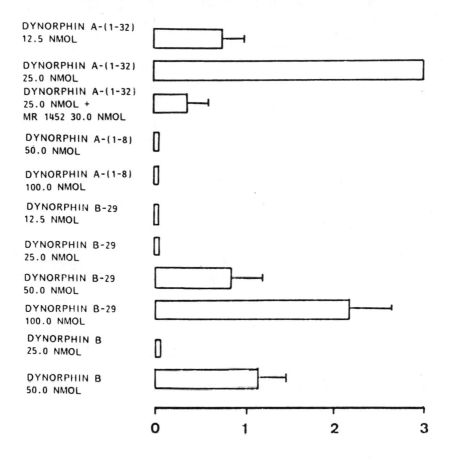

FIG. 4. Effects of dynorphin-related peptides injected intrathecally on motor function in the rat. Motor function was evaluated 15 min after administration. Each *bar* represents the mean and SEM from six to eight animals.

several animals showed a slight motor impairment, but all of them recovered from this effect within less than 1 hr (Fig. 8).

Neurotensin

Intrathecal neurotensin (12.5 and 25 nmol) evoked an increase in the nociceptive threshold which was assessed by the hot plate but not by the vocalization test (Fig. 6) or the tail-flick (data not shown). Animals showed the maximal amplitude response within 5 min after treatment and returned at base-line latencies in 60 min. The peptide did not alter motor function (Fig. 8).

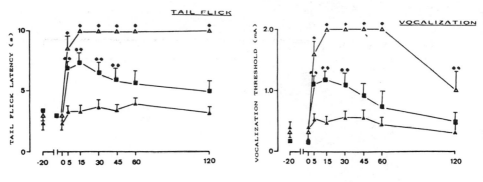

FIG. 5. Time course of the antinociceptive effect of somatostatin-(1–14) injected intrathecally. (▲)Vehicle; (■)somatostatin, 12.5 nmol; (△)somatostatin, 25 nmol. Each curve represents the mean and SEM from six animals; (*) $p < 0.01$; (**) $p < 0.05$ versus vehicle-treated group.

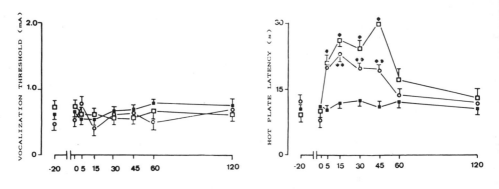

FIG. 6. Time course of the antinociceptive effect of neurotensin injected intrathecally. (■)Vehicle; (○)neurotensin, 12.5 nmol; (□) neurotensin, 25 nmol. Each curve represents the mean and SEM from six to eight animals; (*) $p < 0.01$; (**) $p < 0.05$ versus vehicle-treated group.

s-Calcitonin and CGRP

Similar to neurotensin, s-calcitonin (0.25 and 0.50 nmol) and CGRP (7.5 and 15 nmol) elevated the nociceptive threshold in the hot-plate test, but not in the vocalization test (Fig. 7) or in the tail-flick (data not shown), without producing motor impairment (Fig. 8). Both peptides produced a long-lasting, dose-dependent elevation of the nociceptive threshold. However, the effect elicited by s-calcitonin was duplicated only by a dose of CGRP 30-fold higher.

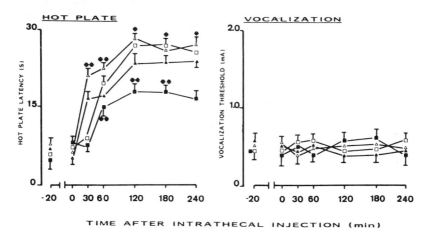

FIG. 7. Time course of the antinociceptive effect of salmon calcitonin (sCT) and calcitonin-gene-related peptide (CGRP) injected intrathecally. (▲)sCT, 0.25 nmol; (△)sCT, 0.50 nmol; (■)CGRP, 7.5 nmol; (□)CGRP, 15 nmol. Each curve represents the mean and SEM from eight to ten animals; (*) $p < 0.01$; (**) $p < 0.05$ versus pretreatment values.

DISCUSSION

The antinociceptive and motor responses to intrathecal dynorphin A-(1-32) in the present study fit a pattern similar to that observed after dynorphin A-(1-17): The peptide caused alterations in nociception and motor function clearly distinguishable in time (18). However, the antinociceptive effect of dynorphin A-(1-32) was longer in duration, as ascertained by the vocalization test.

On the contrary, dynorphin A-(1-8) was much less potent and devoid of remarkable effects on motor behavior. The peptide dynorphin B and its C-terminal extension dynorphin B-29 displayed a low potency in producing effects on nociception and motor function at spinal level. In all, this may be related to a rapid degradation of these peptides (18); alternatively a different affinity may also be suggested of dynorphin-gene-related peptides for the same dynorphinergic receptor (2). Although all the investigated peptides occur in the central nervous system, the significance of the concomitant presence of so many biologically active peptides coming from the same precursor remains obscure. The strong impact that dynorphin A-(1-17) and its C-terminal extension dynorphin A-(1-32) have at spinal level on antinociception and motor function strengthens the possibility of a physiological role for these peptides. The k-type opioid antagonist MR 1452 prevented the observed effects of dynorphin-related peptides. This fact is consistent with *in vitro* and *in vivo* studies suggesting that they have a higher affinity for k-type opioid receptors (3,16).

The intrathecal administration of somatostatin-(1-14) gave a profile of

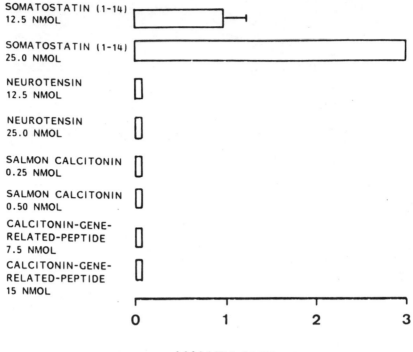

FIG. 8. Effects of nonopioid peptides injected intrathecally on motor function in the rat. Motor function was evaluated 15 min after administration of neurotensin and somatostatin or 1 hr after salmon calcitonin and calcitonin-gene-related peptide. Each *bar* represents the mean and SEM from six to ten animals.

activity similar to that elicited by dynorphin-related peptides, producing distinguishable effects in nociception and motor function. The peptide caused a long-lasting motor weakness or paralysis of hind-limbs after a dose above those eliciting antinociception. Such an effect can interfere with the tail-flick test, as this involves a motor response to the afferent nociceptive input. In fact, the vocalization threshold returned to predrug values within 120 min after injection of somatostatin-(1-14), thus indicating that rats were again reactive to noxious stimuli.

The mechanism underlying the observed effects on motor function is as yet unknown. Further research will be necessary to determine whether this action is simply pharmacological or whether it reproduces a physiological effect of endogenous peptides. Another possibility is that these peptides may produce toxic effects on spinal structures, as hypothesized by Post and Paulsson (14) to explain motor paralysis after intrathecal injection of peptide analogs of substance P. In actual fact, these authors found that these analogs elicited antinociception and caused, at higher doses, an extensive necrosis of neural bodies in both ventral and dorsal horn, with a prolonged paraplegia. Studies on possible neurotoxic effects of the assayed peptides are therefore needed. In any case, data of the present investigations indicate that caution is required in the clinical application of these peptides, since recent reports refer to intrathecal administration of dynorphin A-(1-13) (21) and somatostatin-(1-14) (4) in human beings.

Neurotensin, CGRP, and s-calcitonin did not produce any motor dysfunction after intrathecal administration, although they produced elevation of nociceptive threshold evidenced by the hot-plate test only. These peptides showed a different time-course of the antinociceptive effect: of brief duration (45 min) that of neurotensin, according to Yaksh et al. (23), and long-lasting (more than 2 hr) that of CGRP and s-calcitonin. However, the CGRP antinociceptive activity, on a molar basis, was far below that of s-calcitonin. The different potency displayed by the two peptides may be indicative of a different affinity for the same receptor or, alternatively, as suggested by Seifert et al. (17), CGRP and s-calcitonin may bind to different binding sites.

The lack of effects on tail-flick and vocalization tests of some of the investigated peptides (neurotensin, CGRP, and s-calcitonin) cannot at present be explained. It is possible that they affect different neural circuitry, mediating sensory inputs at spinal level and with discriminative capacities towards behaviorally relevant noxious signals.

In conclusion, examination of the behavioral effects produced by intrathecally injected opioid and nonopioid peptides indicates that they participate in the complex functions mediated by spinal systems. Spinally administered neuropeptides not only play a role in pain processing, but may have an impact on the motor function. However, further investigations seem necessary in this direction, considering the relevance of clinical implications.

ACKNOWLEDGMENTS

This research was supported by grants of MPI and CNR (85.00573.56). We thank Mr. B. Barattini for his expert photographic work and Dr. F. Franch (Sandoz) for a kind gift of salmon calcitonin.

REFERENCES

1. Basbaum, A. I. (1985): Functional analysis of the cytochemistry of the spinal dorsal horn. In: *Advances in Pain Research and Therapy, Vol. 9,* edited by H. L. Fields, R. Dubner, and F. Cervero, pp. 149–175. Raven Press, New York.
2. Chavkin, C., and Goldstein, A. (1981): Specific receptor for the opioid peptide dynorphin. Structure-activity relationships. *Proc. Natl. Acad. Sci. USA,* 78:6543–6547.
3. Chavkin, C., James, I. C., and Goldstein, A. (1982): Dynorphin is a specific endogenous ligand of the k opiate receptor. *Science,* 235:413–415.

4. Chrubasik, J., Meynaidier, J., Blond, S., Scherepreel, P., Ackerman, E., Weinstock, M., Bonath, K., Cramer, H., and Wunsch, E. (1984): Somatostatin, a potent analgesic. *Lancet,* II:1208–1209.

5. Civelli, O., Douglass, J., Goldstein, A., and Herbert, E. (1985): Sequence and expression of the rat prodynorphin gene. *Proc. Natl. Acad. Sci. USA,* 82:4291–4298.

6. DeGroat, W. C., Kawatani, M., Hisamitsu, T., Lowe, I., Morgan, C., Roppolo, J., Booth, A. M., Nadelhaft, I., Kuo, D., and Thor, K. (1983): The role of neuropeptides in the sacral autonomic reflex pathways of the cat. *J. Autonom. Nerv. Syst.,* 7:339–350.

7. Dubner, R. (1985): Specialization in nociceptive pathways: sensory discrimination, sensory modulation and neural connectivity. In: *Advances in Pain Research and Therapy, Vol. 9,* edited by H. L. Fields, R. Dubner, and F. Cervero, pp. 111–137. Raven Press, New York.

8. Gibson, S. J., Polak, J. M., Bloom, S. R., Sabate, I. M., Mulderry, P. M., Ghathel, M. A., McGregor, G. P., Morrison, J. F. B., Kelly, J. S., Evans, R. M., and Rosenfeld, M. G. (1984): Calcitonin gene-related peptide immunoreactivity in the spinal cord of man and eight other species. *J. Neurosci.,* 4:3101–3111.

9. Gibson, S. J., Polak, J. M., Bloom, S. R., and Wall, P. D. (1981): The distribution of nine peptides in the rat spinal cord with special emphasis on the substantia gelantinosa and on the area around the central canal (lamina X). *J. Comp. Neurol.,* 201:65–77.

10. Guidobono, F., Netti, C., Sibilia, V., Olgiati, V. R., and Pecile, A. (1985): Role of cathecolamines in calcitonin-induced analgesia. *Pharmacology,* 31:342–348.

11. Herman, B., and Goldstein, A. (1985): Antinociception and paralysis induced by intrathecal dynorphin. *A.J. Pharmacol. Exp. Ther.,* 232:27–32.

12. Kuraishi, Y., Hirota, N., Sato, Y., Hino, Y., Satoh, M., and Takagi, H. (1985): Evidence that substance P and somatostatin transmit separate information related to pain in the spinal dorsal horn. *Brain Res.,* 325:294–298.

13. Olgiati, V. R., Guidobono, F., Netti, C., and Pecile, A. (1983): Localization of calcitonin binding sites in rat central nervous system: evidence of its neuroactivity. *Brain Res.,* 265:209–215.

14. Post, C., and Paulsson, I. (1985): Antinociceptive and neurotoxic actions of substance P in the rat's spinal cord after intrathecal administration. *Neurosci. Lett.,* 57:159–164.

15. Przewlocki, R., Shearman, G. T., and Herz, A. (1983): Mixed opioid/nonopioid effects of dynorphin and dynorphin-related peptides after their intrathecal injection in rats. *Neuropeptides,* 3:233–240.

16. Przewlocki, R., Stala, L., Greczek, M., Shearman, G. T., Przewlocka, B., and Herz, A. (1983): Analgesic effects of μ- and k-opiate agonists and, in particular, dynorphin at the spinal level. *Life Sci.,* 33 (Suppl. 1):649–652.

17. Seifert, H., Chesnut, J., DeSourza, E., Rivier, J., and Vale, W. (1985): Binding sites for calcitonin gene-related peptide in distinct areas of rat brain. *Brain Res.,* 346:195–198.

18. Spampinato, S., and Candeletti, S. (1985): Characterization of dynorphin A-induced antinociception at spinal level. *Eur. J. Pharmacol.,* 110:21–30.

19. Spampinato, S., Candeletti, S., Cavicchini, E., Romualdi, P., Speroni, E., and Ferri, S. (1984): Antinociceptive activity of salmon calcitonin injected intrathecally in the rat. *Neurosci. Lett.,* 45:135–139.

20. Spampinato, S., and Goldstein, A. (1983): Immunoreactive dynorphin in rat tissues and plasma. *Neuropeptides,* 3:193–212.

21. Wen, H. L., Mehal, Z. D., Ong, B. H., Ho, W. K. K., and Wen, D. Y. K. (1985): Intrathecal administration of Beta-endorphin and dynorphin-(1–13) for the treatment of intractable pain. *Life Sci.,* 37:1231–1220.

22. Yaksh, T. L., and Noueihed, R. (1985): The physiology and pharmacology of spinal opiates. *Annu. Rev. Pharmacol. Toxicol.,* 25:433–462.

23. Yaksh, T. L., Schmauss, C., Micevych, P. E., Abay, E. O., and Go, V. L. W. (1982): Pharmacological studies on the application, disposition and release of neurotensin in the spinal cord. *Ann. NY Acad. Sci.,* 400:228–242.

Advances in Pain Research and Therapy,
Vol. 10. Edited by M. Tiengo et al.
Raven Press, Ltd., New York © 1987.

Comparative Electrophysiological Analysis of Nonsteroidal Anti-inflammatory Drug Activity in Arthritic Rats

*P.C. Braga, **G. Biella, and **M. Tiengo

*Department of Pharmacology, Chemotherapy, and Toxicology, University of Milan, 20129 Milan, Italy; and **Centro Studi Analgesia, University of Milan, 20129 Milan, Italy*

The development of several new nonsteroidal anti-inflammatory drugs (NSAIDs), generally more potent and with a longer duration of action than acetylsalicylic acid and with a specific antinociceptive activity, renewed interest in models for assessment of analgesia.

The common testing procedures in animals used, at present, for detecting drugs with antinociceptive characteristics use nociceptive stimuli considered to be painful for animals because they are known to be painful for humans.

The first approach in investigating the analgesic activity of a drug is usually to use such tests as the tail-flick, hot-plate, Randal-Selitto, etc., which investigate the antinociceptive activity of a drug by studying the nociceptive motor responses.

Generally, drugs able to reduce or abolish sensation of pain at the same time reduce or abolish the spasm of striated muscle induced by the nociceptive reflex (23). Nevertheless, these tests apply only to acute or transient pain because they involve brief exposure to painful stimuli. Chronic pain is the other aspect of the "pain problem" that is equally and possibly more important than acute pain. In the literature there is a discrepancy in that most studies are acute. This is probably because it is more complicated to set up an experimental stable model for investigation of chronic pain.

For this reason the recent reproposal of an old pharmacological model, adjuvant-induced arthritis in the rat but with a new electrophysiological approach, is of interest (17,21). This model has been confirmed to be a good model for the study of chronic pain (8,9,19,31), and moreover has many features of clinical development and biochemical alteration (1,6,18,24,30,39) in common with rheumatoid arthritic disease in man.

In arthritic rats, there are important modifications of the firing behavior of the thalamic ventrobasal neurons to somatic stimulation. The neurons activated by noxious stimuli were found to have different physiological properties from those of neurons in the same region in nonarthritic animals (17,21) and, specifically, it has been shown that there are many neurons with firing activated only by ankle extension, or flexion, or mild stimulation of inflamed fields (17).

This electrophysiological approach is interesting because it may help us understand the problem of chronic pain and suggest pharmacological therapy. Investigations with "behavioral" tests give only a part of the answer, since behavior is only an epiphenomenon of what happens in the CNS when it feels pain and reacts to it.

We have explored the electrophysiological patterns of firing of thalamic neurons in arthritic rats to investigate the antinociceptive activity of different NSAIDs and to compare their characteristics.

MATERIALS AND METHODS

Experiments were performed with male Sprague-Dawley rats weighing 200 to 260 g at the time of the electrophysiological recording. (During the development of arthritis the rats lost weight.)

The arthritic syndrome was induced by intradermal injection of 0.1 ml of a suspension of killed *Mycobacterium butyricum* in heavy mineral oil (concentration 5 mg/ml; Difco) into the plantar surface of the left hind foot (30). The animals were housed in individual cages and given water and food *ad libitum;* the light schedule was 8 hr light, 16 hr dark. The guidelines (10) published on ethical standards for investigations of experimental pain in animals were followed.

Electrophysiological investigations were performed between the eighth and sixteenth days after the adjuvant administration, using rats exhibiting clearly visible evidence of arthritis (i.e., erythema, swelling to twice normal size of the paws and tibiotarsal joint) and related behavior (vocalization, reduced motility).

Animals were anesthetized with 1 g/kg urethane, i.p., a lower dosage than normal because arthritic rats are more sensitive to anesthesia than normal rats. After the animal was placed in a stereotaxic frame, a small hole (3-mm diameter) was drilled in the skull and the dura mater was carefully removed to allow stereotaxic positioning of the micropipette in the thalamus. The exposed cortical surface was covered with warm mineral oil. The animals were kept warmed on a hot plate maintained at 37 to 38° C.

The color and the vascularization of the extremities and their ability to return quickly to their previous state after application of pressure or joint movement was checked, and whenever it had deteriorated, the experiments were terminated (32).

To record extracellular activity, single-barreled micropipettes were used, the tips were broken back to a tip diameter of 2 to 4 μm and were filled, by the fiberglass technique, with a 2 M NaCl solution saturated with Pontamine sky blue, for subsequent localization. The resistance was 10 to 18 MΩ.

The coordinates for correct electrode placement in the nucleus lateralis and ventrobasalis of thalamus were taken from the atlas of Fifkova and Marsala (15) (AP 2.5–3.0; L 2.5–3.5; H 3.0–4.0 and 4.5–5.0). The recording electrode was connected to an amplifier and the neuronal activity was filtered, displayed on an oscilloscope, and recorded on an FM tape recorder.

A window discriminator was used to differentiate spikes from noise. The output pulses of constant amplitude and duration (TTL) were channeled into an integrator in order to have a continuous analog rate-meter display of the firing.

The noxious test stimuli used were either ankle extension or flexion or mild lateral pressure of the heel (calibrated forceps). These stimuli did not induce any responses in nonarthritic rats. The stimuli were applied for 10 sec and were repeated every 5 or 10 min. Recordings were obtained from neurons that had low basal spontaneous firing rates and reacted to these stimuli with clearly excitatory effects. In arthritic rats it is possible to find neurons with spontaneous "paroxysmal" firing rates (21,22). These neurons were not studied because their irregular high-frequency burst discharges interfered with seeking evoked responses. Care was taken to avoid damage to the skin and sensitization. The drugs used, slowly injected intravenously, were: saline alone in nondrug control rats; lysine acetylsalicylate (aspirin), 54 mg/kg; suprofen at doses of 0.9, 1.8, 3.7, 7.5, 15, 30, and 54 mg/kg; tenoxicam at doses of 0.15, 0.30, 0.60, 1.2, and 2.4 mg/kg.

The drugs were dissolved in saline, the volume of injection was 0.33 ml, and the pH of the solution was between 6.6 and 7.4.

The effects of the drugs were investigated on only one cell for each animal to avoid residual drug effects, and the electrophysiological recording was continued until the return of basal firing, to obtain the time-courses of the effects of the different doses.

RESULTS

Figure 1 shows an example of the effect of aspirin at 54 mg/kg, i.v., investigated in a first group of six arthritic rats. Reduction of the evoked mobilization was evident at 10 min and this effect lasted until 30 min., on the average, and then progressively wore off, with return to normal responses at 55 (± 5) min.

Taking this behavior of aspirin as a reference, the activities of suprofen and tenoxicam, two other NSAIDs recently proposed for their interesting antinociceptive action but with completely different chemical structures, were compared with it. Suprofen is an α-methyl-4- (2-thienylcarbonyl) benzene acetic acid which belongs to the aryl-propionic class of NSAIDs (Fig.

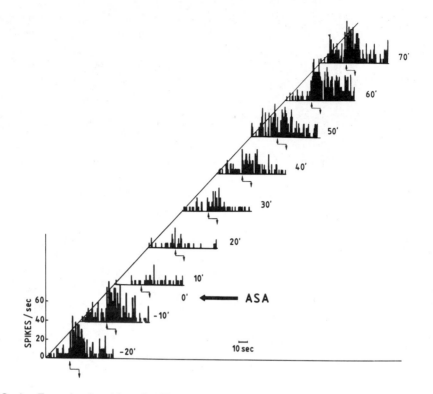

FIG. 1. Example of aspirin action. Rate-meter recordings every 10 min showing a depressive effect with time-course for 54 mg/kg, i. v. Ankle mobilization: start, duration, end (zigzag arrow); aspirin injection (←).

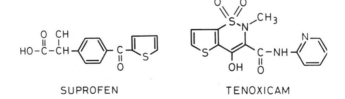

SUPROFEN   TENOXICAM

FIG. 2. Chemical structure of suprofen and tenoxicam.

2), while tenoxicam is a 4-hydroxy-2-methyl-N-pyridyl-2H-thien [2,3-one] 1,2-thiazine-3-carboxamide-1, 1-dioxide, and belongs to the oxicam class of NSAIDs (Fig.2).

Figure 3 shows an example of the effects of 3.7 mg/kg suprofen, i.v. The effect on the evoked neuronal activity (nine neurons) was very rapid, being

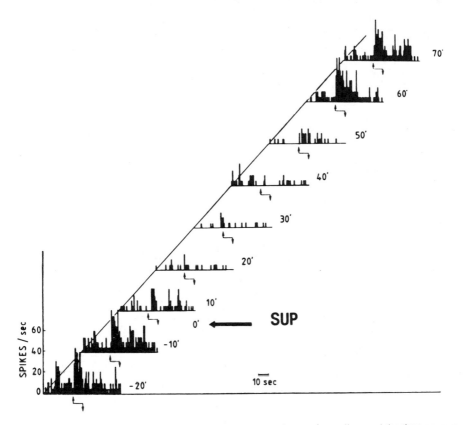

FIG. 3. Example of rate-meter recordings showing the depressive action and the time-course of the effect of 3.7 mg/kg suprofen, i.v. Ankle mobilization: start, duration, end (zigzag arrow); suprofen injection (←).

already evident 5 to 10 min. after administration. Maximal depression was seen between 20 to 50 min, on the average, and then wore off progressively with a return to basal levels at 60 (±7) min.

In comparison with the above, the effects of 0.6 mg/kg tenoxicam, i.v. (ten neurons) were visible at 30 min, on the average, with maximal inhibition of the evoked firing between 30 to 60 min. The effect had worn off by 80 (±12) min (Fig. 4).

After determining the mean doses of tenoxicam and suprofen that induce effects comparable to that of aspirin, we investigated whether increasing doses of NSAIDs produce increasing pharmacological effects. A total of 25 thalamic neurons for tenoxicam and 28 thalamic neurons for suprofen, always located in the nucleus lateralis or ventrobasalis, were investigated. A comprehensive view of the effects and the time-courses of increasing doses of tenoxicam and suprofen are given in Figs. 5 and 6, which are examples of

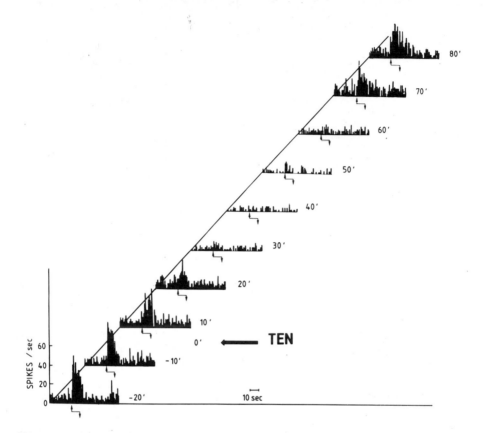

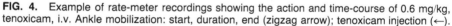

FIG. 4. Example of rate-meter recordings showing the action and time-course of 0.6 mg/kg, tenoxicam, i.v. Ankle mobilization: start, duration, end (zigzag arrow); tenoxicam injection (←).

the peristimulus histograms obtained with increasing doses of the two drugs. For each dose, the mean of the number of spikes for every interval was calculated and the final value was plotted against time to compare the time-courses at the various doses, as shown in Figs. 7 and 8.

The longer time-courses for increasing doses of tenoxicam and suprofen induced us to analyze for linear correlation (Fig. 9).

DISCUSSION

First of all, this new electrophysiological approach gives us the possibility of studying chronic pain directly at the thalamus, an important relay in the pain pathway to the cortex. Since the kind of pain investigated is originated by the arthritic reaction, we can now investigate pharmacologically and

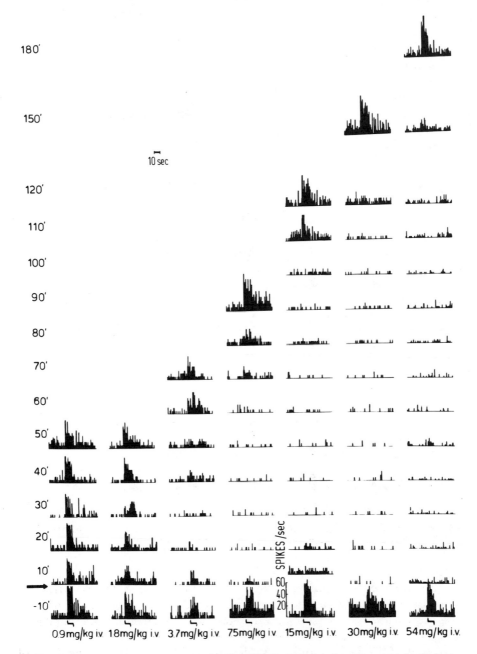

FIG. 5. Comprehensive view of the effects and time-course (rate-meter recordings) for increasing doses of suprofen. See Fig. 3 for identification of symbols.

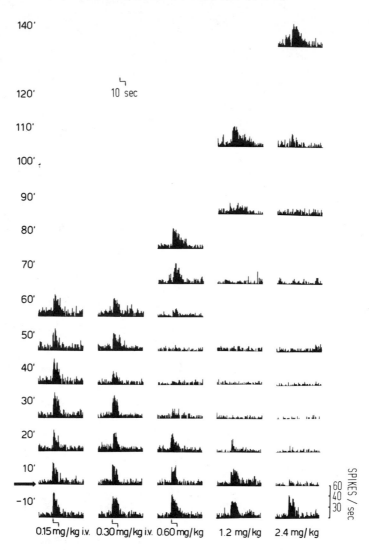

FIG. 6. Comprehensive view of the effects and time-course (rate-meter recordings) for increasing doses of tenoxicam. See Fig. 4 for identification of symbols.

directly the specific antinociceptive effects in the CNS of the NSAIDs, instead of their overall effect, a mixture with different proportions of anti-edema, anti-inflammatory, antiprostaglandin, antipyretic, and antalgesic actions.

A dose of 54 mg/kg aspirin, i.v., is able to definitely reduce the firing of nociceptive thalamic neurons evoked in arthritic rats by articular manipulation, and this is in agreement with the data of Guilbaud (22).

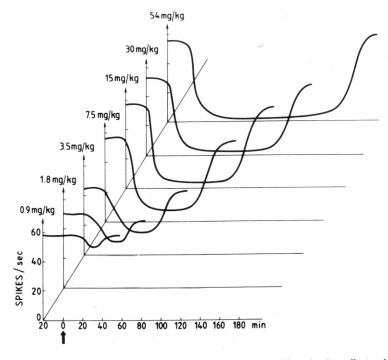

FIG. 7. Schematic overall view of the progressive inhibitory and long-lasting effects of supro-fen increasing doses (↑ = suprofen injection). Each line is the interpolation of the mean firing values for the corresponding time-interval for each dose.

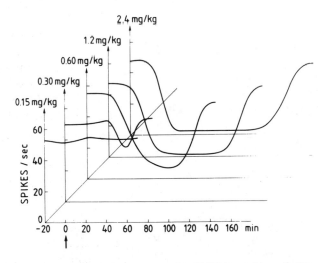

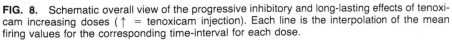

FIG. 8. Schematic overall view of the progressive inhibitory and long-lasting effects of tenoxi-cam increasing doses (↑ = tenoxicam injection). Each line is the interpolation of the mean firing values for the corresponding time-interval for each dose.

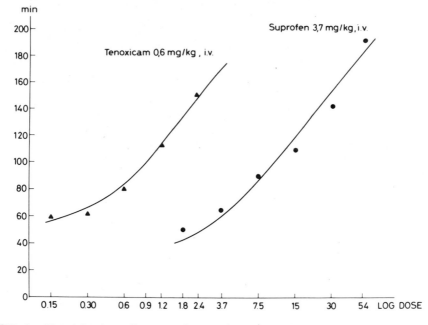

FIG. 9. Plot of the dose-effect curve for suprofen and tenocicam. (x = log dose; y = duration in minutes of the inhitory effect on thalamic-evoked firings (▲——▲) tenoxicam; (●——●) suprofen.

Even suprofen and tenoxicam can give the same result, but at doses of 3.7 mg/kg, i.v., and 0.6 mg/kg, i.v., indicating the greater potency of these NSAIDs. Similar effects (Fig. 10) of isoxicam (0.4 mg/kg, i.v.) and the diclofenac (1 mg/kg, i.v.) were seen always in the thalamus of the arthritic rat, indicating that probably all the compounds of this class can reduce the firing evoked by peripheral painful stimuli. Of additional interest is the dose-effect curves obtained with increasing doses of tenoxicam and suprofen. From a pharmacological point of view, this opens up a new area for investigation of "predictability" of data, obtained with this specific electrophysiological tool: a result that is shown here for the first time.

For the mechanism of action of the effects we have seen, there are many data in the literature (13,14,28,29,38) indicating that during inflammation drastic changes occur in the microenvironment of the peripheral fiber endings, primarily due to the formation and release of such endogenous chemical substances as H^+ ions, bradykinin, histamine, 5-hydroxytryptamine, and prostaglandins, all inducing local sensitization by lowering the thresholds of the nociceptors to nociceptive input, thus causing pain. Since the synthesis of prostaglandins is inhibited by NSAIDs, this has been accepted as the mechanisms of the antinociceptive action of NSAIDs. However, this mech-

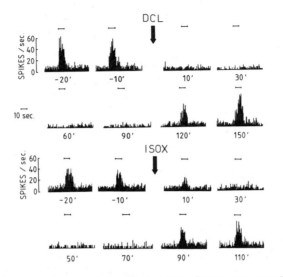

FIG. 10. Example of isoxicam and diclofenac action. Rate-meter recordings showing the effect and the time-course of 0,4 mg/kg, i.v., and 1 mg/kg, i.v., respectively.

anism is not completely satisfactory. There are certain discrepancies, as reported in a previous study (4). In arthritic rats, for instance, aspirin has an analgesic activity at doses well below those required for effective anti-inflammatory and antiarthritic activity (16,33,34). Moreover, even in animals unable to synthesize inflammatory prostaglandins because of essential fatty acid-deficient diets, the analgesic acids have been shown to be effective (3,5).

Ferreira and other investigators (11,12,31) claim that NSAIDs, in addition to their peripheral anti-inflammatory activity, have a central analgesic component. This hypothesis is supported by experimental data. Chen and Chapman (7), for instance, reported that aspirin decreased the evoked potentials in the brain after electric shocks applied to the tooth. Scott (37) described a similar finding: The dentinal receptor in the cat excited by painful stimulation was inhibited by aspirin applied topically to the dentine. Gramov found reversible inhibition by aspirin of discharge activity in the cortical neurons of the rabbit (20). Belcher (2) also reported that the responses of four dorsal horn neurons activated by noxious heat were depressed by aspirin. In our electrophysiological recordings, especially those after increasing doses of tenoxicam and suprofen (Figs. 5,6), it is possible to see that not only is there inhibition of the evoked responses, but also a reduction in spontaneous basal rate. A preliminary comparison of the effects of aspirin and suprofen in nonarthritic rats stimulated by mechanical behavior with those in arthritic rats indicate such an action also against acute pain, but with a decrease in the basal firing also present.

The above-mentioned bibliographic data lead in the same direction and fit our findings that not only is evoked activity inhibited by aspirin, suprofen, tenoxicam, isoxicam, and diclofenac, but spontaneous activity is also reduced, indicating that a neuronal mechanism probably overlaps the antiprostaglandin effects, agreeing with Ferreira's hypothesis.

Neuron membrane hyperpolarization induced by NSAIDs has been postulated by some investigators (35–38) and this would agree with the finding that aspirin enhanced presynaptic inhibition in the cat dorsal horn, thus reducing the effectiveness of incoming sensory stimuli. This enhancement fits into the spinal-gate control theory of pain of Melzach and Wall (27), in which enhancement of presynaptic inhibition is associated with analgesia by reduction of the effectiveness of repetitive input in generating responses in the CNS.

From our electrophysiological recordings of the thalamus, it is not possible at present to answer the question whether NSAIDs acts in the periphery or in the CNS, or in both. Our studies are still in progress and the extension of the electrophysiological characterization to oither NSAIDs makes it possible not only to investigate their antinociceptive effects but also to examine closely their possible mechanisms of action.

ACKNOWLEDGMENTS

This research was partially supported by Centro Nazionale delle Ricerche grant 83.02228.56.115.02380 and by Ministero della Pubblica Istruzione, Italy. We thank C. Panara for technical assistance.

REFERENCES

1. Awouters, F., Lenertes, P. M. H., and Niemegeer S. (1976): Increased incidence of adjuvant arthritis in Wistar rats. *Arzneim Forsch.*, 26:40–43.
2. Belcher, G. (1979): The effects of intra-arterial bradykinin, histaminie, acethilcholine, and prostaglandin E_1 on nociceptive and non-nociceptive dorsal horn neurons of the cat. *Eur. J. Pharmacol.*, 56:385–395.
3. Bonta, I. L., Bult, H., v.d., Ven, L. L. M., and Noorhoek, J. (1976): Essential fatty acids deficiency: a conditions to discriminate prostaglandin and not prostaglandin mediated components of inflammation. *Agents Actions*, 6:154–158.
4. Braga, P. C., Biella, G., Fraschini, F., and Tiengo, M. (1986): Depressive effects of suprofen, a new NSAID, on thalamic evoked neuronal firing in arthritic rats. *Neuropharmacology*, 25:1055–1062.
5. Brune, K., and Lanz, R. (1984): Mode of action of peripheral analgesic. *Arzneim. Forsch.*, 34:1060–1065.
6. Burstein, N.A., and Waksman, B. H. (1964): The pathogenesis of adjuvant disease in the rat. I. A histologic study of early lesions in the joints and skin. *Yale J. Biol. Med.*, 37:177–194.
7. Chen, A. C. N., and Chapman, C. R. (1980): Aspirin analgesia evaluated by event-related potentials in man: Possible central action in brain. *Exp. Brain Res.*, 39:359–364.
8. Colpaert, F. C., Meert, T., De Witte, P., and Schmitt, P. (1978): Further evidence validating adjuvant arthritis as an experimental model of chronic pain in the rat. *Life Sci.*, 31:67–75.

9. De Castro-Costa, M., De Sutter, P., Gybels, J., and Vann Hees; J. (1981): Adjuvant-induced arthritis in rats: a possible animal model of chronic. *Pain,* 10:173–185.
10. Editorial (1980): *Pain,* 9:141–143.
11. Ferreira, S. H., Lorenzetti, B. B., and Correa, F. M. A. (1971): Blockade of central and peripheral generation of prostaglandins explains the antialgic effect of aspirin-like drugs. *Pol. J. Pharmacol. Pharm.,* 30:133–140.
12. Ferreira, S. H., Lorenzetti, B. B., and Correa, F. M. A. (1978): Central and peripheral antialgic action of aspirin-like drugs. *Eur. J. Pharmacol.,* 53:39–48.
13. Ferreira, S. H., Moncada, S., and Vane, J. R. (1971): Indomethacin and aspirin abolish prostaglandin release from spleen. *Nature (New Biol.),* 231:237–241.
14. Ferreira, S. H., Moncada, S., and Vane, J. R. (1973): Prostaglandins and the mechanism of analgesia produced by aspirin-like drugs. *Br. J. Pharmacol.,* 49:85–97.
15. Fifkova, E., and Marsala, J. (1967): Stereotaxic atlases for cat, rabbit and rat. In: *Electrophysiological Methods in Biological Research,* edited by J. Bures, M. Petram, and J. Zachar, pp. 653–731. Academic Press, New York.
16. Fleming, J. S., Bierwagen, M. E., Pircio, A. W., and Pindell, M. H. (1966): A new anti-inflammatory agent 1-(4-chlorobenzoyl)-3-(5-tetrazolylmethyl)-indole. (BL-R743). *Arch. Intern. Pharmacodyn.,* 178:423–436.
17. Gautron, M., and Guilbaud, G. (1982): Somatic responses of ventrobasal thalamic neurones in polyarthritic rats. *Brain Res.,* 237:459–471.
18. Gleen, E. M., and Gray, J. (1965): Adjuvant-induced polyarthritis in rats: biological and histological background. *Am. J. Vet. Res.,* 26:1180–1194.
19. Gouret, C., Macquet, G., and Raynaud, G. (1976): Use of Frend's adjuvant-arthritis test in anti-inflammatory drug screening in the rat: value of animal selection and preparation at the breeding center. *Lab. Anim. Sci.,* 26:281–287.
20. Gromov, A. I. (1982): Spike activity and chemical sensitivity of cortical units under depression of prostaglandin biosynthesis in rabbit. *Neurofiziologiia,* 14:130–134.
21. Guilbaud, G., Gautron, M., and Peschanski, M. (1981): Response electrophysiologiques des neurones du complexe neutrobasal du thalamus a des stimulations cutanees et articulaires chez des rats presentant une polyarthrite inflammatoire. *C.R. Acad. Sci. (Paris),* 292:227–230.
22. Guilbaud, G., Benoist, J. M., Gautron, M., and Kayser, V. (1982): Aspirin clearly depresses responses of ventrobasal thalamus neurons to joint stimuli in arthritic rats. *Pain,* 13:153–163.
23. Journa, J. (1984): Pain-depressing agents and the spinal, nociceptive system. *Arzneim-Forsch.,* 34(II):1084–1088.
24. Katz, L., and Piliero, S. J. (1969): A study of adjuvant polyarthritis in the rat with special reference to associated immunological phenomena. *Ann. NY Acad. Sci.,* 147:515–536.
25. Levitan, H., and Barker, J. L. (1972): Effect of non-narcotica analgesics on membrane permeability of molluscan neurones. *Nature (New Biol.),* 239:55–57.
26. McLaughlin S. (1973): Salicylates and pospholipids bilayer membranes. *Nature,* 243:234.
27. Melzack, R., and Wall, P. D. (1965): Pain mechanism: a new theory. *Science,* 150:971–981.
28. Moncada, S., Ferreira, S. H., and Vane, J. R. (1974): Sensitization of pain receptors of the dog knee joint by prostaglandins. In: *Prostaglandin Synthetase Inhibitors,* edited by H. J. Robinson, and J. R. Vane, p.189. Raven Press, New York.
29. Moncada, S., Ferreira, S. H., and Vane, J. R. (1975): Inhibition of prostaglandin biosynthesis as the mechanism of analgesia of aspirin-like drugs in the dog knee joint. *Eur. J. Pharmacol.,* 31:250–260.
30. Newbould, B. B. (1963): Chemotherapy of arthritis induced in rats by mycobacterial adjuvant. *Br. J. Pharmacol.,* 21:127–136.
31. Okuyama, S., and Aihara, H. (1984): The mode of action of analgesic drugs in adjuvant arthritic rats as an experimental model of chronic inflammatory pain: possible central analgesic action of acidic nonsteroid antiinflammatory drugs. *Jpn. J. Pharmacol.,* 35:95–103.
32. Peschansky, M., Guilbaud, G., Gautron, M., and Besson, J. M. (1980): Encoding of noxious heat messages in neurones of the ventrobasal thalamic complex of the rat. *Brain Res.,* 197:401–413.

33. Pircio, A. W., Bierwagen, M. E., Strife, W. E., and Nicolosi, W. D. (1972): Pharmacology of new non-steroidal anti-inflammatory agent 5-cyclohexylindan-l-carboxylic acid. *Arch. Intern. Pharmacodyn.*, 199:151–163.
34. Pircio, A. W., Fedele, C. T., and Bierwagen, M. E. (1975): A new method for the evaluation of analgesic activity using adjuvant-induced arthritis in the rat., *Eur. J. Pharmacol.*, 31:207–215.
35. Riccioppo Neto, F. (1980): Further studies on the actions of salicylates on nerve membranes. *Eur. J. Pharmacol.*, 68:155–162.
36. Schorderet, M., and Straub, W. R. (1971): Effects of non-narcotic analgesic and non-steroid anti-inflammatory agents upon inorganic phosphates, intracellular potassium and impulse conduction in mammalian nerve fibers. *Biochem. Pharmacol.*, 20:1355–1361.
37. Scott, D. (1968): Aspirin: action on receptor in the tooth. *Science,* 161:180–184.
38. Vane, J. R. (1971): Inhibition of prostaglandin synthesis as a mechanism of action for aspirin-like drugs. *Nature (New Biol.),* 231:232–236.
39. Waksman, B. H., Pearson, C. M., and Sharp, J. T. (1960): Studies of arthritis and other lesions induced in rats by injection of mycobacterial adjuvant. II. Evidence that the disease is a disseminated immunologic response to exogenous antigen. *J. Immunol.,* 85:403–417.

Advances in Pain Research and Therapy,
Vol. 10. Edited by M. Tiengo et al.
Raven Press, Ltd., New York © 1987.

Immediate Muscular Pain from Physical Activity

L. Vecchiet, M.A. Giamberardino, and I. Marini

Institute of Medical Physiopathology, University of Chieti, 66100 Chieti, Italy

Myofascial pain is an experience common to everyone. This pain occurs in many different circumstances as a result of somatically localized pathological events which are primary or secondary to visceral affections (2).

Before dealing with the subject of immediate muscular pain, the clinical aspects of the sensation should be defined. This is possible by means of the findings obtained using experimentally induced physical and/or clinical stimuli, or exercise with occluded circulation. In all circumstances, the pain is always fairly well localized and markedly diffused whether it is obtained by application of a sphygmomanometer armlet to the junction of an exercising limb, or by injection of a hypertonic saline solution into a limited area of the muscle. The only difference is that, in the test in ischemia, pain spreads to the whole muscle area in activity, whereas pain after the hypertonic saline solution is felt only in the involved muscle and is frequently referred to somatic structures in the metameric field. Although muscular pain occurs in various intensities, from slight to maximum, it has very constant qualitative characteristics, being described as bruising, aching, cramping, constrictive, or burning. This pain is also variable in duration, according to its cause, and has a continuous, subcontinuous, or intermittent time pattern.

In the case of particularly severe deep somatic pain, there may be autonomic phenomena which never appear in superficial somatic pain and are also much slighter than those induced by visceral pain. These consist of pallor, sweating, and, occasionally, nausea.

From an objective point of view, painful symptoms can be provoked or increased by means of additional stimuli (muscle compression).

Although myofascial pain is not clinically distinguishable whatever the noxious agent, it can, however, be recognized by the latent period from stimulus to onset. On the basis of this parameter it is possible to distinguish an *immediate* pain arising contemporaneously with the application of a noxious stimulus, a *recurrent* pain, appearing subsequently after a variable interval generally of a few minutes, when the stimulation has been damaging, and a *delayed* pain which occurs many hours after the stimulus.

PAIN FROM PHYSICAL ACTIVITY

Physical activity is a very frequent cause of muscular pain which can appear as a result of different etiological events and physiopathogenetic mechanisms. A well-known pain is that appearing in patients with obstructive arteriopathy of the lower limbs or myocardium when a discrepancy occurs between blood flow and metabolic tissue needs as a result of exercise. Less well known, but very frequent, is the pain that occurs or increases during activity in subjects with trigger points within the myofascial structures (19).

During physical activity there are also other circumstances which may operate via the mechanism of an excess of stimulation damaging the tissue. These circumstances are bruising, strain, or sprain. The most common injury causing pain in the muscle is bruising (29). Although pain from contusive trauma is the most frequent, it is not, however, the most typical as regards the mechanism of its production, since the mechanical stimulus inevitably involves the surface tissues. Typical examples of purely muscular injury are strain or sprain. These are relatively frequent, particularly in sport, and cause two pains. The first is short and sudden and is described by the patient as bruising, lacerating, or lashing; the second occurs at different intervals after the first and is of variable intensity: dull, diffuse, and long-lasting.

Muscular pain during physical activity may also occur in completely physiological conditions. Everyone has experienced how an intense, or at least unusual, physical activity, or even remaining in the same position for a long time, produces a feeling of discomfort, which, in time, may become really painful and eventually intolerable (17,22). In order to study the clinical characteristics of this sensation more thoroughly, ergometric tests were used to reproduce the different types of contraction in free blood-flow or in induced ischemia.

PAIN FROM MUSCULAR CONTRACTION IN ISCHEMIA

It has now been proved in numerous studies that a severe pain occurs when a limb undergoes repeated isotonic and isometric muscular contractions in experimental ischemia (6,7,16,17). It is also well known that algic sensations are not caused if ischemia is provoked in a limb at rest, even for relatively long periods (6). In fact, if the blood flow is interrupted for 20 min by applying a sphygmomanometer armlet to the upper arm and raising the pressure above the systolic blood level, only paresthesic sensations are recorded, which consist of (7): (a) tingling, which occurs after a delay of 1 min 16 sec and lasts approximately 3 min 15 sec; and (b) numbness, which occurs after a delay of 14 min 21 sec and lasts until the end of the test.

If pain occurs during a test in simple ischemia, it reveals a latent algogenic condition involving the structures in the arm. The painful sensation following muscular contraction in ischemia has generally been studied exercising the hand muscles. The most common experimental models involve flexing of the middle finger against a load of 1 to 3 kg for a period of one-half sec or 1 sec. This method has shown that isometric exercise performed in ischemia is asymptomatic for several minutes but provokes pain after 34 to 48 contractions. The sensation arises after the same latent period if ischemia is kept for 20 min before the muscular work, while it occurs noticeably earlier if an exercise is performed before the interruption of blood flow. Once started, the pain increases progressively and becomes intolerable after 60 to 80 contractions; it stops within 3 sec of restored circulation.

When the ischemic condition is maintained after stopping the exercise, according to some authors the painful symptoms not only continue but increase with time, whereas other authors claim that they decrease but do not disappear completely (4,11). Other research has been concerned with the relationship between the physical and metabolic parameters of the contraction and the latent period, and the increase of the symptom with time. Studies using isotonic contractions of the adductor muscles of the finger (hand-grip) have shown a linear relationship between the onset of intolerable pain and the frequency of the contractions (7).

In order to establish further relationships between the above-mentioned parameters and the appearance of pain and its evolution in time, contractions of increasing duration were carried out by the flexing muscles of the forearm against various loads. The results obtained have proved that pain begins after performing a number of contractions, reverses in proportion to the load and to the duration of every single contraction, and increases in intensity (moderate, severe, and intolerable) in close relation to the number of contractions made. It has also been possible to show that the number of contractions performed before pain onset is roughly half the number needed for the pain to become intolerable, that if the circulation is restored the pain disappears in 1 to 2 sec and, finally, that the recovery of the metabolism from the muscular work is complete 10 min after the normalization of blood flow (13).

The relationship between the parameters studied has been codified in this formula:

$$P = C \times L^{1/2} \times D^{1/3}$$

in which P is pain, C is the number of contractions, L is the load against which the muscle is exerted, and D is the duration of each contraction (13,16,17). Recent studies using intermittent isometric contractions performed by the adductor muscle of the thumb have made it possible to establish relationships between the onset of pain and the force, frequency, and duration of the contractions, as well as the energetic expenditure. By varying the force and frequency of the contractions, it has been shown that an exponential increase in pain corresponds to the increase in energy consumed. These relationships can be expressed as follows:

$$P = (F \times t)^k/C$$

In which $(F \times t)$ is the integral of force with time, k an exponent which remains constant in spite of the variations in the contraction frequency, and C is a constant (11). It has been concluded that predominant factors influencing the evolution of pain are the energetic expenditure and the contraction frequency. The force exerted is less important in this sense. It has also been observed that high frequencies induce a stronger pain under the same conditions of energy expenditure and, at a given frequency, the energy consumed and the onset of intolerable pain are independent of the force of the contraction (11). Because pain from exercise in ischemia can easily be reproduced and numerous experimental models can be applied, many intensive studies have been made on this subject. The first suggestion concerning the most complete definition of the physiopathogenetic bases of pain was made by Lewis (6), who considered three factors in the genesis of the sensation, that is, the intermediate metabolism from ischemia, tissue hypoxia, and the compression of nerve elements. The metabolic factor he indicated as being responsible for the evolution of pain was a stable compound "substance P" (Pain), capable of diffusing slowly throughout the extracellular spaces. This substance, produced physiologically during the contraction with occluded blood flow, would accumulate and reach a concentration high enough to stimulate the nociceptors. Concerning the other two factors, the author claimed that tissue hypoxia and pressure exerted on nerve elements did not play any role in determining the sensation (6). The metabolic aspects of pain from contraction in induced ischemia has undoubtedly been the subject of wider research.

Before Lewis, some authors had already indicated lactic, pyruvic, and phosphoric acid as being responsible for pain (5). This hypothesis was not confirmed, since patients affected by muscular phosphorylase deficiency (McArdle's syndrome) felt pain all the same when undergoing exercises in ischemia, despite not being able to produce metabolites and intermediaries of Krebs cycle and, in particular, lactic acid (7).

Other researchers (13,17) have suggested the hypothesis of the production of a pain-inducing metabolite during muscular contraction. Such a substance would gradually diffuse into the extracellular spaces because of its high molecular weight, after being accumulated in contractile muscle cells.

A wide series of research has been carried out to analyze the algogenic capacities of agents such as histamine, acetylcholine, phosphocreatine, serotonin, potassium, hydrogen ions, bradykinin, prostaglandins, leukotrienes, and substance P.

It is now widely acknowledged that numerous products of the intermedi-ate metabolism that accumulate in the interstitium during contraction in ischemia can contribute to the stimulation of algosensitive nerve-endings; the most active of these have been identified as kinins. Prostaglandins do not seem to be directly responsible for pain but it has been noted that they are active in the sensitization of the receptors by reducing their excitability threshold (28).

The hypothesis that insufficient oxygen in the tissue is a cause of pain has recently been reconsidered. Relative research has not revealed any differ-ence between a group of individuals who breathed pure oxygen at 3 atm with partial pressure approximately 2,200 mm Hg (approximately 15 times the normal value) and a group who breathed normal air. The parameters examined in this comparison were the speed of onset and increase in pain and the time needed for a complete metabolic recovery from the exercise (13). It has been noticed that, in both groups, it takes 10 min of muscular inactivity with free blood flow to avoid having to stop the subsequent is-chemic test sooner because of a more rapid onset of intolerable pain (13). The relationship between ischemic damage to the muscle and that to the sensitive fibers has also been studied: This problem has been approached through a series of experiments. In this context, one significant observation was that the stimulation of the muscle by a hypertonic saline solution (which does not induce pain but only a subclinical algogenic condition), followed by the induction of ischemia only in the nerve, gives rise to pain similar to that produced by a more concentrated saline solution in normal circulatory con-ditions. It has, therefore, been concluded that ischemia of the nerve trunk can amplify the latent algogenic condition, thus making it evident.

At present, it is believed that mechanical components associated with muscle contraction also play a role in provoking pain. The fact that pain starts earlier at higher contraction frequencies leads one to suppose that its generation is influenced by rate of change of force developed by the fibers, rather than by absolute force (11). It is not clear how this factor induces the onset of and the increase in pain. It is hypothesized that there is a central interaction of stimuli leaving the chemical and mechanical nociceptors (9,11). This hypothesis could be supported by the analysis of the effects of analgesic drugs with different mechanisms of action. It has, in fact, been proved that NSAIDs have a limited activity in the control of acute ischemic pain which is, however, suppressed using opium derivatives (15). The pe-ripheral receptor units involved seem to be the amyelinic free nerve endings of the perivascular muscle nerves (3).

PAIN FROM CONCENTRIC DYNAMIC CONTRACTION

Concentric dynamic contraction does not usually cause muscular pain (17). Models of this type of contraction have been applied experimentally on limited areas of the body, such as the adductor muscles of the fingers, in order to study the latency of pain onset and the increase in pain with time in relation to the force, frequency, and duration of the contractions.

Particular attention has been paid to establish the connection between the contraction frequency and the onset and intolerability of the symptom. It has been noted that voluntary contractions of the right index finger against a load of 2.5 kg performed at a frequency of 30/min, even for over 35 min, do not induce pain of such intensity that the exercise has to be stopped. However, from a frequency of contractions of 70/min to the highest possible frequency (approximately 90/min), 120 contractions are, on average, enough to elicit intolerable pain (17).

In larger areas of the body, it has also been observed experimentally that pain starts only when the intensity of the exercise is too high for the individual aerobic capacity. Rectangular (22) and triangular ergometric bicycle tests have been performed in order to study this pain. In the rectangular tests it has been observed that (22):

1. With the increase in work-load, there is a critical-effort test for each subject, which provokes an aching, cramp-like, diffuse, poorly localized pain (in one or more muscles) within 10 to 20 min.
2. Lower power levels than those of critical effort never cause pain whatever the duration of the test.
3. Higher power levels, however, give rise to pain with a latent period steadily decreasing in relation to the increasing effort.
4. Control tests performed at different times give similar results as regards the onset of pain under the same conditions of power exerted.

In agreement with other reports it has been shown that even a quite short and not very intensive training period has a clear influence on the behavior of muscle pain during the same effort trials. It has been noted, in fact, that (22):

1. In very few subjects there are no substantial differences.
2. In other cases, however, the latency of pain onset increases slightly, or remains the same, but the subjects manage to continue the test for 30 min: There is, therefore, a decrease in pain intensity.
3. In others, the latency of pain onset is increased when performing the exercise at the same power level.
4. Finally, in most subjects, the painful symptoms appear only for higher work-loads.

Muscular pain arises almost always when performing an exercise of steadily increasing intensity.

It is of common knowledge that, when performing triangular tests up to the maximum effort the test is stopped in most cases because of pain in the involved limbs. In the triangular tests it has been observed that (22):

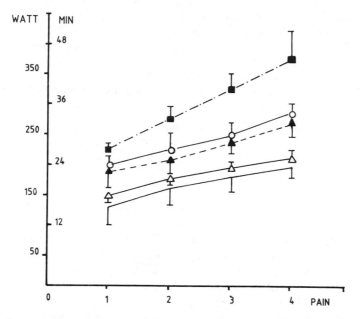

FIG. 1. The muscular pain pattern during triangular ergometric bicycle tests with level increased by 25 watts every 3 min, performed by homogeneous groups of: untrained men (————), untrained football players (△————), trained football players (▲ – – – –), basketball players (○————), cyclists (■—·—·-). The pain is measured by means of a common numerical scale: 0 = no pain; 1 = notable pain; 2 = annoying pain; 3 = severe pain; 4 = intolerable pain.

1. No pain whatsoever is felt up to a certain intensity of work-load.
2. At determinate intensities of the exercise, the same sort of pain starts in the involved limbs as that occurring in the rectangular tests. This pain increases steadily during the tests, sometimes with the same work-load but more often with a progressive increase in the load, until it becomes impossible to continue.
3. In all subjects the test is interrupted because of muscular pain in the limbs involved: Very occasionally there are different reasons for stopping the exercise (dyspnea, muscular exhaustion).
4. The painful response has a very uniform pattern in homogeneous groups of subjects (same age, sex, job, or sport) (Fig. 1).

As has been noted, pain can be induced during concentric dynamic contraction by functionally overloading the involved muscles (13,17). Since the sensation produced has the same characteristics as the pain caused by exercise in ischemia, it has been hypothesized that the physiopathogenetic mechanism is the same in both cases. This consists of the release and accumulation in the extracellular space of algogenic substances secondary to the suffering in the tissue induced by the work-load and the contraction frequency. Muscle work against a determinate resistance provokes, therefore, a relative ischemic condition whose intensity is related to the load; the contraction frequency, on the other hand, causes an insufficient washout of active metabolites because of the reduced free blood flow time. Various studies have been performed in order to verify the hypothesis that algogenic substances are produced during this type of contraction. Investigations have been made into the algogenic capacity of plasma separated from blood coming from the somatic area subjected to the effort and it has been found that this capacity is linked to the presence of algogenic substances, in particular, lactic acid, pyruvic acid, histamine, kinins, and potassium (21). It has also been observed that this property of the blood increases significantly with the onset of pain. The relationship between the onset of pain and the marked increase of the algogenic substances in the plasma suggests that, in this phase, an increased permeability of the microvessels is produced in the area of the striated muscle subjected to the work load. This increase would cause the passage of preactive algogenic substances from the circulatory to the interstitial area and the enzymatic activation of these substances would occur in the interstitium, a percentage of them then passing into the blood coming from the involved area. The metabolites produced would be able to induce pain through the activation of the chemonociceptive fibroreceptor nerve endings (8,9,10).

DYNAMIC ECCENTRIC CONTRACTION

Muscular pain can also be caused by dynamic eccentric contraction. The characteristic of this pain is, however, that it occurs after many hours, and it is therefore not included in this study.

PAIN FROM ISOMETRIC CONTRACTION

Muscular pain can easily be induced by means of isometric contractions. In a series of tests using phases of prolonged isometric contraction against increasing loads on the femoral quadriceps muscle, it has been shown that (24,27):

1. The exercise provokes a burning pain which increases steadily throughout the test.
2. The painful sensation passes through various phases, from simple discomfort to slight pain and to intolerable pain.
3. The test always has to be stopped because of the pain.
4. The painful response to progressive loads is exponential regarding not only its latency but also its maximum level of tolerability.

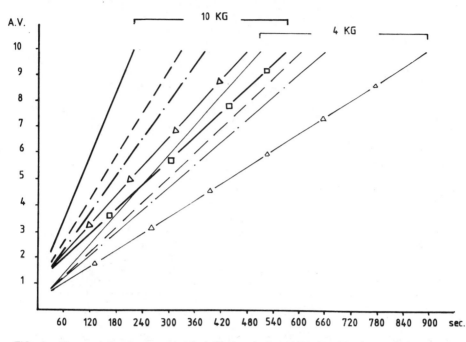

FIG. 2. The evolution in time of pain intensity measured by visual analog scale in a quadriceps muscle performing isometric contractions against 4- and 10-kg loads applied to the ankle joint. Continuous contractions (———), repeated 30 sec contractions with resting periods of 5 sec (– – – –), 10 sec (—·—·—), 15 sec (—△—), and 20 sec (—□—). Contractions with intervals of 20 sec against the 4-kg load do not provoke pain.

5. The latency of pain onset and the time needed to reach the highest intensity are in reverse proportion to the load, the increase in pain being, therefore, linear.

Further findings on muscular pain have been obtained through tests of isometric contractions performed at fixed intervals. The load and the duration of each contraction were kept constant (the latter being 30 sec) while the resting periods were of different length in each test (5, 10, 15, and 20 sec).

In the case of tests interrupted because of intolerable pain it has been observed that:

1. The time of pain onset increases linearly as the resting intervals are increased in duration.
2. The time of pain onset decreases linearly, and is in direct proportion to the resting period in the contractions following relaxation.
3. The intensity of the pain increases linearly both at the beginning and at the end of every contraction period, and this increase declines as the resting period increases (Fig. 2).

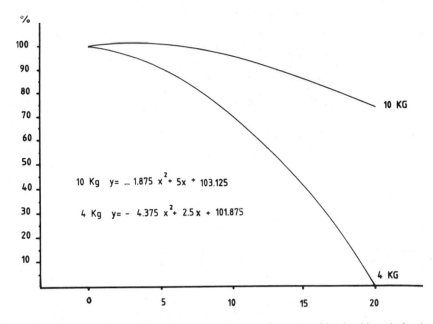

FIG. 3. The percentage of subjects stopping the test because of intolerable pain for 4- and 10-kg loads, respectively, in continuous contractions and repeated 30-sec contractions with resting intervals of 5, 10, 15, and 20 sec.

It has also been observed that when the relaxation period is increased, a progressively higher percentage of subjects are forced to stop the test because of fatigue and not because of pain. The duration of the relaxation period necessary for intolerable pain to disappear is directly related to the load (Fig. 3).

Numerous studies have been carried out to establish the genesis of pain evoked by isometric muscle contraction. It can be hypothesized, also in this case, that at the origin of the sensation there is, on one hand, the release of active metabolites as a result of muscular exercise and, on the other, the accumulation of these metabolites because of the circulation arrest (12). To confirm this, we can mention the many studies investigating the effects of this type of contraction on the blood flow in the skeletal muscle involved.

It has been observed that the blood supply increases during static contractions below 30% of the maximum voluntary contraction (MVC), and decreases when contractions are performed at levels above this value (1). It has also been established that strong contractions of the hand (hand-grip) at 70% of MVC completely arrest the circulation in the forearm (1). The muscle contraction necessary to cause a complete intramuscular blood occlusion has been assessed in percentage at approximately 60% of MVC (1).

The arrest of the circulation could be determined by the increase in intramuscular pressure above the systolic blood level, and also by the interference that the contracted muscular masses and the differently angled joints exert on the blood supply to the muscles by the major arteries (18).

PAIN FROM PHYSICAL ACTIVITY AND MYOFASCIAL TRIGGER POINTS

It is of common knowledge that physical activity is very often conditioned by the pain arising from trigger points in the myofascial structures (19). In order to investigate this pain more thoroughly, experimental algogenic foci have been induced in muscles then subjected to dynamic concentric or isometric contractions.

The trigger points can be produced very easily by injecting a hypertonic saline solution in the tissue. Such an injection causes a painful sensation which lasts 15 min and produces a latent algogenic condition which continues to act locally for several hours or even days, and may become evident through additional stimuli, such as muscle contraction.

Dynamic Concentric Contraction

An experimental algogenic focus has been produced by injecting 1 ml 10% hypertonic saline solution in the distal third of the vastus lateralis of the left quadriceps, rectangular ergometric bicycle tests then being performed at the 70% level of the maximum heart rate predicted for the age (220 minus age) 1 min, and 3, 6, 24, 48, and 72 hr after the injection. It has been found that (23,25,26):

1. The exercise induces a diffuse, steadily decreasing pain in the injection area for up to 48 hr.
2. The pain level curves are similar in shape, but there is a notable difference in pain peak time during the test according to the delay after the trigger.
3. The difference is of high statistical significance and the maximum pain level generally decreases exponentially when the delay increases.
4. On the contrary, the time of appearance of the pain peak increases in relation to the delay. (Fig. 4).

Isometric Contraction

The results obtained by subjecting the femoral quadriceps to an isometric contraction against a constant load have been compared with those found 30 min, and 24 and 48 hr after the production of an algogenic focus in the muscle using the previously described method.

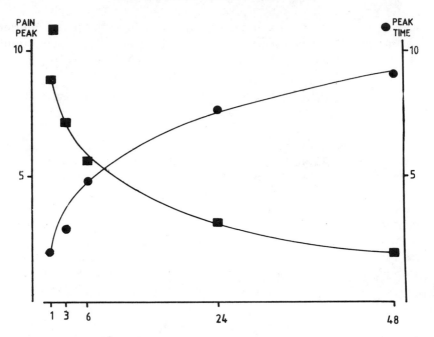

FIG. 4. The averaged pain peak and the time of the peak during the test are plotted versus the delay from trigger to submaximal work: The curves are roughly exponential.

It has so been observed that 30 min after the injection, the pain from isometric contraction, when compared with the basal test (20), (a) starts after a much shorter latent period in all subjects; and (b) intensifies more rapidly so that the test is shorter in duration.

It has also be seen that the experimental algogenic focus causes a significant change in the basal response after 24 hr but ceases to function after 48 hr (Table 1).

TABLE 1. *Results of the statistical analysis before and after the induction of the algogenic focus regarding the latency of pain onset and maximum tolerability level*

Tests performed[a]	Latency of pain onset (sec)	SD	Latency of maximum tolerability level (sec)	SD	t	p
1	103	±27	362	±20	—	—
2	66	±22	275	±17	12.25	0.001
3	73	±11	309	±30	4.16	0.01
4	104	±30	362	±18	0.27	0.9

[a] 1: Basal test; 2, 3, 4: tests performed 30 min, 24 hr, and 48 hr after focus induction.

The particular behavior of the pain from dynamic concentric or isometric contractions after induction of an experimental trigger point can be explained both by the algogenic focus itself and by the biochemical tissue changes produced by the muscular activity. It is well known that during muscle contraction numerous metabolites are released (4,10,28) which, in low concentrations, produce only metabolic effects responsible for cardiocirculatory and respiratory changes in effort and, in high concentrations, activate also high threshold fiber units carrying algogenic signals (4,14,27).

In the presence of latent algogenic foci, the painful sensation may occur as a result of a summation of impulses.

The suggested interpretation would explain not only the location of the pain in the area where the experimental algogenic focus is induced, but also the steady decrease in the sensation after an identical physical effort in relation to the decreasing trigger activity.

CONCLUSIONS

By means of this review of the studies on acute muscle pain from physical effort, it has been possible to prove that the symptom may occur not only during pathological events but also as a frequent consequence of normal concentric or isometric dynamic contraction. Since this pain can be so easily reproduced it represents a particularly suitable experimental model in clinical and physiopathological studies.

Among the numerous findings obtained, some are of particular interest: One is the appearance of pain during concentric dynamic muscular activity using well defined work-loads and the modification of its threshold of onset and intolerability following training. Another is the disappearance of pain during intermittent isometric contractions in relation to the increase in the resting period, by which it is possible to define if the activity is stopped because of pain or because of fatigue.

On the basis of these two findings it is possible to suggest not only a physiopathogenetic interpretation of immediate muscular pain from effort, but also the use of this pain in the functional assessment of the individual performance of the skeletal muscle since the symptom arises during anaerobic activity with lactic acid formation.

REFERENCES

1. Barnes, W. S. (1980): The relationship between maximum isometric strength and intramuscular circulatory occlusion. *Ergonomics,* 4:351–357.
2. Cervero, F. (1980): Deep and visceral pain. In: *Pain and Society,* edited by H. W. Kosterlitz and L. Y. Terenius, pp. 263–282. Verlag Chemie, Weinheim.
3. Iggo, A. (1974): Pain receptors. In: *Recent Advances on Pain,* edited by J. J. Bonica, P. Procacci, and C. A. Pagni, pp. 3–35. Thomas, Springfield, Illinois.
4. Keele, C. A., and Armstrong, D. (1974): Substances producing pain and itch. In: *Monographs of the Physiological Society, Vol. 12,* edited by H. Barcroft, H. Davson, and W. D. M. Paton, pp. 1–374. Edward Arnold, London.

5. Kissin, M. (1934): The production of pain in exercising skeletal muscle during induced anoxaemia. *J. Clin. Invest.*, 13:37–45.
6. Lewis, T. (1942): *Pain.* Macmillan, New York.
7. McArdle, B., and Verell, D. (1955): Responses to ischaemic work in the human forearm. *Clin. Sci.*, 15:305–318.
8. Mense, S. (1977): Nervous outflow from skeletal muscle following chemical noxious stimulation. *J. Physiol. (Lond.)*, 267:75–88.
9. Mense, S. (1977): Muscular nociceptors. *J. Physiol.*, 73:233–240.
10. Mense, S. (1981): Sensitization of group IV muscle receptors to bradykinin by 5-hydroxytryptamine and prostaglandin E_2. *Brain Res.*, 225:95–105.
11. Mills, K. R., Newham, D. J., and Edwards, R. H. T. (1982): Force, contraction, frequency and energy metabolism as determinants of ischaemic muscle pain. *Pain*, 14:149–154.
12. Mills, K. R., Newham, D. J., and Edwards, R. H. T. (1984): Muscle pain. In: *Textbook of Pain*, edited by P. D. Wall and R. Melzack, pp. 319–330. Churchill Livingstone, Edinburgh.
13. Park, S. R., and Rodbard, S. (1962): Effects of load and.duration of tension on pain induced by muscular contraction. *Am. J. Physiol.*, 203:735–738.
14. Peruzzi, G., Tallarida, G., Baldoni, F., Raimondi, G., Massaro, M., and Sangiorgi, M. (1980): Attuali orientamenti sulla regolazione riflessa periferica della funzione cardiocircolatoria durante l'esercizio muscolare. *Recenti Prog. Med.*, 3:278–290.
15. Posner, J. (1984): A modified submaximal effort tourniquet test for evaluation of analgesics in healthy volunteers. *Pain*, 19:143–151.
16. Rodbard, S. (1970): Muscle pain. In: *Pain and Suffering: Selected Aspects*, edited by B. L. Crue, pp. 150–162. Thomas, Springfield, Illinois.
17. Rodbard, S., and Pragay, E. B. (1968): Contraction, frequency, blood supply, and muscle pain. *J. Appl. Physiol.*, 2:142–145.
18. Rohter, F. D., and Hyman, C. (1962): Blood flow in the arm and finger during muscle contraction and joint position changes. *J. Appl. Physiol.*, 17:819–823.
19. Simon, D. G., and Travell, F. G. (1984): Myofascial pain syndromes. In: *Textbook of Pain*, edited by P. D. Wall and R. Melzack, pp. 263–276. Churchill Livingstone, Edinburgh.
20. Vecchiet, L., Colozzi, A., Pardi, V., Flacco, L., Ribaldi, R., and Obletter, G. (1987): Muscular pain from isometric contraction: modifications induced by algogenic focil. *Algologia (in press)*.
21. Vecchiet, L., Dolce, V., and Galletti, R. (1976): Algogenic activity of human plasma following muscular work. In: *Kinins. Pharmacodynamics and Biological Roles*, edited by F. Sicuteri, N. Back, and G. L. Haberland, pp. 177–182. Plenum Press, New York.
22. Vecchiet, L., and Galletti, R. (1979): Muscular pain under effort. In: *First International Congress on Sports Medicine Applied to Football, Vol. 1*, edited by L. Vecchiet, pp. 39–50. D. Guanella, Rome.
23. Vecchiet, L., Marini, I., D'Autilio, A., Feroldi, P., and Rinaldi, A. P. (1985): Muscular pain in submaximal exercise produced by experimental trigger. *Eur. Rev. Med. Pharmacol. Sci.*, 7:449–452.
24. Vecchiet, L., Marini, I., and Feroldi, P. (1983): Muscular pain caused by isometric contraction: evaluation of pain through visual analog scale. *Clin. Ther.*, 5:504–508.
25. Vecchiet, L., Marini, I., and Feroldi, P. (1984): Muscular hyperalgesia from submaximal exercise and experimental triggers. *Pain(Suppl.)*, 2:265.
26. Vecchiet, L., Marini, I., Feroldi, P., and D'Autilio, A. (1984): Relationship between pain and changes in HR, VE, and VO_2 during isometric tests. *Eur. Rev. Med. Pharmacol. Sci.*, 6:429–436.
27. Vecchiet, L., Marini, I., and Zucchi, P. L. (1982): Il dolore muscolare da contrazione isometrica: correlazione con alcuni parametri cardiorespiratori. *Algologia*, 2:247–260.
28. Yaksh, T. L., and Hammond, D. L. (1982): Peripheral and central substrates involved in the rostral transmission of nociceptive information. *Pain*, 13:1–85.
29. Yates, A., and Smith, M. A. (1984): Musculo-skeletal pain after trauma. In: *Textbook of Pain*, edited by P. D. Wall and R. Melzack, pp. 234–239. Churchill Livingstone, Edinburgh.

Advances in Pain Research and Therapy,
Vol. 10. Edited by M. Tiengo et al.
Raven Press, Ltd., New York © 1987.

Nature of Exercise-Induced Muscle Pain

*D.A. Jones, *D.J. Newham, **G. Obletter, and
**M.A. Giamberardino

*Department of Medicine, University College London, London WC1, England; and
**Institute of Medical Physiopathology, University of Chieti, Chieti, Italy

Muscular pain during and after exercise must be one of the most commonly experienced sensations of discomfort in everyday life yet very little is known about its causes. Of the two main types of pain associated with exercise we only briefly consider pain arising during activity, but concentrate on the possible causes of delayed onset pain and the relationship between this and muscle damage.

PAIN DURING EXERCISE

During high-intensity exercise discomfort develops rapidly in the muscles and is similar in sensation to ischemic pain, the main characteristics of which were first documented by Lewis and co-workers (20,21). They suggested that during muscular activity with the circulation occluded, some factor, possibly a metabolite, is released from the fibers and accumulates giving rise to pain. When the circulation is restored this substance is dispersed and the pain rapidly decreases. The pain is related to the metabolic cost of the contraction with a positive exponent, but mechanical activity also contributes to the sensation (24). For the same integrated force, exercise in which there is a rapid contraction and relaxation cycle is more painful than contractions at a lower frequency (Fig. 1). It is not clear whether this is because of different energetic costs, whether the mechanical activity causes potentiation of the peripheral receptors, or there is some process of central summation. The identity of the algesic substance also remains unknown: Potassium, inorganic phosphate, and various nucleotides may all be released from active muscle and could separately or together activate pain fibers. However, lactate and hydrogen ions are unlikely to be major causes of pain since patients with myophosphorylase deficiency who cannot produce lactate, develop pain during ischemic contractions to the same, if not greater, extent than normal subjects.

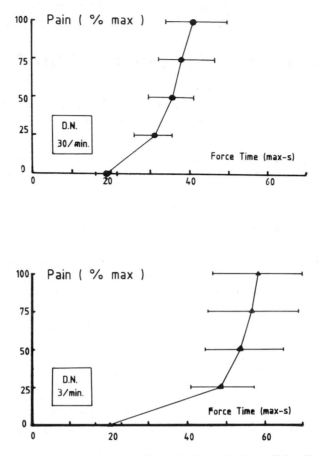

FIG. 1. Pain as a function of integrated force in the adductor pollicis with the circulation occluded. Subject held repetitive 50% maximum isometric force for either, (*below*) 10 sec contraction with 10 sec rest or (*above*) 2 sec contraction with 2 sec rest. Note that pain developed more rapidly with contractions at the higher frequency.

PAIN DEVELOPING AFTER EXERCISE

It is common experience that heavy or unaccustomed exercise is associated with a type of pain that becomes evident some hours after the end of exercise and may persist for several days (13,14). Asmussen (3) was the first to note that this form of pain was caused mainly, if not exclusively, by movements in which the active muscle is stretched, such as in walking down hill, or when lowering weights. This type of movement is often referred to as "eccentric exercise" or "negative work." The work described here is based on our observations of three muscle groups exercised in this way. They are the quadriceps stretched during stepping (26), the calf muscles exercised by walking backwards down an inclined treadmill (27), and the forearm flexors stretched by forcibly extending the forearm (16). In every case muscle pain developed in those muscles that had been stretched.

During the exercise the subject is aware of high forces generated in the muscle and tendons, but there is no ischemic pain such as associated with high force concentric or isometric contractions. After 10 to 20 min of eccentric exercise the subject usually notices difficulty in controlling the movement; there is considerable tremor and loss of force and altered contractile properties, the latter being slow to recover (30). Another notable feature is difficulty in fully flexing and extending the affected limb. These sensations are generally described as "unusual" but never as painful. In the next 6 to 12 hr discomfort develops in the exercised muscle. Typically the subject who exercises one day will go to bed with minor discomfort only to wake the next morning with severe and, in some cases, almost disabling pain felt while trying to get out of bed. At rest there is little or no discomfort and it is not until the muscle is moved or touched that the pain is experienced. There are a number of sensations of which the two most prominent are discussed below.

MUSCULAR STIFFNESS

This sensation is most evident after a period of rest, such as sitting in a chair when, on attempting to rise, difficulty and pain is experienced stretching the affected muscles. There is a sensation of mechanical stiffness which feels as if the muscle had become shorter. After eccentric exercise of the forearm flexors there is difficulty straightening the elbow and if this is done forcibly there is a painful stretching sensation in the belly of the muscle much as experienced when overstretching a normal muscle. With continuing activity the sensations diminish and after a few minutes of warmup, movements become fairly normal. At the end of exercise, however, when the muscle is again rested the sensations return with, as far as can be judged in the absence of objective measurements, a similar intensity.

Stiffness has not yet been quantitatively assessed but seems to be worse 2 to 3 days after the exercise and can still be felt by the subjects 7 to 10 days later.

MUSCLE TENDERNESS

Tenderness is a feeling of discomfort elicited by pressure. In the tender muscle the feeling is similar, if not identical, to that around a bruise or tendon sprain. With no movement and nothing touching the muscle there is no pain. Isometric contractions are relatively pain-free, but when the affected muscle is contracted at a shortened length, the tenderness is most acute. While making many actions unpleasant, such as sitting if the gluteal muscles are affected, there is little indication that the tenderness inhibits activation of muscles, at least for isometric contractions with muscles at resting length.

Of the various sensations, tenderness has been most extensively studied since it can be quantified by pressing on the muscle and measuring the force required to elicit a painful response (9). This technique also allows the distribution of pain over the surface of the muscle to be determined. After stepping exercise, pain develops in the quadriceps used to step down in the distal/medial and lateral areas with the midportion over the rectus femoris being relatively pain-free. It has been suggested that the pain is associated with the musculotendinous junctions but in a complex muscle such as the quadriceps the attachments are so ubiquitous that it is difficult to assess this. For the forearm flexors, tenderness in the biceps developing after exercise is generally most severe along the midline in the proximal region. On palpation the pain can generally be localized to the medial aspect of the long head of the biceps, which is probably the tendon attachment.

The tenderness, which in some cases can make the muscle acutely sensitive to touch, is maximum 1 to 2 days after eccentric exercise and is generally absent or much reduced by 5 days (see later).

CAUSES OF MUSCLE TENDERNESS

It has become almost a truism to suggest that muscle pain is a result of damage; the important questions, however, are whether it is muscle fibers or connective tissue that is damaged and what is the nature of the signal from the damaged tissue. Hough (14) suggested that disruption of muscle fibers was the cause, but since then most workers have favored damage to connective tissue as the most likely explanation (4,13,19). There is, however, only limited evidence for this (1), and recently it has become apparent that eccentric exercise can cause considerable damage to muscle fibers (2,10,18,23,28,29) reviving speculation that these could be the source of the algesic substance.

Inflammation and Muscle Tenderness

The sensations of swelling and tenderness developing after eccentric exercise are similar to those of classical inflammation and as such should be amenable to treatment with anti-inflammatory agents. Our own experience with aspirin, however, is that this produces little or no effect at doses of 1,200 to 2,400 mg/day (C. Grieg, *unpublished observations*), and Janssen et al. (15) also found that nonsteroidal anti-inflammatory agents were without effect on muscle pain. The rapid training effect which lasts for many weeks (17) makes cross-over trials difficult, but recently we have carried out a trial of a steroidal anti-inflammatory agent, prednisolone (10 mg/day), using stepping exercise in which the pain developed in one leg with the subject taking placebo or prednisolone, was compared 3 weeks later with pain in the opposite leg while taking the other substance (11).

Nine subjects took prednisolone or placebo for 7 days and on the third day carried out 20 min of stepping exercise. Pain developing in the quadriceps that had been stretched was measured on the following days. There was no significant difference between the pain scores when the subjects were taking prednisolone or placebo.

The nonsteroidal anti-inflammatory agents inhibit the enzyme cyclooxygenase preventing the formation of prostaglandins while, presumably, leaving the formation of leukotrienes unaffected. Steroidal agents are thought to prevent the liberation of arachadonic acid from phospholipids, thereby preventing the formation of all the metabolites. Our results suggest that the arachadonic acid cascade is not involved in the development of delayed onset muscle tenderness. Other indices of inflammation such as white cell counts, have also proved to be negative (5).

Tissue edema

Many subjects experiencing delayed onset muscle pain complain of "tightness and swelling" in the affected muscle. The muscle may appear swollen and we have measured increases in circumference of 5 to 10% in the calf and biceps. Small increases in volume have been reported by Talag (32) and Bobbert et al. (5), although the latter point out that nonpainful swelling can be seen after other forms of exercise.

Increased intramuscular pressure is well known to give rise to painful sensations in the anterior tibial compartment (22), and tissue edema with a consequent rise in pressure has been suggested as a cause of delayed onset muscle pain (5,6). We have measured intramuscular pressure in painful and pain-free biceps muscles after performing eccentric contractions of the forearm flexors for 20 to 40 min (25). The contralateral muscle served as a control in some cases, and in others serial measurements were made on the same muscle during and after the painful period. A 21-gauge needle was inserted 2 cm into the midline position in the belly of the biceps and connected to a pressure transducer. The system was filled with sterile saline which was very slowly infused to ensure that the needle tip remained open. The resting pressure was found to be 10.4 ± 2.6 mm Hg in the painful muscles and 10.3 ± 2.1 in the pain-free muscles. When serial measurements were made there was no tendency for higher pressures to occur when muscles were painful.

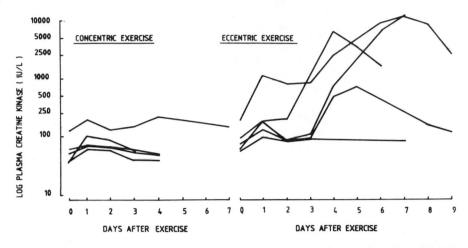

FIG. 2. Plasma creatine kinase after concentric and eccentric exercise. *Left:* Subjects walked forward up an inclined treadmill for 1 hr and plasma CK and calf muscle tenderness were measured on subsequent days. *Right:* Subjects walked backwards down the same incline for 1 hr. (From ref. 26.)

In addition to these experimental findings there are other observations that make it unlikely that increased intramuscular pressure is the cause of pain. During isometric contractions the intramuscular pressure can rise to several hundred mm Hg (12), but this is not perceived as painful in the same way as muscle tenderness and even in an already tender muscle isometric contractions do not aggravate the pain. We have also noticed that when a tender muscle is biopsied, the presence of a relatively large needle in the muscle, which must distort the tissue and increase pressure locally, does not produce any additional pain.

Release of Soluble Material from Damaged Muscle Fibers

A good indication of muscle damage is the release of soluble muscle proteins into the circulation, the most commonly measured being creatine kinase (CK). There are two types of response following activity. The first is a one- or twofold increase in plasma level with a peak occurring approximately 24 hr after the exercise (7), and this corresponds well with the muscle tenderness suggesting that some algesic substance is released from damaged muscle. However, this extent and time course of CK release is a common response to many forms of exercise whether or not the muscles subsequently become painful (e.g., ref. 31). In a study in which subjects walked up an inclined treadmill (i.e., concentric exercise where muscles are shortening) a small rise in plasma CK was seen 24 to 48 hr after exercise (Fig. 2) at a time

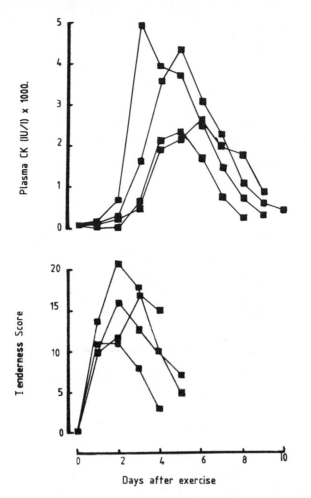

FIG. 3. Tenderness and plasma creatine kinase after eccentric exercise of the forearm flexors. Subjects performed 20 min of maximum eccentric exercise (contractions: 4/min) and plama CK (*above*) and muscle tenderness were evaluated at daily intervals.

when there was no pain in the muscles. When the subjects walked backwards down the same incline thereby stretching their muscles, a similar small peak was seen at 24 hr (Fig. 2) when the calf muscles were very painful. In the next 7 days the plasma CK showed a second peak reaching levels of 5,000 to 10,000 IU/liter 4 to 6 days after the exercise. This second large release of CK was at a time when the muscles were no longer tender (27).

The time course of pain development in the biceps and CK release after eccentric exercise of the forearm flexors is shown in Fig. 3.

Tenderness was maximum 1 to 2 days after the exercise, whereas the peak

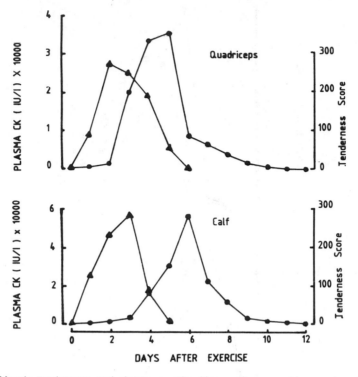

FIG. 4. Muscle tenderness and plasma creatine kinase after eccentric exercise of quadriceps and calf muscles. Quadriceps (*above*) exercised by 20 min stepping; calf muscles exercised by 2 hr walking backwards down an inclined treadmill. Tenderness (▲); CK (●).

CK release occurred after 4 to 6 days. A similar time course has been found with the calf and quadriceps (Fig. 4). The release of CK and pain are thus seen to be dissociated in time. However, CK is a large molecule and we have preliminary data showing that myoglobin, a smaller protein, is released one day sooner than CK. In a muscle that is clearly damaged even smaller proteins and peptides could be released at a time when the muscle is painful. In this case, a relationship might still be expected between the extent of the muscle damage, as indicated by the subsequent CK release, and the severity of the muscle pain. In cases where there is a large CK release there is always considerable pain, but the reverse is not always true. There have been many occasions when subjects have reported painful muscles yet they have shown no evidence of muscle damage as judged by plasma CK levels. The peak pain and plasma CK levels for two female subjects after exercise of the forearm flexors are shown in Fig. 5. One had a high plasma CK, while the other had a smaller CK response but reported greater pain. It is, however, notoriously difficult to compare scores between subjects since reporting of pain is subjec-

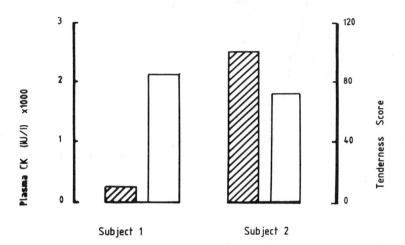

FIG. 5. Muscle pain and plasma creatine kinase in two subjects after eccentric exercise. Both subjects performed 20 min eccentric exercise of the forearm flexors and muscle tenderness and plasma CK were measured at daily intervals. Peak values are shown for each subject. CK (crosshatched area); muscle tenderness (open area).

tive, but there are occasions when it is possible to compare different levels of pain and damage within the same subjects. One of the features of eccentric exercise is the rapidity with which the muscle adapts to repeated exercise (17). Quadriceps tenderness and plasma CK are shown in Fig. 6 for a subject who performed stepping exercise at weekly intervals. During the first week there was a large release of CK which was much reduced the second week and there was no significant release on subsequent weeks. Although a little reduced, the pain was still appreciable in the second and third weeks when there was no evidence of further muscle fiber damage.

Further evidence that muscle fiber damage is not the direct cause of muscle pain comes from work in which technetium pyrophosphate has been used to localize the damaged muscle. After stepping exercise, the pain and discomfort is felt in the quadriceps, gluteal, and adductor muscles of the leg that has been used to step down, and in the contralateral calf that is stretched as the subject lands on an extended foot. Technitium scanning has shown that damage is restricted to the adductor and gluteal muscles, while the quadriceps, which feels very painful, shows no additional uptake of technetium (28).

The experimental evidence demonstrates that eccentric exercise can cause both pain and extensive damage to muscle fibers, however the time course and the magnitude of these two events are poorly coordinated and it seems unlikely that substances released from damaged muscles are the cause of the delayed onset muscle tenderness. The relationship is therefore seen to be coincidental rather than causal.

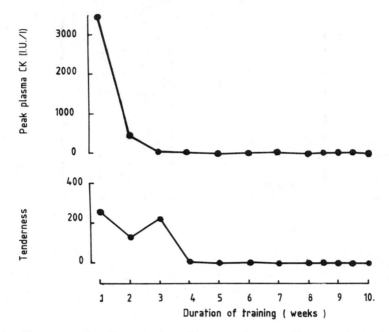

FIG. 6. Plasma creatine kinase and quadriceps tenderness with repeated exercise. One subject performed 20 min stepping exercise once a week for 10 weeks, and peak values for muscle pain and CK are shown for each week. Note the rapid training effect for plasma CK but a slower reduction in pain.

Reflex Activity

On the basis of electromyograph (EMG) recordings from painful muscles DeVries (8) suggested that damage may result in increased reflex contraction of the muscle and consequent local areas of painful ischemia. More recent studies (1,5) have found no evidence to support this view, and in our own experience painful muscles are electrically silent. It also seems an unlikely explanation as ischemic pain is not the same sensation as tenderness.

Local Anesthetics and Tenderness

Subjects who have had needle biopsies of tender muscles have commented that when the needle is inside the muscle there is no greater feeling of discomfort than when sampling from a pain-free muscle. When taking biopsies the procedure is to infiltrate local anesthetic down to the muscle fascia, and when this is done sensations of tenderness are much reduced suggesting that pain arises in the fascia rather than the muscle tissue. These observations must be treated with some care, as it is possible that sensory nerves from the muscle may run through the fascia where it is anesthetised, but it is consistent with the evidence that damage to the muscle fibers themselves is not the cause of pain. This is in keeping with the various suggestions that pain may be due to connective tissue injury.

SUMMARY AND CONCLUSIONS

Delayed onset muscle pain takes two main forms, a feeling of mechanical stiffness with pain when the muscle is extended, and, second, a tenderness experienced on moving or touching the muscle. Both are the result of eccentric exercise in which the muscle is stretched. Although many of the sensations are similar to those of inflammation there is no evidence that pain is due to increased intramuscular pressure or the formation of prostaglandins or leukotrienes. Eccentric exercise can result in the release of large quantities of soluble proteins from muscle, but the extent and time course of this does not correlate well with the muscle pain. These observations point to damage of the connective tissue as the most probable cause of the muscle pain although direct evidence for this is limited to the findings of Abraham (1) for hydroxyproline excretion after exercise. There is clearly a need for more detailed studies of muscle connective tissue morphology and metabolism in relation to exercise. As far as algesic substances are concerned, there is little indication as to the identity of these. It is unlikely that metabolites of arachadonic acid are involved, and consequently techniques for measuring the tissue content, or for blocking the action of substances such as bradykinin and histamine need to be developed.

Exercise-induced muscle pain remains an enigma but one that is particularly interesting since it is such a common feature of everyday life. It is also fascinating in that it is one area of research where personal observations and introspection play an important role alongside experimental studies.

ACKNOWLEDGMENTS

Much of this work has been supported by the Wellcome Trust and the Muscular Dystrophy Group of Great Britain.

REFERENCES

1. Abraham, W. M. (1977): Factors in delayed muscle soreness. *Med. Sci. Sports*, 9:11–26.
2. Armstrong, R. B., Ogilvie, R. W., and Schwane, J. A. (1983): Eccentric exercise induced injury to rat skeletal muscle. *J. Appl. Physiol.*, 54:80–93.
3. Asmussen, E. (1953): Positive and negative muscular work. *Acta Physiol. Scand.*, 28:364–382.
4. Asmussen, E. (1956): Observations on experimental muscle soreness. *Acta Physiol. Scand.*, 28:364–382.

5. Bobbert, M. F., Hollander, A. P., and Huijing, P. A. (1986): Factors in delayed onset muscular soreness of man. *Med. Sci. Sports Exer.,* 18:75–81.
6. Brendstrup, P. (1962): Late edema after muscular exercise. *Arch. Phys. Med. Rehabil.,* 43:401–405.
7. Byrnes, W. C., Clarkson, P. M., White, J. S., Hsich, S. S., Frykman, P. N., and Maughan, R. J. (1985): Delayed onset muscle soreness following repeated bouts of down hill running. *J. Appl. Physiol.,* 59:710–715.
8. DeVries, H. A. (1966): Quantitative electromyographic investigation of the spasm theory of muscle pain. *J. Phys Med.,* 45:119–134.
9. Edwards, R. H. T., Mills, K. R., and Newham, D. J. (1981): Measurement of severity and distribution of experimental muscle tenderness. *J. Physiol.,* 317:1–2P.
10. Friden, J., Sjostrom, M., and Ekblom, B. (1983): Myofibrillar damage following intense eccentric exercise in man. *Int. J. Sports Med.,* 4:170–176.
11. Headley, S. A. E., Newham, D. J., and Jones, D. A. (1987): The effect of prednisolone on exercise induced muscle pain and damage. *Clin. Sci.,* 70:85P.
12. Hill, A. V. (1948). The pressure developed in muscle during contraction. *J. Physiol.,* 107:518–526.
13. Hill, A. V. (1951): Mechanics of voluntary muscle. *Lancet,* ii:947–951.
14. Hough, T. (1902): Ergographic studies in muscular soreness. *Am. J. Physiol.,* 7:76–92.
15. Janssen, E., Kuipers, H., Verstappen, F., and Costill, D. (1983): Influence of an anti-inflammatory drug on muscle soreness. *Med. Sci. Sports Exer.,* 15:165.
16. Jones, D. A., and Newham, D. J. (1985): A simple apparatus for exercising the biceps muscle. *J. Physiol.,* 365:10P.
17. Jones, D. A., and Newham, D. J. (1985): The effect of training on human muscle pain and damage. *J. Physiol.,* 365:76P.
18. Jones, D. A., Newham, D. J., Round, J. M., and Tolfree, S. E. J. (1986): Experimental human muscle damage: morphological changes in relation to other indices of damage. *J. Physiol.,* 375:435–448.
19. Komi, P. V., and Buskirk, E. R. (1972): Measurement of eccentric and concentric conditioning on tension and electrical activity of human muscle. *Ergonomics,* 15:417–434.
20. Lewis, T. (1942); In: *Pain,* pp. 96–104. MacMillan, New York.
21. Lewis, T., Pickering, G. W., and Rorthschild, P. (1931): Observations on muscular pain in intermittent claudication. *Heart,* 15:359–383.
22. Matsen (1979). Compartmental syndromes. *New Engl. J. Med.,* 300:1210–1211.
23. McCully, K. K., and Faulkner, J. A. (1985): Injury to skeletal muscle fibres of mice following lengthening contractions. *J. Appl. Physiol.,* 59:119–126.
24. Mills, K. R., Newham, D. J., and Edwards, R. H. T. (1982): Force, contraction frequency and energy metabolism as determinants of ischaemic muscle pain. *Pain,* 14:149–154.
25. Newham, D. J., and Jones, D. A. (1985): Intra-muscular pressure in the painful human biceps. *Clin. Sci.,* 69:27P.
26. Newham, D. J., Jones, D. A., and Edwards, R. H. T. (1983): Large and delayed plasma creatine kinase changes after stepping exercise. *Muscle Nerve,* 6:36–41.
27. Newham, D. J., Jones, D. A., and Edwards, R. H. T. (1986): Plasma creatine kinase after concentric and eccentric contractions. *Muscle Nerve,* 9:59–63.
28. Newham, D. J., Jones, D. A., Tolfree, S. E. J., and Edwards, R. H. T. (1986): Skeletal muscle damage: a study of isotope uptake, enzyme efflux and pain after stepping. *Eur. J. Appl. Physiol.,* 55:106–112.
29. Newham, D. J., McPhail, G., Mills, K. R., and Edwards, R. H. T. (1983): Ultrastructural changes after concentric and eccentric contractions. *J. Neurol. Sci.,* 61:109–122.
30. Newham, D. J., Mills, K. R., Quigley, B. M., and Edwards, R. H. T. (1983): Pain and fatigue following concentric and eccentric muscle contractions. *Clin. Sci.,* 64:55–62.
31. Shumate, J. B., Brooke, M. H., Caroll, J. E., and Davies, J. E. (1979): Increased serum CK after exercise: a sex linked phenomenon. *Neurology,* 29:902–904.
32. Talag, T. S. (1973): Residual soreness as influenced by concentric, eccentric and static contractions. *Res. Q.,* 44:458–469.

Advances in Pain Research and Therapy,
Vol. 10. Edited by M. Tiengo et al.
Raven Press, Ltd., New York © 1987.

A Mesolimbic Neuronal Loop of Analgesia

Ji-Sheng Han

Department of Physiology, Beijing Medical University, Beijing 100083, China

There is a growing body of evidence showing that the analgesic effect of morphine is mediated not only by its direct action on opioid receptors, but also by the subsequent activation of some other neurotransmitter systems, such as serotonin (5-HT) (38) and endogenous opioids (5,17,47,48). The importance of 5-HT in the descending nociceptive control from brainstem to the spinal cord has been well documented (10,12,52). In the forebrain, 5-HT may also play a role in mediating morphine analgesia (1,20 40), although the exact sites of action are far from clear.

In order to characterize its sites of action we have injected cinanserin, a 5-HT antagonist, into discrete brain areas of the rabbit and monitored its effect on the analgesia induced by intravenous injection of morphine (5 mg/kg). It was found that there are four brain areas in which microinjection of cinanserin attenuated morphine analgesia by more than 50%, i.e., periaqueductal grey (PAG) (33), nucleus accumbens (51), habenula (51), and amygdala (49). It should be noted that it is the same brain nuclei in which microinjection of naloxone blocked morphine analgesia by more than 75% (54). Since systematically administered morphine can act on multiple brain sites, and activation of raphe system will release 5-HT in multiple sites of the forebrain area, blocking one neurotransmitter in one nucleus would be expected to lose only a small fraction of the effect of morphine, rather than one-half or three-fourths of its total effect, provided that these nuclei are connected in a parallel fashion. We therefore made a conjecture that 5-HT and morphine or endogenous opioids may work in series to form a neuronal loop, so that blocking one site at any part of the loop breaks the whole system.

Based on these preliminary findings, the present study was performed to clarify: (a) Is there a neuronal loop in the brain modulating nociception or pain perception? (b) What are the neurotransmitters used by this neuronal circuitry?

Nucleus accumbens is a limbic structure with possible involvement in morphine analgesia (11,57). It is innervated with nerve terminals containing 5-HT and enkephalin-like immunoreactivity (31,43). While enkephalins are contained mostly in short axoned interneurons located within the nucleus accumbens (31,32), 5-HT is contained in nerve terminals originated most probably from midbrain raphe nuclei located in or near the PAG area (2,6). We therefore decided to explore the possible interactions of 5-HT and opioids in the PAG and nucleus accumbens.

METHODS

Experiments were performed in rabbits. Nociception was measured by the latency of the escape response (withdrawal of the head) induced by strong radiant heat focused on the nostril region (25). Stainless steel guide cannulae were implanted stereotaxically, directing to both sides of the PAG (P9.5; L1.0; H10.5) and the nucleus accumbens (A, 6.0; L1.2; H8.5) (16,41). During the experiment of brain microinjections, a stainless steel tubing of 0.3 mm was inserted into, and extended 2 mm beyond, the tip of the guide cannula to reach the target nucleus. A slow-injection apparatus (Palmer) was used to infuse 1 μl of solution in a period of 8 min (in PAG) or 4 min (in the nucleus accumbens). The injection cannula was left *in situ* for another 2 min. Injection was made once a week for a maximum of 5 weeks.

The chemicals used in this study were: morphine HCl (Shengyang Drug Company, or Qin-Hai Drug Company, China), naloxone HCl (Endo Laboratories), (+)naloxone HCl (a gift from Dr. Jacob, NIH), cinaserin (Squibb), bestatin (Sigma), thiorphan (a gift from Drs. Berger and Chipkin). They were dissolved in 0.9% NaCl (NS) for intracerebral injection.

At the conclusion of the experiment the rabbit was sacrificed and the head was removed and fixed in 10% formalin for 1 week. Methylene blue solution, 0.1 μl, was injected into the brain through the same injection cannula previously used for drug administration. The sites of injection were verfied in serial 0.4 mm cryostat sections.

Data of the nociceptive tests from different animals were grouped according to the sites of brain injection determined at the end of the study by an independent experimenter. Data from animals with injection sites placed within the nucleus were designated the drug group, and those from animals with incorrect placement of the injection sites (located in the vicinity of the target nucleus) were designated the drug control group. Data from animals with injection of NS into the nucleus were designated NS control group. All the data are expressed as mean ± SEM. Student's *t*-test was used for determining the significance of difference between two groups. Details of the methodology can be found in the previous publications (22,24,30,50).

ACTIVATION BY MORPHINE OF A SEROTONERGIC PATHWAY FROM PERIAQUEDUCTAL GRAY TO THE NUCLEUS ACCUMBENS

Microinjections of morphine, 10 μg, into PAG of the rabbit produced an increase in the escape response latency (ERL) by 136 ± 14% in 40 min, and remained at the high level within the observation period of 1 hr. Reduction of the dose of morphine to 5 μg resulted in an increase of ERL by 83 ± 20%. This effect can be repeatedly demonstrated at 1-week intervals for a total of 5 weeks without significant decrease in efficacy (24). In control experiments 1 μl NS was injected into PAG, and the changes in ERL in a period of 60 min were within the limits of −1 ± 5% to 13 ± 6% that are not significantly different from the preinjection level.

To investigate whether the ascending serotonergic pathway directing to nucleus accumbens plays a role in mediating the analgesic effect induced by intra-PAG injection of morphine, we injected 5-HT antagonist cinanserin bilaterally into the nucleus accumbens and found that the analgesic effect was dose-dependently attenuated (Fig. 1). The results indicate that the ascending serotonergic pathway is indeed involved in mediating the analgesia induced by intra-PAG injection of morphine. This was supported by another experiment where 5-hydroxytryptophan (5-HTP), the direct precursor of 5-HT, was injected into the nucleus accumbens (2 μg in each side), and the effect of morphine analgesia was significantly prolonged. Direct injection of 5-HT (10 μg in each side) into nucleus accumbens resulted in a marked increase of the nociceptive threshold with a peak effect of 83 ± 14% 30 min after its administration (24).

A SEROTONIN-ENKEPHALIN INTERACTION IN THE NUCLEUS ACCUMBENS

Since nucleus accumbens contains both 5-HT and endogenous opioids (31), and both are involved in morphine analgesia (51,54), one would ask what is the possible relation between 5-HT and opioids in this nucleus? Are they functioning in parallel, or connected in series? It was reasoned that if 5-HT activates the release of opioids, then the analgesic effect of 5-HT should be blocked by the opioid antagonist naloxone. If the reverse is true, the analgesic effect of opioids should be blocked by the 5-HT antagonist cinanserin. Fig. 2 shows that the analgesia induced by injecting 5-HT into nucleus accumbens was significantly reduced by naloxone injected into the same site (via the same cannula). In this experiment, (+) naloxone, which has no affinity with opioid receptors, was used as control for naloxone. In another experiment it was shown that the analgesic effect produced by the enkephalin analog [D-Ala^2, D-Leu^5]enkephalin (DADLE) was not affected by cinanserin injected into the same site (50). The results favor the hypothesis that 5-HT released from the ascending serotonergic pathways activates some opioid-containing interneurons.

To test the role of the endogenous opioids in this system, we have adopted an antibody microinjection technique (19,23). Figure 3 shows that the analgesia produced by intra-PAG injection of morphine was markedly

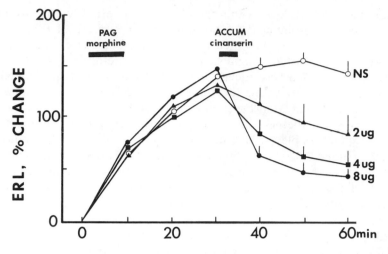

FIG. 1. The analgesic effect induced by intra-PAG injection of morphine (10 μg) was antagonized by cinanserin administered bilaterally to the nucleus accumbens. The doses of cinanserin used in each side are shown at the *right* side of the panel; n = 8–10 in each group. ERL: escape response latency in seconds; PAG: periaqueductal gray; ACCUM: nucleus accumbens; NS: normal saline. *Vertical bars* indicate SEM.

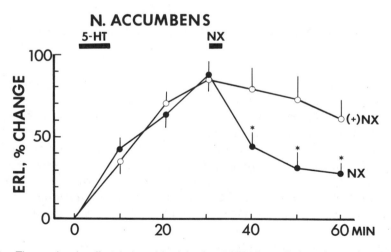

FIG. 2. The analgesic effect induced by injecting 5-HT bilaterally into the nucleus accumbens was blocked by naloxone (NX) injected into the same sites. The doses administered in each side were: 5-HT, 10 μg; naloxone or (+)naloxone, 4 μg; injection volume, 1 μl; n = 14 in naloxone group; n = 8 in (+)naloxone group; (*) $p < 0.05$.

suppressed by immunoglobulin G (IgG) against [Met]enkephalin (ME), microinjected into the nucleus accumbens. IgG obtained from nonimmunized rabbit was without effect. The degree of suppression produced by enkephalin antibodies was comparable to that produced by a large dose of naloxone, 8 μg in each side of the nucleus accumbens (50). We therefore concluded

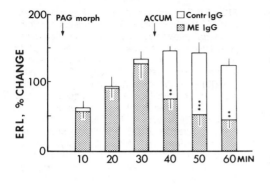

FIG. 3. The analgesic effect induced by injecting morphine (10 μg) into PAG was blocked by [met]enkephalin (ME)IgG administered bilaterally in the nucleus accumbens (7.5 μg in each side, $n = 6$), IgG from normal rabbit serum was used as control ($n = 8$). ME antiserum (titer 1:800) was a gift from Professor L. Terenius, Uppsala University.) This antiserum has a 100% cross-reactivity with [leu]enkephalin and Tyr-Gly-Gly-Phe. Cross-reactivity with α-, β-, and γ-endorphin were < 5%. Normal rabbit serum (NRS) was prepared in this laboratory. Purification of IgG from antiserum or NRS was performed by ammonium sulfate precipitation, followed by affinity chromatography in a Protein A Sepharose CL-4B column (Pharmacia), with a yield of 9–11 mg IgG/ml serum. Significance of difference between two groups is shown as (**) $p<0.01$, (***) $p<0.001$.

that ME may play a key role in the nucleus accumbens to mediate the analgesic effect induced by intra-PAG injection of morphine.

NEURONAL PATHWAY FROM NUCLEUS ACCUMBENS TO PAG

Since the current knowledge does not implicate nucleus accumbens as a strategic site in the pain perception pathways, it is not yet clear how enkephalin in the nucleus accumbens could exert an analgesic effect. From the hypotheses put forward in the introduction, one would think that ME released from the interneurons in the nucleus accumbens may trigger other

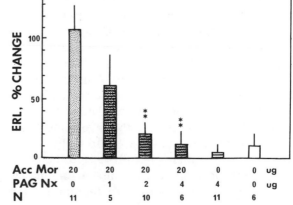

FIG. 4. The analgesic effect produced by unilateral injection of morphine (20 μg) into nucleus accumbens was dose-dependently blocked by intra-PAG injection of naloxone which was given 30 min after morphine administration. *Column height* indicates changes in ERL 20 min after the injection in PAG. Doses of naloxone are shown as the total amount injected into both sides. (**)$p<0.01$ compared to the NS control group (*first column*).

Acc Mor	20	20	20	20	0	0	ug
PAG Nx	0	1	2	4	4	0	ug
N	11	5	10	6	11	6	

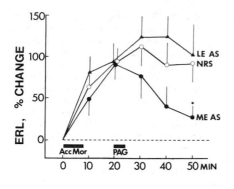

FIG. 5. The analgesia induced by microinjection of morphine (20 μg) into nucleus accumbens was antagonized by intra-PAG injection of [Met]enkephalin antiserum (ME AS), 1 μl in each side, but not by LE antiserum (LE AS) or normal rabbit serum (NRS). ME AS (titer 1:6000) was obtained by immunizing the rabbit with ME in this laboratory. Cross-reactivities with LE, β-endorphin, dynorphin, and ME-Arg^6-Phe^7 were 1.1%, 0.8%, 0.2%, and 0.1%, respectively. LE AS (titer 1:8000) was also prepared in this laboratory. Cross-reactivities with ME, β-endorphin, and dynorphin were 3.7%, 0.09% and 0.05%, respectively. NRS was obtained from nonimmunized rabbit; n = 6–7 in each group. (*) $p < 0.01$ compared to the NRS group.

neuronal structures to project back to the PAG, thus forming a neuronal loop.

Figure 4 shows that the analgesia produced by morphine administered in nucleus accumbens can be blocked by naloxone injected into PAG. This effect is dose-dependent: when the dose of naloxone injected into PAG was increased to 4 μg, the effect of morphine was almost totally abolished. Similar blocking effect was obtained when ME antiserum was injected into PAG, but not by [Leu]enkephalin (LE) antiserum (Fig. 5), suggesting that ME may serve as the terminal link of the descending pathway.

Neurons of the nucleus accumbens project via the medial forebrain bundle to lateral hypothalamic areas, ventral tegmental area, substantia nigra, and retrorubral field (9). No histological evidence is available for an enkephalinergic pathway projecting from nucleus accumbens to PAG. However, morphological and functional studies have suggested a possible indirect connection between nucleus accumbens and PAG, through a relay in the habenula (29,45). Preliminary results supporting this possibility are illustrated in Fig. 6.

In conclusion, the analgesic effect of exogenously administered morphine depends very much on the normal functioning of the brain's own 5-HT and opioids, especially the serotonergic and enkephalinergic transmission subserving the mesolimbic neuronal circuitry between PAG, nucleus accumbens, and habenula. Moreover, peripheral stimulation such as electroacupuncture (EA) has been shown to be very effective in activating the 5-HT and opioid systems in the central nervous system (21), and the analgesic effect of EA are known to be significantly suppressed by the microinjection of cinanserin or naloxone into PAG, nucleus accumbens, and habenula (33,51,54). Therefore, the involvement of the putative mesolimbic loop in mediating EA analgesia is also highly suggestive.

If the hypothesis put forward in the present study is true, then facilitation of enkephalinergic transmission in the nucleus accumbens would be expected to potentiate and/or prolong the analgesic effect produced by syste-

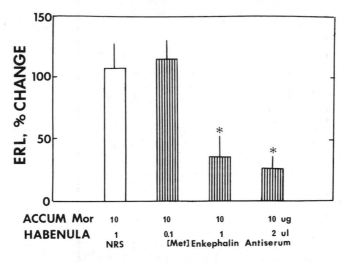

FIG 6. The analgesic effect produced by intra-accumbens injection of morphine (20 μg) was antagonized by ME antiserum (ME AS) injected bilaterallly into habenula at a dose of 1 μl (n = 9) or 2 μl (n = 6) in each side. No significant antagonism was observed when the dose of ME AS was reduced to 0.1 μl (made up to 1 μl with NS, n = 5). Normal rabbit serum (NRS), 1 μl in each side, was used as control (n = 8). ME AS and NRS were the same batches as described in Fig. 5. Intrahabenular injection was given 30 min after the intra-accumbens injection of morphine, and the data shown in the figure were taken 20 min after the intrahabenular injection.

matically administered morphine or by EA stimulation. This has been tested in the following experiments.

POTENTIATION OF MORPHINE ANALGESIA AND ELECTROACUPUNCTURE ANALGESIA BY INHIBITORS OF ENKEPHALIN DEGRADING ENZYMES

More than five enzymes have been characterized that are known to be involved in the degradation of enkephalins, among which the aminopeptidase and dipeptidyl carboxypeptidase (enkephalinase) seem to be the most important ones (28,42). Bestatin (7) and thiorphan (39) are powerful inhibitors of the aminopeptidase and enkephalinase, respectively. We have reported that intracerebroventricular (i.c.v.) injection of bestatin (0.6 μmol) or thiorphan (0.4 μmol) in rabbits increased the ERL by more than 100%, an effect completely reversed by a small dose of naloxone (0.125 mg/kg) (55). The results suggest that inhibition of enkephalin degradating enzymes in the brain may result in an accumulation of enkephalins to manifest a prolonged analgesic effect.

In the present study, bestatin or thiorphan at doses of 1, 2, and 4 μg was injected into the nucleus accumbens. Table 1 shows that unilateral injection of 2 or 4 μg bestatin or thiorphan produced marked increase in ERL, lasting

TABLE 1. *Analgesic effect of thiorphan and bestatin administered to the nucleus accumbens*

		In[c]	n	Basal ERL[a] (S)	% Change of ERL after intracerebral injection				
					10 min	20 min	30 min	40 min	50 min
NS[b]	1 µl	In[c]	8	5.4 ± 0.4	1 ± 1	4 ± 3	1 ± 2	3 ± 1	1 ± 2
Thiorphan	1 µg	In	7	6.0 ± 0.2	44 ± 22	21 ± 16	-3 ± 5	-2 ± 5	2 ± 3
		Out[c]	1	6.3	-16	-21	-8	-21	3
	2 µg	In	8	6.8 ± 0.4	32 ± 3[d]	46 ± 10[d]	103 ± 24[e]	51 ± 19[f]	8 ± 9
		Out	5	6.4 ± 0.6	-6 ± 3	5 ± 9	-5 ± 3	17 ± 17	12 ± 12
	4 µg	In	7	6.4 ± 0.7	94 ± 19[e]	97 ± 21[e]	117 ± 21[e]	77 ± 19[d]	49 ± 13[d]
		Out	5	6.6 ± 0.8	18 ± 4	26 ± 18	17 ± 19	13 ± 6	1 ± 2
Bestatin	1 µg	In	7	6.0 ± 0.9	38 ± 11[d]	28 ± 6[d]	15 ± 7	4 ± 2	2 ± 2
		Out	1	5.6	4	23	29	21	7
	2 µg	In	10	6.2 ± 0.6	74 ± 17[e]	85 ± 23[d]	33 ± 23	20 ± 18	6 ± 3
		Out	4	5.4 ± 0.8	-1 ± 8	14 ± 17	2 ± 11	9 ± 17	-2 ± 4
	4 µg	In	8	7.0 ± 0.5	88 ± 21[e]	140 ± 23[e]	81 ± 23[d]	78 ± 22[d]	45 ± 14
		Out	3	5.8 ± 0.8	15 ± 10	12 ± 3	5 ± 8	1 ± 2	4 ± 6

[a]ERL; escape response latency.
[b]NS, 0.9% NaCl.
[c]In, the site of injection is within the nucleus; Out, the injection site is outside the nucleus.
[d]$p < 0.01$ as compared to the NS control group.
[e]$p < 0.001$ as compared to the NS control group.
[f]$p < 0.05$ as compared to the NS control group.

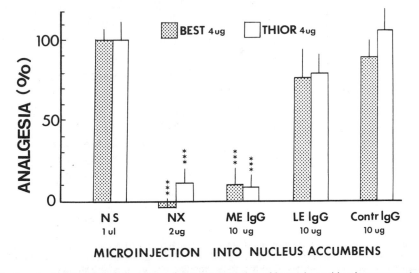

FIG. 7. Analgesia elicited by intra-accumbens injection of bestatin or thiorphan was antagonized by naloxone and ME IgG, but not by LE IgG, administered in the same site 10 min after bestatin or thiorphan. The analgesic effect represents the average of three measurements taken after the second injection. The results are normalized for comparison between the two enzyme inhibitors thiorphan and bestatin, and between the five different treatments. ME AS, LE AS, and NRS were the same as described in Fig. 5. The IgG, purified with Protein A Sepharose CL-4B column, showed the same immunoreactivity as the authentic antisera in the radioimmunoassay system.

for 30 to 50 min. No significant analgesia was detected when the same amount of thiorphan was injected in the vicinity of the nucleus accumbens, showing site specificity of the action. One µg thiorphan or bestatin produced only a marginal analgesia lasting for 10 to 20 min. Fig. 7 shows that the analgesic effect of bestatin or thiorphan (4 µg) administered into nucleus accumbens can be blocked by naloxone (2 µg), or IgG obtained from ME antiserum, but not by IgG purified from LE antiserum.

To assess the effect of bestatin on morphine analgesia, morphine (1 or 2 mg/kg, i.v.) was injected after the intra-accumbens injection of bestatin (1 µg). As can be seen from Fig. 8, 1 mg/kg morphine, which was noneffective by itself, becomes strongly analgesic when used in combination with bestatin. In animals injected with 2 mg/kg morphine, bestatin doubled the analgesic effect. Similar results were obtained when thiorphan was used instead of bestatin. No significant potentiation of morphine analgesia was found when bestatin or thiorphan was injected outside of the nucleus (data not shown).

In another experiment, the effect of thiorphan or bestatin on EA analgesia was tested. One µg thiorphan or 1 µl of NS was administered in nucleus accumbens during the period of EA stimulation. The results are shown in Fig. 9A. In the NS control group EA stimulation produced a 150% increase in ERL, which faded away after the cessation of EA stimulation, and ap-

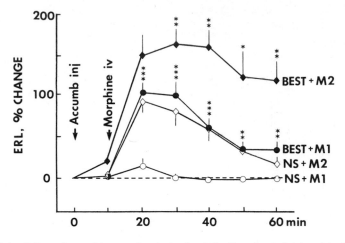

FIG. 8. Potentiation of morphine analgesia by bestatin (1 μg) administered to the nucleus accumbens. M1, morphine 1 mg/kg, i.v.; M2, morphine 2 mg/kg. The significance of the difference between the bestatin and the corresponding NS group is shown as (*) $p<0.05$, (**) $p<0.01$, and (***) $p<0.001$; $n = 16$ in M1 groups, and $n = 8$ in M2 groups.

proached the base-line level in 50 min. In animals given thiorphan (1 μg), the after-effect of EA analgesia was markedly potentiated. Similar results were obtained when bestatin (1 μg) was used instead of thiorphan (Fig. 9B).

DISCUSSION

A well-established mechanism for morphine analgesia is the activation of a descending serotonergic system from the brainstem raphe nuclei to the dorsal horn to suppress nociceptive transmission (12,15,38,52). The involvement of enkephalins (26,27,48) and dynorphins (48) in the descending inhibitory system has also been suggested. Compared to the extensive studies performed at the spinal level, the cerebral neuronal circuits subserving morphine analgesia are poorly understood.

To evaluate the possible role of the ascending serotonergic pathways in morphine analgesia, we started our study by microinjection of morphine into PAG, since PAG (44,53), especially its ventral portion (53,56), has long been shown to be a strategic site for morphine analgesia. Clusters of serotonergic neurons have been demonstrated not only in the ventral portion of the PAG [nucleus raphe dorsalis (NRD)], but also in a wide area ventrolateral to the aqueduct (13,18), which constitutes a structural basis for morphine-serotonin interaction. That an ascending serotonergic pathway from PAG to the nucleus accumbens is involved in morphine analgesia is suggested by the findings that the analgesic effect induced by morphine administered to the PAG could be blocked by cinanserin, a 5-HT blocker (Fig.1), and potentiated by 5-HTP, the direct precursor of 5-HT (24), administered bilaterally

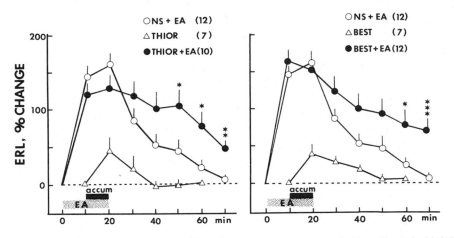

FIG. 9. Potentiation of the aftereffect of EA analgesia by thiorphan (**left**) and bestatin (**right**) administered bilaterally to nucleus accumbens at a volume of 1 μl in each side. The *dark bar* indicates the period of microinjection (1 μl); the *shaded box* indicates the period of electroacupuncture (EA) stimulation (0.3 msec, 1 V 2–15 Hz; see ref. 25 for details). The significance of the difference between the thiorphan (or bestatin) plus EA group, and the NS plus EA group is shown as (*) $p<0.05$, (**) $p<0.01$, and (***) $p<0.001$.

to the nucleus accumbens; and that direct administration of 5-HT in the nucleus accumbens resulted in a marked analgesia (24) comparable to that produced by intra-PAG injection of morphine.

Further studies revealed that the analgesic effect elicited by intra-PAG injection of morphine is blocked not only by cinanserin (24), but also by the narcotic antagonist naloxone (50) administered in the nucleus accumbens in a dose-dependent manner, suggesting that an opioid mechanism is also involved in this effect.

Immunohistochemical studies have shown that nucleus accumbens is innervated by nerve terminals containing opioid peptides derived from all three precursor systems [proenkephalin, prodynorphin, and pro-opiomelanocortin (POMC)] (32). However, neuronal perikarya found in the nucleus accumbens contain proenkephalin-related peptides (31), but not prodynorphin- or POMC-related opioid peptides (32). We therefore examined whether enkephalinergic neurons located in the nucleus accumbens were involved in this reaction. An antiserum recognized ME and LE (proenkephalin-related peptides), but not the longer-chain endorphins (POMC-related peptides), was microinjected into the nucleus accumbens. The effect of morphine was decreased by at least 50%, which favors the hypothesis that immunoreactive enkephalins are released in nucleus accumbens for mediating morphine effects (Fig. 3). This was substantiated by the findings that morphine analgesia was potentiated by intra-accumbens injection of bestatin and thiorphan, potent inhibitors of enkephalin-degrading enzymes, that facilitated enkephalinergic transmission (Fig. 8). It should be pointed out that while these results suggest proenkephalin-related opioid peptides as the most probable candidates for these analgesic mechanisms operative in the nucleus accumbens, they do not rule out the possible participation of other opioids mediating morphine effects in this nucleus.

Concerning the putative interrelationship between 5-HT and enkephalins in the nucleus accumbens, there are at least three possibilities: (a) The existence of enkephalins in approximately one-third of the neurons located in NRD (36) suggests that 5-HT and enkephalins may act as cotransmitters in the synaptic events; (b) 5-HT released in the nucleus accumbens may activate the enkephalinergic interneurons within the nucleus, as was seen in the caudate-putamen where 5-HT plays an excitatory role (37); (c) Enkephalins may accelerate the release of 5-HT, although no evidence is yet available in favor of this possibility. That the effect of 5-HT could be blocked by opioid antagonist naloxone (see Fig. 2) seems to support the idea that serotonergic terminals may activate the enkephalinergic neurons. Since naloxone was injected into the same site as was 5-HT, one would anticipate that the enkephalins are released from short axoned interneurons.

In relation to the possible mechanisms for the nucleus accumbens to exert an analgesic effect, it is worth mentioning that electrical stimulation of the nucleus accumbens in the rat was reported to accelerate the neuronal discharges of the nucleus raphe magnus, This effect was blocked by naloxone microinjected into the PAG (34), suggesting a neuronal pathway from the nucleus accumbens to the PAG, using opioids as mediators. To avoid stimulating fibers of passage, we have adopted microinjection of morphine into the nucleus accumbens instead of electrical stimulation. The results shown in Fig. 4 and 5 indicate that the descending pathway emanating from nucleus accumbens to PAG started with opioceptive neurons and ended with enkephalinergic nerve terminals, and that ME seems to play a more important role than LE in mediating the descending pain control from nucleus accumbens to PAG.

The possible involvement of habenula in the descending pathway from nucleus accumbens to PAG is suggested by the notions that (a) habenula has been regarded as the major link between forebrain structures and midbrain raphe nuclei (29,45); and (b) electrical stimulation of nucleus accumbens was shown to modulate the discharges of pain-related neurons in the PAG, and this modulatory effect was almost totally abolished after lesioning of the habenula (46). Results shown in Fig. 6 indicate that a [Met]enkephalinergic relay may be involved in the pathway from nucleus accumbens to the PAG.

A hypothetical diagram of the mesolimbic neuronal loop of analgesia is shown in Fig. 10. Exogenously administered or endogenously released opioids (e.g., during EA stimulation) may act on the opioceptive neurons located in PAG, nucleus accumbens, and habenula to push the loop into action. When the neuronal loop is set into function, it may send efferent

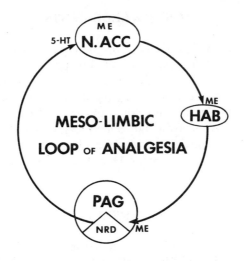

FIG. 10. Diagram showing the putative mesolimbic neuronal loop of analgesia. HAB, habenula; N.ACC, nucleus accumbens; NRD, nucleus raphe dorsalis; PAG, periaqueductal grey; ME, [Met]enkephalin. For details, see text.

fibers to neuronal structures implicated in pain perception. For example, efferents from PAG may project to nucleus raphe magnus and the neighboring reticular formation (3,4), and further downward to the spinal cord (14,35,48) to form a descending inhibitory control for nociception (15); or may project rostrally to the thalamus to suppress the transmission of nociceptive information in nucleus parafascicularis and other medial thalamic nuclei (8).

The present hypothesis may help to explain why the analgesic effect produced by morphine or EA stimulation can be blocked more than 75% by the focal injection of naloxone into PAG, nucleus accumbens, or habenula (54), or by injection of cinaserin into the nucleus accumbens (51). Once the neuronal loop is activated by exogenously administered morphine or endogenously released 5-HT or opioids, the excitation would be expected to reverberate for certain period. This may explain the phenomenon that the effect of EA analgesia outlasts the period of EA stimulation as seen in Fig. 9. In certain chronic pain patients, in whom the endogenous serotonergic and enkephalinergic systems might have been activated by the noxious stimuli, the effect of EA analgesia may last for hours or days.

The neuronal loop shown in this study might have represented only a small part of the complicated interconnection between the lower brainstem and the limbic system. More study is needed to explore the detailed picture of the putative mesolimbic loop of analgesia, which may prove to be a powerful mechanism for pain modulation on top of the medullospinal pain control system.

ACKNOWLEDGMENTS

The author thanks his colleagues for their participation in the work described: Z. F. Zhou, Y. T. Xuan, W. Q. Jin, L. C. Yu, and Y. S. Shi. The author also thanks Dr. P. L. Zhang, Professor of Anatomy, for help in identifying the sites of injection. The gifts of naloxone from Endo Laboratories, cinanserin from Squibb and Sons, thiorphan from Drs. J. Berger and R. Chipkin, (+) naloxone from Dr. Jacob (NIH), and ME antiserum from Dr. L. Terenius are highly acknowledged. The work was supported by research grants from the Ministry of Health and the Academia Sinica, the People's Republic of China.

REFERENCES

1. Alder, M., Kostowski, W., Recchia, M., and Samanin, R. (1975): Anatomical specificity as the critical determinant of the interrelationship between raphe lesions and morphine analgesia. *Eur. J. Pharmacol.,* 32:39–44.
2. Azmita, E. C., Jr., and Segal, M. (1978): An autoradiographic analysis of the differential ascending projections of the dorsal and median raphe nuclei in the rat. *J. Comp. Neurol.,* 179:641–668.
3. Behbehani, N. M., and Fields, H. L. (1979): Evidence that an exitatory connection between the periaqueductal grey and nucleus raphe magnus mediates stimulation produced analgesia. *Brain Res.,* 170:85–93.
4. Beitz, A. Z., Mullett, M. A., and Weiner, O. L. (1983): The periaqueductal grey projects to the rat spinal trigeminal, raphe magnus, gigantocellular pars alpha and paragigantocellular nuclei arise from separate neurons. *Brain Res.,* 288:307–314.
5. Bergman, F., Altsteller, R., and Weissman, B. A. (1978): *In vivo* interaction of morphine and endogenous opiate-like peptides. *Life Sci.,* 23:2601–2608.
6. Bobillier, P., Seguin, S., Petijean, F., Salvert, D., Touret, M., and Jouvet, M. (1976): The raphe nucleus of the cat brain stem: A topographical atlas of their efferent projections as revealed by autoradiography. *Brain Res.,* 113:449–486.
7. Chaillet, P., Marcaiscollado, H., Castentin, J., Yi, C. C., Delabaume, S., and Schwartz, J. C. (1983): Inhibition of enkephalin metabolism by, and antinociceptive activity of, bestatin, an aminopeptidase inhibitor. *Eur. J. Pharmacol.,* 86:329–336.
8. Chang, K. L., Wei, C. P., Lin, Y. M., Chou, L. H., Lo, C. L., and Chang, T. C. (1979): Effect of stimulation of midbrain raphe nuclei on the discharge of pain sensitive cells in nucleus parafascicularis of thalamus and its significance in acupuncture analgesia. *Acta Physiol. Sin.,* 218:209–218.
9. Chronister, R. B., Sikes, R. W., Trow, T. W., and DeFrance, J. F. (1981): The organization of nucleus accumbens. In: *The Neurobiology of Nucleus Accumbens,* edited by R. B. Chronister and J. F. DeFrance, pp. 97–146. Hear Institute, Brunswick.
10. Deakin, J. F. W., and Dostrosky, J. O. (1978): Involvement of periaqueductal grey matter and spinal 5-hydroxytryptaminergic pathways in morphine analgesia—Effects of lesions and 5-hydroxytryptamine depletion. *Br. J. Pharmacol.,* 63:159–165.
11. Dill, R. E., and Costa, E. (1977): Behavioural dissociation of the enkephalinergic system of nucleus accumbens and nucleus caudatus. *Neuropharmacology,* 16:323–326.
12. Du, H. J., Kitahata, L. M., Thalhammer, J. G., and Zimmermann, M. (1984): Inhibition of nociceptive neuronal response in the cat's spinal dorsal horn by electrical stimulation and morphine microinjection in nucleus raphe magnus. *Pain,* 19:249–257.
13. Felton, D. C., and Cummings, J. P. (1979): The raphe nuclei of the rabbit brain stem. *J. Comp. Neurol.,* 187:199–244.
14. Fields, H. L., Basbaum, A. I., Clanton, C. H., and Anderson, S. D. (1977). Nucleus raphe magnus inhibition of spinal cord dorsal horn neurons. *Brain Res.,* 126:441–453.

15. Fields, H. L. (1984): Brainstem mechanisms of pain modulation. In: *Neural Mechanisms of Pain,* edited by L. Kruger and J. C. Liebskind, pp. 241–252. Raven Press, New York.

16. Fifkova, E., and Marsala, J. (1967): Stereotaxic atlas for the cat, rabbit and rat. In: *Electrophysiological Methods in Biological Research,* edited by J. Bures, M. Petran, and J. Zachar, pp. 65–90. Academic Press, New York.

17. Fu, T. C., and Dewey, W., L. (1979): Morphine antinociception: Evidence for the release of endogenous substance(s). *Life Sci.,* 25:53–60.

18. Geyer, M. A., Dawsey, W. J., Knapp, S., Bullard, W. P., and Mandell, A. J. (1976): histologic and enzymatic studies of the mesolimbic and mesostriatal serotonergic pathways. *Brain Res.,* 106:241–256.

19. Han, J. S. (1984): Antibody microinjection technique as a tool to clarify the role of opioid peptides in acupuncture analgesia. *Pain (Suppl.),* 2:667.

20. Han, J. S., Chou, P. H., Lu, C. H., Yang, T. H., and Jen, M. F. (1979): The role of central 5-hydroxytryptamine in acupuncture analgesia. *Sci. Sin.,* 22:91–104.

21. Han, J. S., and Terenius L. (1982): Neurochemical basis of acupuncture analgesia. *Annu. Rev. Pharmacol. Toxicol.,* 22:193–220.

22. Han, J. S., Yu, L. C., and Shi, Y. S. (1986): A mesolimbic loop of analgesia III. A neoronal pathway from nucleus accumbens to periaqueductal grey. *Asia Pacific J. Pharmacol.,* 1:17–22.

23. Han, J. S., Xie, G. X., Zhou, Z. F., Folkesson, R., and Terenius, L. (1984): Acupuncture mechanisms in rabbit studied with microinjection of antibodies against β-endorphin, enkephalin and substance P. *Neuropharmacology,* 23:1–5.

24. Han, J. S., and Xuan, Y. T. (1986): A mesolimbic loop of analgesia I. Activation by morphine of a serotonergic pathway from periaqueductal grey to nucleus accumbens. *Int. J. Neurosci.,* 29:109–118.

25. Han, J. S., Zhou, Z. F., and Xuzn, Y. T. (1983): Acupuncture has an analgesic effect in rabbits. *Pain,* 15:83–91.

26. Hokfelt, T., Ljundahl, A., Terenius, L., Elde, R., and Nilsson, G. (1977): Immunohisto-chemical analysis of peptide pathways possibly related to pain and analgesia: Enkephalin and substance P. *Proc. Natl. Acad. Sci. USA,* 74;3081–305.

27. Hokfelt, T, Terenius, L., Kuypers, H. G., and Dann, O. (1979): Evidence for enkephalin immunoreactive neurons in the medulla oblongata projecting to the spinal cord. *Neurosci. Lett.,* 14:55–60.

28. Hughes, J. (1983): Biogenesis, release and inactivation of enkephalins and dynorphins. *Br. Med. Bull.,* 39:17–24.

29. Ito, M., Kadakaro, M., and Sokoloff, L. (1985): Effects of lateral habenula lesion on local cerebral glucose utilization in the rat. *Brain Res.,* 377:245–254.

30. Jin, W. Q., Zhou, Z. F., and Han, J. S. (1986): Electroacupuncture and morphine analgesia potentiated by bestatin and thiorphan administered to the nucleus accumbens of the rabbit. *Brain Res.,* 380:317–324.

31. Johansson, O., and Hokfelt, T. (1981): Nucleus accumbens: Transmitter histochemistry with special reference to peptide-containing neurons. In: *The Neurobiology of the Nucleus Accumbens,* edited by R. B. Chronister and J. F. DeFrance, pp. 147–172. Hear Institute, Brunswick.

32. Khachaturian, H., Lewis, M. E., Schafer, M. K.-H., and Watson, S. J. (1985): Anatomy of the CNS opioid systems. *Trends Neurosci.,* 8:111–119.

33. Kon, B. E., Zhou, Z. F., and Han, J. S. (1983): The involvement of serotonergic transmission in periaqueductal grey for electroacupuncture analgesia and morphine analgesia in rabbits. *Kexue Tongbao,* 28:888–891.

34. Liu, X., and Zhu, B. (1983): Influence of stimulating the nucleus accumbens on the activities of nucleus raphe magnus in the rat. *Physiol Sci.,* 3:16–18.

35. Mantyh, P. W., and Peschanski, M. (1982): Spinal projection from the PAG and dorsal raphe in the rat, cat and monkey. *Neuroscience,* 7:2769–2776.

36. Moss, M. S., Glazer, E. J., and Basbaum, A. I. (1981): Enkephalin-immunoreactive perikarya in the cat raphe dorsalis. *Neurosci. Lett.,* 21:33–337.

37. Park, M. K., Gonzales-vegas, J. A., and Kitai, S. T. (1982): Serotonergic excitation from dorsal raphe stimulation recorded intracellularly from rat caudate-putamen. *Brain Res.,* 243:49–58.

38. Rivot, J. P., Weil-Fugazza, J., Godefroy, F., Bineau-Thurotte, M., Ory-Lavollee, L., and Besson, J. M. (1984): Involvement of serotonin in both morphine and stimulation-produced analgesia: Electrochemical and biochemical approaches. In: *Neural Mechanisms of Pain*, edited by L. Kruger and J. C. Liebeskind, pp. 135–166. Raven Press, New York.

39. Roques, B. P., Fournie-Zaluski, M. C., Soroca, E., Lecomte, J. M., Malfroy, B., Llorens, C., and Schwartz, J. C. (1980): The enkephalinase inhibitor thiorphan shows antinociceptive activity in mice. *Nature (Lond.)*, 288:286–288.

40. Samanin, R., Gumulka, W., and Valzelli, L. (1970): Reduced effect of morphine in midbrain raphe lesioned rats. *Eur. J. Pharmacol.*, 10:339–343.

41. Sawyer, C. H., Everett, J. W., and Green, J. D. (1954): The rabbit diencephalon in stereotaxic coordinates. *J. Comp. Neurol.*, 101:801–824.

42. Schwartz, J. C. (1983): Metabolism of enkephalins and the inactivating neuropeptidase concept. *Trends Neurosci.*, 6:45–48.

43. Simantov, R., Kuhar, M. J., Uhl, G. R., and Snyder, S. H. (1977): Opioid peptide enkephalin: immunohistochemical mapping in rat central nervous system. *Proc. Natl. Acad. Sci. USA*, 74:2167–2171.

44. Tsou, K., and Jang, C. S. (1964): Studies on the site of analgesic action of morphine by intracerebral microinjection. *Sci. Sin.*, 13:1099–1199.

45. Wang, R. Y., and Aghajanian, G. K. (1977): Physiological evidence for habenula as major link between forebrain and midbrain raphe. *Science*, 197:89–91.

46. Wang, S., Fang, J. Z., and Xa, Y. H. (1984): The effect of stimulating nucleus accumbens on the discharge of pain-related neurons in the periaqueductal grey. *Acta Physiol. Sin.*, 36:38–43.

47. Wu, S. X., Wang, F. S., Zhang, Z. X., and Zou, G. (1984): Effect of morphine on methionin enkephalin content in rabbit brain and cerebrospinal fluid. *Kexue Tongbao*, 29:840–841.

48. Xie, G. X., Xu, H., and Han, J. S. (1984): Involvement of spinal met-enkephalin and dynorphin in descending morphine analgesia. *Acta Physiol. Sin.*, 36:457–463.

49. Xu, D. Y., Zhou, Z. F., and Han, J. S. (1985): Amygdaloid serotonin and endogenous opioid substances (OLS) are important for mediating electroacupuncture analgesia and morphine analgesia in the rabbit. *Acta Physiol. Sin.*, 37:162–171.

50. Xuan, Y. T., Shi, Y. J., Zhou, Z. F., and Han, J. S. (1986): Studies on the mesolimbic loop of antinociception. II. A serotonin-enkephalin interaction in the nucleus accumbens. *Neuroscience*, 19:403–409.

51. Xuan, Y. T., Zhou, Z. F., Wu, W. Y., and Han, J. S. (1982): Antagonism of acupuncture analgesia and morphine analgesia by cinanserin injected into nucleus accumbens and habenula in the rabbit. *J. Beijing Med. Coll.*, 14:23–26.

52. Yaksh, T. L. (1979): Direct evidence that spinal serotonin and noradrenaline terminals mediate the spinal nociceptive effects of morphine in the periaqueductal grey. *Brain Res.*, 160:180–185.

53. Yaksh, T. L., Yeung, J. C., and Rudy, T. A. (1976): Systemic examination in the rat brain sites sensitive to the direct application of morphine: Observation of differential effects within the periaqueductal grey. *Brain Res.*, 114:83–103.

54. Zhou, Z. F., Du, M. Y., Jian, Y., and Han, J. S. (1981): Effects of intracerebral microinjection of naloxone on acupuncture and morphine analgesia in the rabbit. *Sci. Sin.*, 24:1166–1178.

55. Zhou, Z. F., Jin, W. Q., and Han, J. S. (1984): Potentiation of electroacupuncture analgesia and morphine analgesia by intraventricular injection of thiorphan and bestatin in the rabbit. *Acta Physiol. Sin.*, 36:175–182.

56. Zhou, Z. F., Xie, G. X., and Han, J. S. (1985): Substance P produces analgesia by releasing enkephalin in periaqueductal grey of the rabbit. *Kexue Tongbao*, 30:69–73.

57. Zhou, Z. F., Xuan, Y. T., and Han, J. S. (1984): Analgesic effect of morphine injected into habenula, nucleus accumbens or amygdala of rabbits. *Acta Physiol. Sin.*, 5:150–153.

Advances in Pain Research and Therapy,
Vol. 10. Edited by M. Tiengo et al.
Raven Press, Ltd., New York © 1987.

Pain and Motility Disorders in Lumbar Disk Disease: A Computer-Aided Study of 161 Surgically Treated Cases

Roberto Villani and Giuseppe De Benedittis

Pain Research and Treatment Unit, Institute of Neurosurgery, University of Milan, 20122 Milan, Italy

During the past 50 years, following the pioneering studies by Mixter and Barr (1) in 1934, the surgical treatment of lumbar disk herniation (LDH) has been generally accepted as the treatment of choice. However, notwithstanding the progressive improvement in both diagnostic and surgical approaches, the initial enthusiasms have been partially reduced by the findings of frequent and persisting pain sequelae, as well as by the not negligible incidence of recurrences or pseudorecurrences.

To evaluate the efficacy of surgical treatment, it is therefore essential to analyze long-term results. The presence of numerous variables able to remarkably influence prognosis prompted the opportunity of a computerized data elaboration.

To our knowledge, few computer-aided studies have been reported so far (2–5). The aim of the present chapter is to analyze immediate and long-term results of lumbar disk surgery, with particular emphasis on pain and motility disorders.

MATERIAL AND METHODS

One hundred and sixty-one patients, who had undergone surgery in the Neurosurgical Institute, University of Milan, entered the study. The relevant data have been coded into six main sectors (sociodemographic data, risk factors, clinical picture, instrumental diagnostics, surgical treatment, reoperations, long-term results) and 67 segments for a total number of 262 items/patient. Coding as well as data processing have been accomplished by a personal computer (Olivetti M24).

One hundred and one patients were male (62.7%); 60 (37.3%) were female; the ratio M/F was 1.7. The mean age (± SD) was 46 ± 0.8 years (M = 47 ± 0.9; F = 44 ± 1.3).

Sex and age distributions are shown in Fig. 1: The highest incidence was

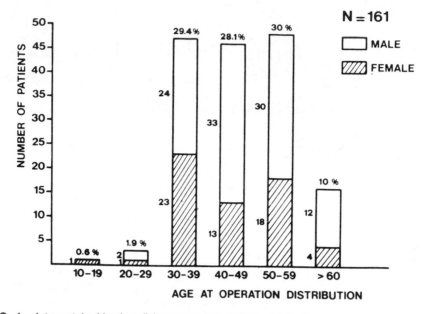

FIG. 1. Intervertebral lumbar disk surgery: sex and age distributions.

found in the fourth to sixth decades (29.4%, 28.1%, and 30%, respectively). With regard to sex, the relative prevalence was in the fourth (38.9%) and fifth (32.7%) decades for women and men, respectively.

With reference to occupation: 40.1% of the patients were blue collar workers, 22.3% housewives, 14.1% white collar workers; pensioners, craftsmen, and traders were in minor percentages.

Primary Risk Factors

The following parameters were analyzed: (a) preexisting pain symptoms; (b) repetitive microtraumas; (c) continuous driving; (d) occupation; and (e) psychosomatic concomitant factors.

Nearly half of the patients (45.6%) had a previous history of pain, mainly lumbar and sciatic. Recurring microtraumas (e.g., lifting of heavy things, anomalous posture, etc.) were found in 18% of cases. The 52.8% of patients who were continuous drivers were usually employed as such.

Work conditions were light in 34.8%, sedentary in 24.8%, moderate (occasional efforts) in 18.6%, and heavy in 21.8%; work accidents accounted for 6.2%. Finally, nearly one-quarter of patients (23.7%) suffered from psychosomatic disorders, mainly gastroenteric ones.

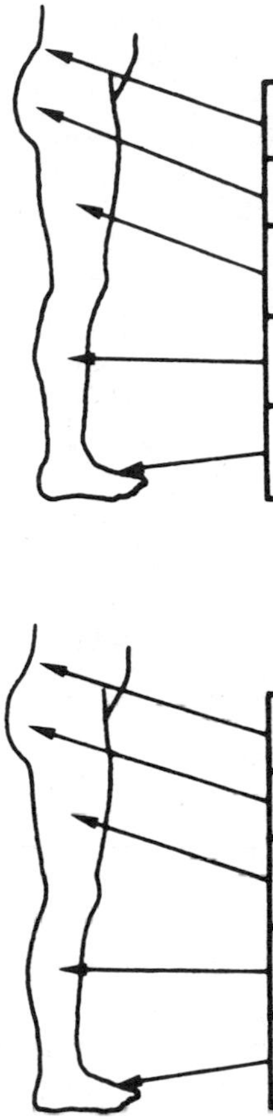

L₄–L₅	N=90		
LUMBAR–SACRAL	**77.8**		
GLUTEAL–HIP	**67.8**		
THIGH	ANT. **22.2**	LAT. **44.4**	POST. **68.9**
CALF	ANT. **66.7**	LAT. **65.6**	POST. **78.8**
FOOT TOES	1° TOE MED. FOOT **2.2**	DORSUM OF FOOT **30.0**	2-5th TOE LAT. FOOT **5.5**

L₅–S₁	N=50		
LUMBAR–SACRAL	**74.0**		
GLUTEAL–HIP	**56.0**		
THIGH	ANT. **18.0**	LAT. **38.0**	POST. **84.0**
CALF	ANT. **66.0**	LAT. **36.0**	POST. **86.0**
FOOT TOES	1° TOE MED. FOOT **6.0**	DORSUM OF FOOT **12.0**	2-5th TOE LAT. FOOT **24.0**

FIG. 2. Pain distribution at the two main intervertebral lumbar disk localizations (L4-L5; L5-S1).

CLINICAL PICTURE

Pain was the predominant symptom at the onset of the disorder (97.5%), as well as thereafter. In most cases (67%), the pain was lumbosciatalgic, in 22.9% in the lumbar region, and in 9.6% in the sciatic region only. The pain event was unique in 51%, recurrent in the remaining cases. Lateralization of pain was right in 44.9%, left in 42.4%, and bilateral in 13.3%.

Pain distribution, with respect to the two main localizations (L_4–L_5 and L_5–S_1), is reported in Fig. 2. It can be noticed that nearly three-fourths of of the patients complained of lumbar pain, both sites being involved in the

TABLE 1. *Intervertebral lumbar disk surgery: Preoperative clinical features*

Signs	No. of cases	%
Spinal	140	87.0
Tension	132	82.0
SLR[a] positive	105[b]	65.2
CSLR[b] "	27	16.8
Neurological		
Reflex		
Abnormal	132	82.0
Sensory	102	63.3
Hypoalgesia and Hypoesthesia	89	55.3
Anesthesia	4	2.5
Paresthesia	22	13.7
Motor	77	47.8
EHL[c]-FHL[d] Weakness	63	39.1
Severe weakness, paraparesis	14	8.7
Trophic	23	14.3
Sphincter	13	8.0

[a]SLR, straight leg raising.
[b]CSLR, crossed straight leg raising.
[c]EHL, extensor allucis longus m.
[d]FHL, flexor allucis longus m.

same ratio. Gluteal hip pain was complained of more frequently when the protrusion was in L_5 (67.8%) than in S_1 (56%). Pain in the crural region and legs was mainly posterior without significant differences between the two roots. The involvement of the dorsum of the foot seemed typical of L_4–L_5 level, while that of the heel, lateral side, and last two toes was more frequent in the L_5–S_1 level.

Physical examination (Table 1) demonstrated a high incidence of spinal signs [reduced motility, antalgic scoliosis, pain (87%)] and tension signs [straight-leg raising and/or crossed straight-leg raising (82%)]. Neurological examination showed: (a) abnormal reflexes (reduced or absent): 82%; (b) sensory deficits (mainly hypoalgesia and hypoesthesia): 63.3%; (c) motor deficits: 47.8% [the muscles involved were mainly the extensor hallucis longus (EHL) and the flexor hallucis longus (FHL), less frequent were cases of severe weakness or paraparesis]; (d) trophic disorders: 14.3%; and (e) sphincter disorders: 8%.

On the basis of the above-stated clinical features, preoperative patients' conditions were classified as follows: (a) grade I (hyperalgesic and paresthetic syndrome): 34.2%; (b) grade II (mild to moderate sensory-motor deficits): 44.7%; and (c) grade III (severe sensory-motor and sphincter deficits): 21.1%.

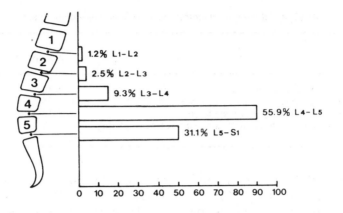

LEVEL OF DISC PROTRUSION AT OPERATION

FIG. 3. Intervertebral lumbar disk surgery: levels of disk lesions.

Instrumental Diagnostics

All the patients underwent static and dynamic X-rays of the lumbosacral spine. Radiographic findings were normal in 50% of them. Within pathological radiograms, the most significant one included: (a) reduction of the intersomatic space (22.4%); (b) osteophytosis associated to arthrosic lesions (37.9%); (c) transitional anomalies, lumbar stenosis, spondylolysis (6%).

All the patients were submitted to sacculoradiculography with positive contrast medium. The relative findings were abnormal in 98.1%: In 67.1% it was a discal bulge; in 20.5% a contrast block; in 11.2% an amputation of the radicular pocket.

Thirty-one percent of cases underwent CT-scanning: A protrusion or discal herniation was revealed in 82% of them.

SURGICAL TREATMENT

Main indications for surgery were: (a) painful symptomatology lasting more than 3 months and resistant to conservative treatment (78.7%); (b) progressive neurological impairment (65.8%); (c) positive contrastographic and tomographic findings (99%).

Within 6 months of the clinical onset, 85.7% of patients were operated on. With respect to the surgical techniques, laminectomy was performed in 15.6%, hemilaminectomy in 47.5%, and interlaminectomy in 36.9%. In the intraforaminal and nerve root encroachment cases (5.6%), a foraminotomy was also performed.

TABLE 2. *Intervertebral lumbar disk surgery: Immediate results*

Grade	No. of cases	%
Grade 1: excellent (asymptomatic)	118	73.3
Grade 2: good (episodic and minor neurological deficits)	25	15.5
Grade 3: Fair (improved signs and symptoms)	13	8.1
Grade 4: Failure (unchanged or worsened signs and symptoms)	5	3.1

The levels of discal lesions found at the time of surgery are shown in Fig. 3: L_1-L_2: 1.2%; L_2-L_3: 2.5%; L_3-L_4: 9.3%; L_4-L_5: 55.9%; L_5-S_1: 31.1%.

With regard to the type of lesion, a simple discal protrusion was found in 27.5%, a partially herniated disc associated with fissuration of the fibrous annulus or subligamentous extrusion in 28.1%, and an extruded disc in 44.4%. This last group may show migrant herniated discs as well as free or sequestrated fragments. With reference to the nervous root, the hernia localization was lateral in 82.4%, medial in 14.8%, anterior or central in 4.3%.

Short-Term Results

Postoperative results (Table 2) were graded according to the following rating scale: grade 1 (excellent: symptom-free): 73.3%; grade 2 (good: moderate, episodic pain associated to residual, limited neurological deficits): 15.5%; grade 3 (fair: improved neurologic symptoms and signs): 8.1%; grade 4 (failure: unmodified or worsened neurologic deficits): 3.1%. A positive correlation between preoperative neurologic conditions and postoperative results was found (Table 3). In fact the patients in the worst neurologic conditions at admission had the highest risk of failure or only moderate therapeutic benefits. No case of intraoperative death was observed.

Thirteen percent of patients complained of postoperative complications.

TABLE 3. *Intervertrebral lumbar disk surgery: Correlation of preoperative conditions and postoperative results*

Preoperative grade			Postoperative grade			
Grade	n	%	1	2	3	4
I	55	34.2	51 (92.8%)	2 (3.6%)	1 (1.8%)	1 (1.8%)
II	72	44.7	53 (73.6%)	14 (19.4%)	3 (4.2%)	2 (2.8%)
III	34	21.1	14 (41.2%)	9 (26.5%)	9 (26.5%)	2 (5.8%)
Total	161	100.0	118 (73.3%)	25 (15.5%)	13 (8.1%)	5 (3.1%)

TABLE 4. *Intervertebral lumbar disk surgery: Reoperations*

Patient status	No. of cases	%
Overall recurrence rate	18	11.2%
Operative findings		
True recurrence	8	44.4
Pseudo-recurrence	5	27.7
Other	5	27.7
Indications		
Persisting pain	16	88.9
Same level	12	66.7
Different level	4	22.3
Neurological deficits	2	11.2
Disk level		
L_4–L_5	13/90	14.4
L_5–S_1	3/50	6.0

In little less than half of the cases (42.8%), they were cicratization disorders (i.e., wound dehiscence or diastase, healing by second intention, etc.); in three cases there was infection of the surgical wound. Other complications (thrombophlebitis of the lower limbs, pulmonary embolism, infection of the urinary tracts, etc.) were less frequent.

The incidence of reoperations due to recurrence of symptoms was 11.2% (Table 4). In 88.9%, pain was the main indication for surgery. In most cases (66.7%), pain was complained of in the same site; in 22.3%, in a different one.

Operative findings showed: (a) a "real" recurrence in 44.4%; (b) a pseudo-recurrence (herniation at a different level) in 27.8%; (c) other causes (arachnoepidural inflammation, arachnoid cysts, peridural fibrosis, etc.) in 27.8%. With regard to site, L_4–L_5 localization showed a recurrence risk more than double than the L_5–S_1 site (14.4% versus 6%). No patient was further operated on for the same symptomatology.

LONG-TERM RESULTS

One hundred and two out of 161 patients operated on for LDH (63.4%) were clinically re-examined in a 1- to 15-year follow-up (70% after more than 3 years following surgery). Assessment of treatment efficacy was done (always directly and never by questionnaire) on the basis of the following parameters: (a) pain symptoms; (b) neurologic sequelae; (c) performance status; and (d) patient's subjective assessment.

Pain Symptoms

Nearly half of the patients (46.1%) were completely pain-free and only a minor percentage (5.4%) complained of unmodified .or worsened pain

TABLE 5. *Intervertebral lumbar disk surgery late results: Pain symptoms*

Symptoms	No. of cases	%
No pain	47	46.1
Pain	55	53.9
Distribution		
Low back and lower limb	25	45.5
Low back	24	43.6
Lower limb	6	10.9
Intensity		
Mild	18	32.7
Moderate	34	61.9
Severe	3	5.4
Frequency		
Episodic	26	47.3
Recurrent	14	25.4
Persistent	15	27.3

(Table 5) as compared with the preintervention pain. Half of the patients (53.9%) went on complaining of pain in the lumbar or lumbosciatic region, mainly of an episodic nature (47.3%), although continuous in 27.3%. Pain intensity was mild in 32.7%, moderate in 60.9%, high in 5.4% only. In 71% of cases pain was markedly exacerbated by movements (incident pain). These data are in agreement with those from the literature (2,5,6).

Neurologic Sequelae

Neurologic sequelae (other than reflex modifications) persisted in 43.1% of cases (Table 6). In most patients (95.4%) they were sensory deficits, generally of moderate entity. Motor deficits, they too usually not validating, were present in 29.5%. Persistent sphincter disorders (incontinence) occurred in four cases (9.1%).

Performance Status

It is worth noting that most patients (80.4%) resumed their working activity, 57.3% within 3 months after the operation, and more than two-thirds (69.5%) maintained the same work as before. Assessment of the performance status was done according to the following classification (Table 7): grade 1 (excellent: performance as before the operation): 63.7%; grade 2 (good: partial and/or late resumption of the same work with good social and

TABLE 6. *Intervertebral lumbar disk surgery late results: Neurologic sequelae*

Neurologic sequelae	No. of cases	%
Negative	58	56.9
Positive	44	43.1
Sensory disturbances	42	95.4
+	38	
++	4	
Motor disturbances	13	29.5
+	11	
++	2	
Sphincter disturbances	4	9.1

occupational adaptability): 16.7%; grade 3 (fair: reduction or significative modification of the working activity with difficult adaptability): 9.8%; grade 4 (inadequate: absolute inability and social withdrawal) 9.8%.

Patient's Subjective Assessment

A group of patients (42.2%) felt "cured", complaining of no clinical symptom or sign; 42.2% were "improved", that is satisfied with operation for the consequent persistent benefits even if complaining of some moderate episodic pain or minor neurologic sequelae; 10.7% were "transiently improved"; and only 4.9% declared themselves to be unmodified or worsened compared to preintervention conditions (Table 8). Consequently, 84.4% of patients submitted to surgery acknowledged a substantial benefit after operation.

Integrated Assessment

Aiming both to unify and quantify the data obtained on the basis of the above-mentioned parameters, a decimal integrated rating scale was formed.

TABLE 7. *Intervertebral lumbar disk surgery late results: Performance status*

Grade	No. of cases	%
1	65	63.7
2	17	16.7
3	10	9.8
4	10	9.8

TABLE 8. *Intervertebral lumbar disk surgery late results: Patient's subjective assessment*

Patient's assessment	No. of cases	%
Cured	43	42.2
Improved	43	42.2
Transiently improved	11	10.7
Unchanged and worsened	5	4.9

A score from 1 to 4 was assigned to each main parameter (pain symptoms and neurological sequelae, performance status, and patient's assessment): the higher the involvement of the selected parameter, the higher was the score. The outcome index for LDH (intervertebral lumbar disk surgery outcome: ILDSO index) was obtained dividing the sum of the scores obtained for the three main parameters into the maximum possible score (12), expressed as a decimal. The lower the outcome index (e.g., 0.25), the better was the long-term result.

On the basis of the outcome index, the following results were obtained (Table 9): (a) excellent (ILDSO index 0.25): 29.4%; (b) good (index 0.33–0.50): 47.1%; (c) fair (index 0.58–0.75): 18.6%; (d) failure (index 0.83–1.00): 4.9%. On the whole, more than three-fourths of the operated patients (76.5%) maintained over a period of time excellent or good results, confirming the validity of the surgical treatment.

Outcome Predictors

The influence of several factors as possible outcome determinants was assessed by means of a multifactorial analysis.

The following factors were considered (Table 10): (a) general factors (age at admission, socio-economic conditions, occupation, pain antecedents, compensation); and (b) clinical factors (preoperative conditions, level and type of

TABLE 9. *Intervertebral lumbar disk surgery: Integrated rating scale*

Rating	ILDSO index	No. of cases[a]	%
Excellent	0.25	30	29.4
Good	0.33–0.50	48	47.1
Fair	0.58–0.75	19	18.6
Failure	0.83–1.00	5	4.9

[a] $n = 102$.

TABLE 10. *Intervertebral lumbar disk surgery: Outcome predictors*

Outcome predictors	p value
General factors	
Age at operation	< 0.9
Social condition	< 0.9
Occupation	< 0.10
Pain history	< 0.09
Compensation	< 0.06
Clinical factors	
Preoperative conditions	< 0.05
Disk level	< 0.06
Type of lesion	< 0.05
Site of lesion	< 0.005
Surgical procedures	< 0.08
Age at follow-up	< 0.005
Concomitant degenerative spine lesions	< 0.001

lesion, surgical procedures, age at follow-up, and concomitant degenerative spinal lesions). Data were statistically elaborated (Mann-Whitney U-test). Results, expressed as probability coefficient (p), showed that the type of lesion (extruded disk) as well as the site (central) of the herniation, together with the severity of preoperative conditions, were statistically significant negative outcome predictors. Above all, the age and the concomitant presence of degenerative lesions (arthrosis) were the main factors able to negatively modify the clinical outcome ($p < 0.005$). On the contrary neither the lesion level, nor the surgical technique, nor psycho-social features of patients were significant outcome predictors. Finally, it is noteworthy that the outcome of patients submitted to reoperation was not significantly different from that medium in the standard population.

In conclusion, computerized and multifactorial analysis of patients operated on for LDH, contrary to timorous or even too circumspect expectations, confirms the long-term validity of the surgical treatment, which still remains, in our opinion, the treatment of choice.

REFERENCES

1. Mixter, W. J., and Barr, J. S. (1934): Rupture of the intervertebral disk with involvement of the spinal canal. *N. Eng. J. Med.,* 211:210–215.
2. Spangfort, E. V. (1972): Lumbar disc hernation. A computer aided analysis of 2504 operations. *Acta Orthop. Scand. (Suppl.):* 142:1–95.
3. Lecuire, J., Bret, P., Dechaume, J. P., Deruty, R., Bellauvir, A., and Berger-Vachon, C. (1973): A propos de 641 interventions pour neuralgie sciatiques par hernie discales. *Neurochirurgie* 19:501–512.

4. Oppel, F., Schramm, J., Schirmer, M., and Zeitner, M. (1977): Results and complicated course after surgery for lumbar disc herniation. *Adv. Neurosurg.,* 4:36–51.
5. Weir, D. K. A. (1979): Prospective study of 100 lumbosacral discectomies. *J. Neurosurg.,* 50:283–289.
6. Thomalske, G., Galow, W., and Ploke, G. (1977): Critical comments on a comparison of two series (1000 patients each) of lumbar disc surgery. *Adv. Neurosurg.,* 4:22–27.

Advances in Pain Research and Therapy,
Vol. 10. Edited by M. Tiengo et al.
Raven Press, Ltd., New York © 1987.

Wrist Antalgic Reflexes in Arthropathies and Neuropathies and Their Behavior Under Transcutaneous Electrical Nerve Stimulation

*Paolo Pinelli, **Beatrice Crespi, and **Angelo Villani

*First Neurological Clinic, University of Milan, 20129 Milan, Italy; and **Department of Neurology, "Clinica del Lavoro" Foundation, Medical Centre of Rehabilitation, 28010 Veruno (No), Italy

Pain is a protective experience occurring together with motor activity which in the most elementary conditions is represented by the withdrawn reflex, while at higher levels of integration develops as antalgic reaction: The conscious control may eventually elaborate a more adapted purposeful behavior.

Electrical stimulation of a nerve with a threshold intensity for group III and unmyelinated afferents elicits spinal polysynaptic reflexes and painful sensations. These reflexes and reactions have been studied in man mainly at the level of the lower limb. In the early neurophysiological research they have been investigated, particularly in the spinal animal, where the withdrawal reflexes are enhanced while the upward afferences are abolished. In man the reflexes elicited in short biceps femori muscle by the electrical stimulation of the sural nerve (RA II and RA III) have been the object of extensive studies in normal subjects (2–4,9,10).

Stereotyped antalgic reactions are less known to occur in man at the upper limb; in fact, the hand is rather released from postural functions and it is more modulated by manipulation-neurons (5). The nociceptive reflex elicited in flexor carpi redialis muscle by the electrical stimulation of the ulnar nerve at the wrist, described by Pinelli since 1955, has been until now rather neglected in clinical neurophysiology.

A more comprehensive analysis of all muscular reflexes in wrist muscles with torque motor and computerized recording of biomechanical and electromyographical variables has been carried out in our laboratory (6). With this methodology we were able to investigate the changes in both postural and nociceptive reflexes in patients with painful wrist alterations of different kinds. On the frame of this experimental work we have planned to reconsider the changes in the motor behavior consequent to nociceptive patho-

TABLE 1. *Pain sensation at different degrees of hand passive movement*

Patient	Age	Sex	Duration of disease (months)	Pain sensation[a] 0°	30°	45°	60°
G.G.	68	F	12	−	+	+ +	+ + +
C.R.	64	F	15	−	−	+ +	+ + +
S.B.	72	M	18	−	−	+	+ + +
C.O.	74	F	21	−	−	+	+ + +
M.M.	68	F	1	−	−	+	+ + +
P.A.	65	F	16	−	−	+ +	+ + +
B.G.	64	M	5	−	+	+ + +	+ + +
C.M.	66	F	15	−	−	+	+ +

[a]−Absent; (+) slight; (++) moderate; (+++) intense.

logical conditions. Three main attitudes and reactions to nociceptive stimuli have been found to occur:

1. Limb withdrawal is a suitable way to move away from the nociceptive stimuli;
2. Limb immobilization is the most effective modality to avoid the source of painful stimulation from arthropathic joints; this goal is achieved by increasing the joint stiffness through a coinnervation of both agonistic and antagonistic muscles;
3. A most active defense could be represented by driving out the external nociceptive stimulus which impacts the limb. In fact, the scratching itself, which can be considered an equivalent of "spinal nociceptive sensations" (8) is an intersegmental reflex of alternating flexion (withdrawn) and extension movement (driving out). This reflex is modulated not only by afferent input but also by higher brain centers which are continuously informed by the spinocerebellar tract and the spinoreticularcerebellar pathway on the limb movement (1).

The central modulation or tuning of wrist reflexes in man in both normal and pathological conditions has been found to play a substantial role on the threshold and the type of muscular reflexes (7).

MATERIALS AND METHODS

The experiments reported in this chapter were performed on eight patients (six females), whose ages ranged from 64 to 74 years. Six patients suffered from wrist arthropathies of different natures; two patients, on the contrary, were affected by cervical (C_7–D_1) radiculopathies. The painful

TABLE 2. *Pain evaluation, stretch and shortening reflexes before and after TENS*

Patient	Pain evaluation[a]		Stretch reflex		Shortening reflex	
	$T_0{}^a$	$T_1{}^c$	T_0	T_1	T_0	T_1
G.G.	+++	−	50	50	200	100
G.R.	+++	−	150	50	150	50
S.B.	+++	+	50	50	100	200
C.O.	+++	+	50	50	100	200
M.M.	+++	+	100	150	50	100
P.A.	+++	+	50	50	100	200
B.G.	+++	++	50	50	50	50
C.M.	++	+	100	150	150	150

[a]Evaluation of pain: (−) absent; (+) slight; (++) moderate; (+++) intense.
[b]T_0: basal condition.
[c]T_1: after TENS.

symptoms occurred for 1 to 5 months in two cases (M.M., B.G.), and more than 1 year in the other six cases (Table 1).

The pain intensity was evaluated on Scott-Huskisson's analog visual scale; the influence of passive limb movement on eliciting pain sensation was also evaluated (Table 1). Besides pain, occurrence of paresthesias was included in clinical assessment.

Wrist muscle reflexes were elicited with movement induced by torque motor at 0 to 40°/sec, and electromyographical surface recordings were carried out in relaxed and preinnervated agonistic and antagonistic wrist muscles. Polysynaptic reflex of flexor carpi radialis muscle was elicited with iterative lateral wrist skin stimulation at subthreshold intensity for a hypothenar M response.

All of these investigations were carried out before and after 1 month of transcutaneous electrical nerve stimulation (TENS) (rectangular pulses with exponential rising phase, at 100 Hz, with duration of single pulse of 0.1 msec).

Two further patients (F.L. and D.L.) with akinesia algera occurring after traumatic lesions of the hand underwent the same neurophysiological investigations.

RESULTS

In Table 2 we reported the findings (pain evaluation, shortening, and stretch reflexes) evaluated before (T_0) and after (T_1) TENS treatment.

Stretch Reflexes

The flexor stretch reflexes were elicited with a wrist extension induced by a torque of $1.2N \times m$. The responses, evaluated as mean values of the

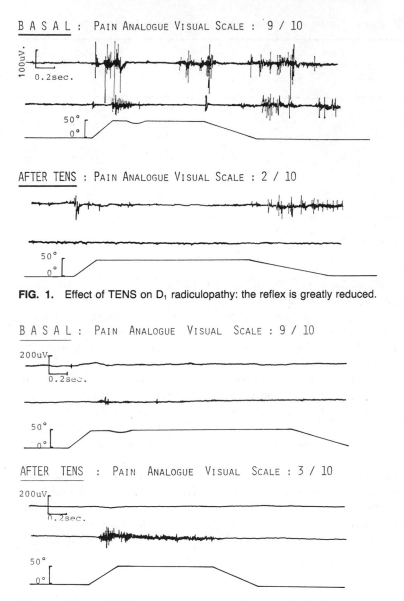

B A S A L : Pain Analogue Visual Scale : 9 / 10

AFTER TENS : Pain Analogue Visual Scale : 2 / 10

FIG. 1.   Effect of TENS on D₁ radiculopathy: the reflex is greatly reduced.

B A S A L : Pain Analogue Visual Scale : 9 / 10

AFTER TENS : Pain Analogue Visual Scale : 3 / 10

FIG. 2.   Effect of TENS on wrist arthropathy: the reflex is slightly increased.

rectified and filtered electromyograph (RFEMG), were in the range of normal values. This result was in good agreement with the ability of the patients to relax the wrist muscles. On the contrary, in the two patients with akinesia algera, both flexor and extensor groups of muscles were coinnervated with increased stretch reflex; however, the difference between the reflex RFEMG and the preinnervation RFEMG still gave values of normal range.

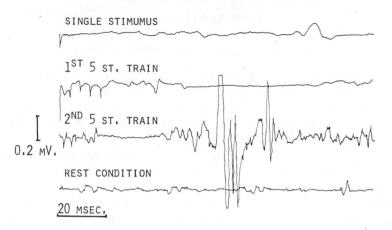

SINGLE STIMUMUS

1ST 5 ST. TRAIN

2ND 5 ST. TRAIN

0.2 MV.

REST CONDITION

20 MSEC.

FIG. 3. Response from flexor carpi radialis elicited by repetitive stimulation at the lateral side of the wrist (third trace).

Shortening Reflexes

In the six patients with a longer duration of the painful condition, the shortening reflexes were significantly increased. This was particularly evident for the tonic reflex with an interfering motor units (M.U.s) activity lasting for more than 10 sec.

TENS Effects

The TENS was markedly efficacious in reducing the pain in the patients with radiculopathy; in the same subjects the shortening reflexes were reduced toward normal values (Figs. 1 and 2). A quite different effect was shown in the patients with the wrist arthropathies; the pain experience was reduced a slight degree, but the shortening reflexes were increased.

Flexor Carpi Radialis Exteroceptive Reflex

The intensity of the train of stimuli able to elicit the exteroceptive reflex was within the normal range in the patient with cervical radiculopathy (Fig. 3). To the contrary, it was 30% decreased in the four patients with long-lasting, painful arthropathy. The TENS treatment lowered the excitability towards normal values.

DISCUSSION

Our neurophysiological investigation clearly shows that the motor reactions of the wrist muscles in patients with different kinds of painful disorders greatly differ according to the corresponding pathological process.

Wrist Arthopathies

In the wrist arthropathies two types of motor reactions have been seen:

1. In some cases the subject presents a tonic coinnervation which fixates the hand and opposes any muscular stretching. This movement-preventing active fixation occurs in the patients with arthropathy, where the pain arises particularly from the affected tendons and muscles even in rest conditions.
2. In other cases the passive movement can be started from relaxed conditions and the subject coinnervates the wrist muscles just at the end of the hand displacement in such a way that it remains fixated in the final position. This type of reaction occurs in the cases where the inflammatory process mainly affects the articular surfaces and painful stimuli arise during the displacement of the hand.

Cervical Radiculopathies

In the cervical radiculopathies we can observe both hand motor reactions previously described. At variance with the patients suffering from arthropathy, the preventive coinnervation developed in successive passive hand movements and the shortening reflexes were often more marked than the stretch reflexes.

TENS and Motor Reactions

The effects of TENS on motor reactions were proportional to the reduction of the painful sensation only in patients with radiculopathy: the fixation reflexes were proportionally decreased. On the contrary, an unexpected increase in postural reactions could occur in some patients with arthropathy in spite of a release from the pain. This particular dissociation could be explained on the basis of an improvement of autonomic pain reflexes previously responsible for muscular ischemia; as a consequence of this improvement the muscular receptor and nerve fiber excitability can be restored.

The identification of these differences in antalgic reactions seems to offer useful criteria for a correct therapeutic approach to these patients. The fixating reflexes and the contractures may prolong the vicious circle responsible for chronic pain. On the other hand, not only the painful stimuli but also the paresthesias due to ectopic endogenous impulses may continuously impinge, through direct or reflex pathways, on the spinal and central neurons; consequently, they can induce some kindling effects; certainly, they release neuro-messengers like substance P; calcitonin, gene-linked peptides (11), and somatostatin (8). Our methodology allows the assessment of the actual state of reflex activity and motor reactions in the single patient; therefore, suitable criteria can be drawn to facilitate the best postural set and motor presetting.

REFERENCES

1. Arshavsky, Y. I., Berkinblitt, M. B., Fukson, O. I., Gelfand, I. M. and Orlovsky, G. N. (1972): Recordings of neurones of the dorsal spinocerebellar tract during evoked locomotion. *Brain Res.,* 43:272–275.
2. Delwaide, P. J., and Crenna, P. (1983): Exteroceptive influence on lower limb motoneurons in man: spinal and supraspinal contributions. In: *Motor Control Mechanisms in Health and Disease, Vol. 39,* edited by J. E. Desmedt, pp. 797–807. Raven Press, New York.
3. Hugon, M. (1973): Exteroceptive reflexes to stimulation of the sural nerve in normal man. In: *New Developments in Electromyography and Clinical Neurophysiology, Vol. III,* edited by J. E. Desmedt, pp. 713–729.
4. Meinck, H. M., Kuster, S., Benecke, R., and Conrad, B. (1985): The flexor reflex— Influence of stimulus parameters on the reflex response. *Electroencephalogr. Clin. Neurophysiol.,* 61:287–298.
5. Mountcastle, U. B. (1978): An organizing principle for cerebral function: the unit module and distributed system. In: *The Mindful Brain,* edited by G. M. Endelman and U. B. Mountcastle, pp. 7–50. MIT Press, Cambridge, Massachusetts.
6. Pinelli, P., and Villani, A. (1984): The central modulation of stretch and shortening reflexes in human wrist muscles. In: *Neurophysiological Contributions for Assessing Rehabilitation in Upper and Lower Motoneuron Diseases,* edited by P. Pinelli, C. Pasetti, and G. Mora, pp. 123–144. *Liviana, Padua.*
7. Pinelli, P., Villani, A., Pasetti, C., and Di Lorenzo, G. (1985): La neurofisiologia clinica nella valutazione della mano emiplegica e del suo trattamento con feedback. In: *Neurologia Riabilitativa,* edited by M. M. Formica. Marrapese Demi, Rome.
8. Wiesenfield-Hallin, Z. (1985): Intrathecal somatostatin modulates spinal sensory and reflex mechanisms: behavioural and electrophysiological studies in the rat. *Neurosci. Lett.,* 62:69–74.
9. Willer, J. C. (1977): Comparative study of perceived pain and nociceptive flexion reflex in man. *Pain,* 3:69–80.
10. Willer, J. C. (1983): Nociceptive flexion reflexes as a tool for pain research in man. In: *Motor Control Mechanisms in Health and Diseases, Vol. 39,* edited by J. E. Desmedt, pp. 809–827. Raven Press New York.
11. Woolf, C. J. (1983): Evidence for central component of post-injury pain hypersensitivity. *Nature (Lond.),* 308:686–688.

Advances in Pain Research and Therapy,
Vol. 10. Edited by M. Tiengo et al.
Raven Press, Ltd., New York © 1987.

Cognitive and Emotional Aspects of Pain

Carlo Lorenzo Cazzullo and Costanzo Gala

State University of Milan, Institute of Psychiatry, 20122 Milan, Italy

The term pain may apply both to an unpleasant experience linked to a physical damage and to the feeling of emotional suffering accompanying anxiety and depression. Having ascertained the multivalent meaning of this etymon, we are immediately brought to the heart of the matter: Pain is a phenomenon, the definition of which may not be easily confined—either in quality or in quantity—to a purely somatic or merely psychic field. Actually, it always stands as the expression of the synergism and of the possibilities of mutual vicariousness between the two realities.

As a symptom, pain is thus, both for the physician and for the patient, the clearest experience of the possible interchangeability between the psychic level and the physical level.

The various definitions of pain (3,6,7) underlie the subjective nature of the painful experience, which is characterized first of all by the concept of nociceptive perception through the nervous system. Nevertheless, an experience of pain may be reported in the absence of stimulation, or else a nociceptive stimulus may not be accompanied by an experience of pain. Thus, pain is an aspecific answer of the body to internal or external stimuli. It is allied to somatic alterations modulated by the ideo-affective component, which is often the most important variable.

Pain is thus considered as a multifactor phenomenon in which biochemical-humoral, neurophysiological, and psychological factors are integrated.

From the neurophysiological point of view, pain is a specific sensorial experience, mediated through nervous structures differing from those that convey other sensations such as touch, pressure, and the thermal sensations of cold and heat. Undoubtedly, any stimulus inducing one of these sensations may induce pain too, but only through a mobilization contemporarily affecting both the mechanisms of pain and those of the above-mentioned sensations.

As regards thermal stimuli, for instance, this phenomenon has been demonstrated by partially blocking a peripheral nerve by means of procaine in order to eliminate the pain sensation, without preventing the thermal sensation of cold from being felt.

On the contrary, when a partial block is induced by ischemia, the sensation of cold disappears before that of pain.

All these somatic aspects are critical, but not essential, per se. However, they involve a series of subtle distinctions, which are essential to the understanding of pain—at least based on our current knowledge.

PSYCHOSOMATIC REACTION TO PAIN

The reaction to pain varies according to the highest cognitive functions, and is at least partly dependent on what a certain sensation *means* for an individual, in the light of his past life experiences.

As it were, the simple distinction between *the perception of pain* and the *response to the experience of pain* may be considered as the dividing line between and the meeting point of the neurophysiological and the psychological factors of pain.

Evidence of the syncretic aspect of the question has already been detected in the expressive manifestations involved in the response to pain. In other words, the feeling of pain involves the body as a whole. Evidence of this was found primarily in distress and *anxiety reactions,* accompanied by patient behaviors and mimic attitudes such as vocal expressions or facial grimaces, perspiration, tachycardia, and an apprehension leading to escape, as may be observed in panic attacks.

It may be stated that, in the history of pain, such *"strong feeling states"* may be predominant in the experience of pain and acquire a fundamental importance in the algesic experience. Thus, although the sensory perception and the feeling state are clearly two different phenomena, they are both fundamental aspects of the experience of pain.

SENSORY-PERCEPTIVE EXPERIENCE OF PAIN

Let us now examine the sensory-perceptive experience in the light of its integrations with the emotional-cognitive experience.

The neurophysiological component of pain may be satisfactorily integrated with its psychophysiologic counterpart. According to Walker (9), there are three levels of integration in pain: the mesencephali tectum, the thalamus, and the cortex. The first stage is surely linked to all the afferent pathways of the encephali trunk. In practice, from the psychophysiological point of view, it represents the activation of the *arousal state,* which enables the peripheral stimulus to be assessed. At this stage, a greater or lesser increase in arousal, due to personal or environmental factors alike, is already affecting the perception of pain. Indeed, *sensations* are usually regarded as generic life experiences with ill-defined delimitations, which lead to a modification of the Self. *Perception,* on the contrary, is regarded as a dynamic, gnosic experience, which, being directly linked to a stimulus, is an effect of the stimulus itself. Perception is characterized by sensory and bodily features alike and it is experienced through a mechanism which is not only direct—in its link with the stimulus—but also indirect—in the referential use of past experiences.

This process is effected through *association* or *conditioning*. A common experience is that of a subject who starts complaining before being affected by the stimulus, for he bears in mind the memory of previous stimulations, linked to environments, objects, and people that are representative of a pain he has already suffered in the past.

Generally speaking, as Sechenov had previously pointed out and Pavlov (5) later demonstrated, conditioned associations and, consequently, conditioned responses are possible up to a certain limit, defined as the terminal link, at which the associations themselves are adopted by the two signaling systems. This theory is in line with the opinion that when a previous experience, even one of pain, is correlated or associated with a more significant later experience, its reappearance no longer induces an attitude of response to pain.

While proceeding in the analysis of the various levels of integration in pain, we must consider the *thalamus* in its twofold aspect. Actually, it is precisely in the thalamus that the "feeling tone," or better, the *personalization of pain*, becomes effective.

EMOTIONAL-COGNITIVE EXPERIENCE OF PAIN

First of all, the emotive component is linked to all acquisitions that are specific to the visceral brain Papez circuit, owing to which the state of excitement produced either by viscera or by the autonomous system may lower the feeling-tone threshold. Second, we must analyze in depth the value of the emotive component and its features. This component is expressed by two basic emotions—*anxiety* and *depression*—which are induced by internal or external stimuli. According to Lazarus, they belong to the category of complex experiences, for they are a way of experiencing the process of reality, in which there is a mutual integration of sensations, perceptions, emotions, ideas, and motor or gestural manifestations. According to this model, which has been adopted and followed by our School, the *process of reality*, or *cognitive process*, is the mental activity through which the effects of all the functions syncretically described above are processed, so that an emotion may be replaced by a motor expression and vice versa. Obviously, this pattern applies conveniently to pain, too.

Let us now examine the third level of integration in pain, that is, the cognitive level that comes into effect in the cerebral cortex. At this stage, it becomes evident that anxiety and depression are complex experiences and not, as it were, emotions merely relevant to the thalamus-hypothalamus. Evidence of this can be found in the progression of these phenomena, which are strictly linked to the experience of pain. It should be noted that also the suppression and the scotomization of pain are strictly linked to this experience, seen in its progression. Indeed, anxiety develops in the face of a *threat* to one's somatopsychic integrity, becomes more marked with a sense of insecurity in the face of danger, and gets worse with a sense of being unfit to tackle the stimulus when it constitutes an attack to the integrity of the personality. As a matter of fact, the fundamental instability of a subject, along with his/her unresolved inner conflicts, may induce responses of greater or lesser quickness and intensity to any kind of stimulus, the painful one included. The expressivity of the response may be manifest and consists primarily in the very *motility* that can be expressed in various ways or forms, which, in turn, are liable to introduce painful peripheral responses.

For instance, think of the incongruous behavior of the head or the trunk as a result of even the slightest painful stimuli, triggering off a painful circuit that finds its origin in the abruptly stimulated segments of the body. Depression is the final stage in the development of anxiety and may be defined as a self-pitying affection leading either to passive attitudes and states of inaction, or to unsuitable, nonphysiological behaviors, which are liable to produce abrupt defensive responses. It is essential to remember that anxiety and depression are always intermingled, and are a possible explanation of some paradoxical responses.

The representation of pain is always central, for the perception of a painful stimulus is completed only when the perceptive function acquires a gnosic character, which lies in the recognition of the stimulus itself. The same applies to the qualitative, intrinsic, or conditioned features linked to the stimulus as an object, as well as to what is generally defined as the *orientation reflex in the face of a danger.*

According to an integrated conception of psychodynamics and psychology, an emotion is always associated with an idea. Therefore, on the one hand, anxiety has always a cognitive aspect, while, on the other hand, it also has a physical, effector or motor aspect.

As a prototype of the sensory-perceptive and ideo-emotional experience, pain provides a rather constant motor response. Every time we feel a pain, we experience a change in our physical life, which implies a preparation in view of new experiences of that kind, as well as a positive or negative planning, according to the way our unconscious has assimilated the original experience.

Another main issue pertains to the *voluntariness and finalism* of the real-life situation in which a subject finds himself when confronted to pain.

It is well known that an appropriate preparation may allow even internal painful stimuli to be assimilated, whereas, in other cases, even the slightest stimuli may induce intense responses, which are a mere expression of *aversion* and refusal on the part of the subject who is confronted with a real-life situation he does not accept.

Having assumed the existence of a constant cognitive component, increased by a greater or lesser emotive participation, and by a greater or lesser activity of the *arousal* functions, let us now try to examine this phenomenon. In our analysis, we shall resort to psychoneurophysiology, a discipline that contributes to the study of cognitive processes, that is, of the way in which a subject experiences his relationship to the inner and environmental reality.

CONTRIBUTIONS OF PSYCHONEUROPHYSIOLOGY TO THE STUDY OF PAIN

The following model is the result of studies carried out at the Neurophysiology Institute of Bristol University, with which our own Institute is twinned. The research guidelines we shall deal with are a model that may be applied to our subject, too.

According to Bernstein (1) the achievement of a self-determined, more or less purposeful motor performance consists of three phases. The first one is the *preparation for movement,* which consists in devising appropriate strategies aimed to the *accomplishment of the movement* itself. The second phase consists in *making the movement.* The third consists in the *acknowledgement* of the result and in its assessment.

This series of phenomena is not merely confined to the sphere of muscular and kineto-articular activities. On the contrary, it is deeply linked to certain activities of the central nervous system, the *brain macropotentials,* which precede, coincide with and follow the motor act. Actually, as Papakostopoulos (4) observed (Fig. 1) in the premotor phase, when there is still no electromyographic activity, the electroencephalographic tracing shows a slow, negative deflection. The upper curve (BP), which represents an average of various motor responses, is defined as "readiness potential" or "Bereitschaft-potential."

In actual fact, the upper trace is marked by two curves: The upper one refers to a self-determined purposeful motor act, whereas the lower shows a self-determined, incorrectly targeted motor act.

In the translation of the central nervous system, the Bereietschaft-potential represents the implementation of the planned operational strategies required for the achievement of the motor performance.

The second phase, which consists of the "motor sensory period" and the "motor completion period," is characterized by the "motor cortez potential" (MCP) and by the P_{200}. The MCP appears in the cortex 80 msec after the beginning of the electromyographic muscular activity. It is an indicator of the efferent activity of the somatosensory system, by which the periphery informs the cerebral cortex of the movement that has been effected.

The knowledge and the assessment of the results of the motor act are two

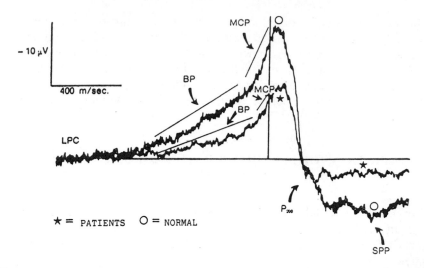

FIG. 1. Brain macropotentials and the motor act.

essential and decisive factors for learning correct performances. Actually, when a subject is engaged in a purposeful motor act implying the improvement of his performance, remarkable modifications in the above-mentioned patterns may be observed, both during the premotor and the postmotor period.

As we have already seen, the width of the Bereitschaft-potential is doubled and a positive wave appears in the postmotor period (see Fig. 1, SPP wave). This wave, defined as "skilled performance positivity," seems to represent the very cognitive moment in the event, that is, the acknowledgement and the assessment of results.

The series of neurophysiological events that have been detected is a supporting evidence of the links existing between *motor* and *mental* activities. It proves that, no matter how it was stimulated—even by means of painful stimuli—the motor act involves the brain as a whole. The purposeful movement is accompanied by highly refined functions of abstraction, which are, at the same time, its prerequisites and its consequences.

Further information on this subject is provided by studies on the expectation wave, discovered by Grey Walter (9) in 1964 and defined as contingent negative variation (CNV) (Fig. 2).

This wave is recorded in the interval between expectation (S_1) and the accomplishment (S_2) of a performance, during which a slow negative wave appears in the cerebral cortex.

The CNV is part of a *cognitive strategy* that is organized in time. It is the result of the ability of two significant stimuli, which are the expression of the cognitive process, *to associate in a temporal link*.

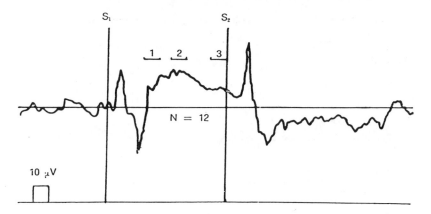

FIG. 2. Contingent negative variation (CNV) and motor performance.

There is a close relationship between the width of the CNV and the levels of attention and arousal: the latter being an essential element in the first phase of appreciation of pain.

As may be seen in Fig. 3, the increase in width of the CNV is directly proportional to the increase in the level of attention. Thus, there is a linear relation between attention and CNV width. On the contrary, there is no monotonic relation between arousal and CNV width in the sense that both a low and a high level of arousal cause a reduction of CNV width (2). Moreover, psychic activity is indeed bidirectional, but, for certain functions, it is by no means monotonic.

Let us now examine the different responses of two subjects—one normal and the other with a high anxiety level—to the same situation, either with or without distractions (Fig. 4).

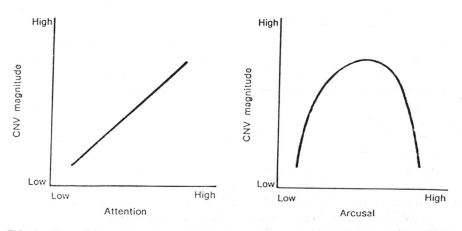

FIG. 3. The effects of attention and distraction on the contingent negative variation (CNV).

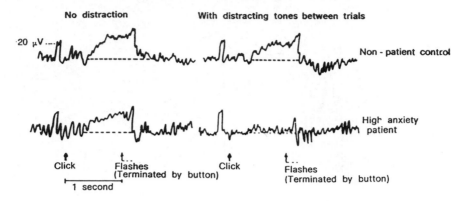

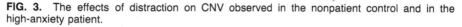

FIG. 3. The effects of distraction on CNV observed in the nonpatient control and in the high-anxiety patient.

In the first tracing (normal subject) only slight variations in CNV width may be detected while the subject is in a situation of distraction. On the contrary, the CNV disappears from the second tracing (highly anxious subject) in the same situation (8).

CONCLUSIONS

The data stated above introduce a factor we had previously mentioned: *emotion.*

The most typical kind of emotion is *anxiety,* which may be defined as an active organization of defense mechanisms, a reaction to an internal or external danger, and a threat to the integrity of the personality, consisting of mind and body.

A stimulus may be either physical (being originated in the outer or inner world, i.e., one's own body and viscera) or psychic (arousing from the environment or from within the sphere of one's thoughts) so that even a painful, nonobjective representation may produce anxiety. Liminal expressive effects are always twofold: both physical (vegetative disorders, tremors, etc.) and psychic (feeling of insecurity, fear, and aggressiveness).

However, the primary effect is a modification of the cognitive process, leading to a supremacy of the mind, peculiar to human beings, which is effective not only in the sphere of pragmatic reality, but also in that of symbolic and imaginary reality.

In the case of the experience of pain, the process is triggered off by objective elements, which, as we have seen, are one of the sources of the pain phenomenon. Only through the cognitive experience, which is peculiar to the individual in a precise moment and in a particular life period, will the general phenomenon of pain acquire a specifically human character.

REFERENCES

1. Bernstein, H. (1967): *The Coordination and Regulation of Movement.* Pergamon Press, New York.
2. Mc.Callum, W. C., and Walter, G. W. (1968): The effects of attention and distraction on the contingent negative variation in normal and neurotic subjects. *Electroencephalogr. Clin. Neurophysiol., 25:319–329.*
3. Merskey, A., and Spear, F. G. (1967): The concept of pain. *J. Psychosom. Res., 11:59–68.*
4. Papakostopoulos, D. (1978): *Neurophysiology of Skilled Performance.* Burden Neurological Institute, Report April 1977.
5. Pavlov, J. P. (1955): *Selected Works.* Foreign Lang Publishing House, Moscow.
6. Sternbach, R. H. (1974): *Pain Patients: Traits and Treatment.* Academic Press, New York.
7. Sternbach, R. H. (1978): *The Psychology of Pain.* Raven Press. New York.
8. Tecce, J. J., Savignano Bowman, J., and Cole, J. O. (1978): Drug effects on contingent negative variation and eyeblinks: the distraction-arousal hypothesis. In: *Psychopharmacology: A Generation of Progress,* edited by M. A. Lipton, A. DiMascio, and F. Killam, pp. 94–102. Raven Press, New York.
9. Walker, A. E. (1943): Central representation of pain. *Proc. A. Res. Nerv. Dis., 23:63–71.*

Advances in Pain Research and Therapy,
Vol. 10. Edited by M. Tiengo et al.
Raven Press, Ltd., New York © 1987.

Conditioned Inhibitory Effects (Freezing) of Painful Stimuli on Voluntary Motility in Two Strains of *Rattus norvegicus*

Carlo Ambrogi Lorenzini, Corrado Bucherelli, and Aldo Giachetti

Department of Physiological Sciences, Università degli Studi di Firenze, 50134 Florence, Italy

In the rat, pain interferes dramatically with voluntary locomotion. One of the most characteristic responses to pain is freezing: The main aspect of this response is the immobile posture of the animal, but the response in itself is to be understood as a complex and coordinate innate behavioral pattern. Freezing may appear as an unconditioned response to fear (e.g., to visual stimuli, like the simulacre of a predator) or as a conditioned response to pain (6). In the second instance, this response is under the control of Pavlovian processes and can be easily elicited by the administration of painful electric stimuli (punishment). Once the animals have received such a punishment inside a given type of experimental apparatus, they readily exhibit freezing when again placed inside the same apparatus (7). On the other hand, it is well known that several strains of *Rattus norvegicus* which are currently employed for experimental work differ considerably, especially in their capacity of reacting to stress. The aim of the present work is to ascertain if there are significant differences in conditioned freezing between Wistar and Long-Evans strains of *R. norvegicus*.

MATERIALS AND METHODS

Forty-two naive male Long-Evans rats, and 36 naive male Wistar rats, all aged 60 days, were employed. The animals were individually housed in stainless steel cages, at a room temperature of $20 \pm 1°C$, natural illumination. Cages were cleaned, and food troughs and water bottles were refilled after the testing session. The animals always received food and water *ad libitum.* The apparatus employed was a light-dark box (1) consisting of a light chamber made of white opaque plastic with a transparent lid (30 × 21 × 15 cm), and of a dark chamber, made on five sides of dark opaque plastic (30 × 21 × 15 cm). The two chambers were connected by a guillotine door (9-cm cross-section).

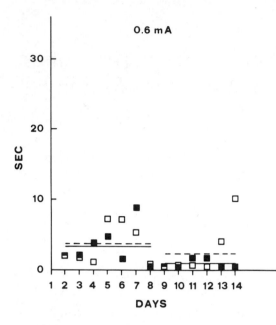

FIG. 1. Duration of initial freezing, for 0.6 mA shocks. (□) Wistar Ss; (■) Long-Evans Ss. Symbols indicate trial mean values. Horizontal lines (*stippled*, Wistar Ss; *solid*, Long-Evans) give mean weekly value.

The floor of both chambers was made of stainless steel rods (2-mm thick, spaced 1 cm); that of the dark chamber could be electrified. The apparatus was placed in an acoustically isolated room, kept at a constant temperature of 20 ± 1°C. Illumination inside the light chamber was 60 lux. The experiment consisted of 14 consecutive daily trials. Every day the animals were manually placed, one by one, in the light box, starting at 9 a.m. During the first week, the animals, following either spontaneous entering in the dark chamber (after which the door was closed), or the direct placement of the animals inside the dark chamber with door closed after a maximal 180-sec step-through latency, received one inescapable electric shock. After the shock the animals were returned to the home cage. Long-Evans and Wistar subjects (Ss) were divided in three equal groups, respectively, of 14 Ss and 12 Ss. For each strain, the groups received, respectively, shocks of 0.6, 0.9, and 1.4 mA (3 sec). During the second week, the Ss did not receive electric shocks. Duration of the initial freezing (i.e., the first freezing exhibited by the animals as soon as they were placed inside the light chamber) was measured for all Ss, freezing being defined as complete immobility, ending when voluntary movements were performed. Freezing data were grouped as follows: days 2 to 8, and days 9 to 14. This because freezing, if present in the first trial, was not due to the electric shock, and, in the same way, because freezing of trial 8 was measured before the omission of punishment. One-way ANOVA was performed on the grouped data.

RESULTS

0.6 mA

As shown in Fig. 1, during the first week freezing duration of Long-Evans and Wistar Ss was very short. No significant differences were found between the two groups [$F(1,180)=0.01$]. During the second week, freezing duration became shorter in both groups of Ss. No significant differences were found between groups [$F(1,154)=1.51$].

Within groups, there were significant differences only between the values of the first and second week of Long-Evans Ss [$F(1,180)=4.05$, $p < 0.05$].

0.9 mA

As shown in Fig. 2, during the first week freezing duration was quite longer than for 0.6 mA shocks in both groups of Ss. Long-Evans exhibited a significantly longer duration of freezing than Wistar Ss [$F(1,180)=4.00$, $p < 0.05$]. During the second week freezing duration became much shorter in both groups of Ss. There were no significant differences between groups [$F(1,154)=2.33$]. Within groups, there were significant differences between weeks for Long-Evans Ss [$F(1,180)=14.35$, $p < 0.001$] and for Wistar Ss [$F(1,154)=8.40$, $p < 0.01$].

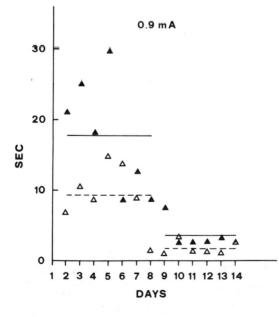

FIG .2. Duration of initial freezing, for 0.9 mA shocks. (△) Wistar Ss; (▲) Long-Evans Ss. For explanations see Fig.1.

1.4 mA

As shown in Fig. 3, during the first week freezing duration became even longer in Long-Evans Ss, while it remained almost constant in Wistar Ss. A significant difference was found between the two groups of Ss [F(1,180)=13.1, $p < 0.001$]. During the second week, freezing duration of Long-Evans Ss remained high, while that of Wistar Ss became much shorter. There were significant differences between groups [F(1,154)=9.98, $p < 0.01$]. Within groups, there were no significant differences between weeks for Long-Evans Ss [F(1,180)=0.57], while there were significant differences between weeks for Wistar Ss [F(1,154)=12.00, $p < 0.001$].

DISCUSSION

The results show that, during the conditioning week (the first one), when the animals received painful punishments, Ss of both strains exhibited similar time-course of freezing. In fact, for 0.6 mA shocks freezing duration was very short, and for 0.9 mA and 1.4 mA shocks freezing durations were almost the same. Nevertheless, a closer scrutiny of the time-course of freezing duration in the whole experiment (conditioning and extinction) shows several interesting differences between strains. During the first week, in Long-Evans Ss, besides the longer duration of conditioned freezing due to the increase of shock intensity from 0.6 to 0.9 mA, there is also a further

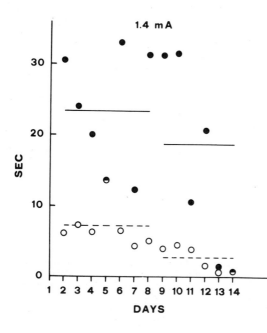

FIG. 3. Duration of initial freezing, for 1.4 mA shocks. (o) Wistar Ss; (●) Long-Evans Ss. For explanations see Fig.1.

lesser increase for 1.4 mA shocks. During extinction, only the highest punishment appears to be well remembered. On the other hand, during the conditioning week, Wistar Ss exhibited a longer duration of freezing for increases of shocks intensity from 0.6 to 0.9 mA. For 1.4 mA shocks not only there was not a further increase, but, instead, a trend towards a decrease could be observed. During extinction, freezing disappeared almost completely in all groups, without correlation with shock intensity. For what concerns Long-Evans Ss, our findings confirm other data obtained by employing the same strain of rats, supporting the conclusion of Fanselow (8) that freezing is an index of fear system activation and that, therefore, the more shock, the more fear, the more freezing. On the other hand, for what concerns albino Ss, our findings appear to confirm rather well the data of Fanselow and Bolles (9): In these animals, for shocks larger than 1 mA no further increase of freezing duration can be obtained; also they confirm the data of Leaton and Borszcz (10) who report that in albino rats freezing duration is shorter for 3 mA shocks than for 1 mA shocks. Therefore, the already described differences in freezing responses of the two strains are confirmed by the results of a single experiment. At this point it may be interesting to underline that between startle reflex and freezing there appears to be a fairly strict correlation.

For instance, we have seen that in the albino rat the increase of shock intensity does not cause an automatic increase of freezing duration. In fact, for 1 mA or 1.5 mA shocks freezing duration may not increase, or may instead decrease (10).

This is a pattern quite similar to the inverted U-shaped relationship described between shock intensity and startle reflex in the same strain (5). On the contrary, in the Long-Evans strain, at least freezing appears to follow much more closely shock intensity (8,9). These differences between Long-Evans and albino rats are only an aspect of the amply described behavioral differences between the two strains (2–4,11–13). In general, the behavioral differences so far described in a variety of experimental situations may be related to the better response to stress and fear of Long-Evans rats. In the present work, only with one intensity of pain stimulation, and only in the Long-Evans strain, motor inhibition persisted during extinction: Also, these findings may be interpreted as due to the higher responsivity to stress of Long-Evans rats.

REFERENCES

1. Ambrogi Lorenzini, C., Bucherelli, C., and Giachetti A. (1986): Some factors influencing conditioned and spontaneous behaviour of rats in the light-dark box test. *Physiol. Behav.,* 36:97–102.
2. Anisman, H., and Waller, T. G. (1972): Facilitative and disruptive effects of prior exposure to shock on subsequent avoidance performance. *J. Comp. Physiol. Psychol.,* 78:113–122.

3. Blanchard, R. J., Blanchard, D. C., Takahashi, T., and Kelley, M. J. (1977)): Attack and defensive behaviour in the albino rat. *Anim. Behav.*, 25:622–634.
4. Broadhurst, P. L. (1958): Determinants of emotionality in the rat: III. Strain differences. *J. Comp. Physiol. Psychol.*, 51:55–59.
5. Davis, M., and Astrachan, D. I. (1978): Conditioned fear and startle magnitude: effects of different footshock and backshock intensities used in training. *J. Exp. Psychol. Behav. Proc.*, 4:95–103.
6. Fanselow, M. S. (1980): Conditional and unconditional components of post-shock freezing. *Pavl. J. Biol. Sci.*, 15:177–182.
7. Fanselow, M. S. (1982). The postshock activity burst. *Anim. Learn. Behav.*, 10:448–454.
8. Fanselow, M. S. (1984): What is conditioned fear? *TINS*, 7:460–462.
9. Fanselow, M. S., and Bolles, R. C. (1979): Naloxone and shock-elicited freezing in the rat. *J. Comp. Physiol. Psychol.*, 93:736–744.
10. Leaton, R. N., and Borszcz, G. S. (1985): Potentiated startle: its relation to freezing and shock intensity in rats. *J. Exp. Psychol. Anim. Behav. Proc.*, 11:421–428.
11. Takahashi, L. K., and Blanchard, R. J. (1982): Attack and defense in laboratory and wild Norway and black rats. *Behav. Proc.*, 7:49–62.
12. Wahlsten, D. (1972): Genetic experiments with animal learning: a critical review. *Behav. Biol.*, 7:143–182.
13. Wilcock, J., and Broadhurst, P. L. (1967): Strain differences in emotionality: open-field and conditioned avoidance behavior in the rat. *J. Comp. Physiol. Psychol.*, 63:335–338.

Subject Index

Subject Index